Hepatocellular Carcinoma: An Issue of Clinics in Liver Disease

Hepatocellular Carcinoma: An Issue of Clinics in Liver Disease

Editor: Arthur Saunders

MURPHY & MOORE
www.murphy-moorepublishing.com

www.murphy-moorepublishing.com

MURPHY & MOORE

Cataloging-in-Publication Data

Hepatocellular carcinoma : an issue of clinics in liver disease / edited by Arthur Saunders.
p. cm.
Includes bibliographical references and index.
ISBN 978-1-63987-300-5
1. Liver--Cancer. 2. Liver--Diseases. 3. Liver--Cancer--Treatment. 4. Liver--Cancer--Diagnosis. I. Saunders, Arthur.
RC280.L5 H47 2022
616.994 36--dc23

Murphy & Moore Publishing,
1 Rockefeller Plaza,
New York City, NY 10020, USA

ISBN 978-1-63987-300-5 (Hardback)

Contents

Preface

Hepatocellular carcinoma is the most common type of liver cancer and occurs in people who have a history of chronic liver diseases such as cirrhosis caused by hepatitis C or hepatitis B infection. Some other diseases such as alpha 1-antitrypsin deficiency and hemochromatosis, and exposure to toxins such as aflatoxin, pyrrolizidine alkaloids and alcohol can increase the risk of developing hepatocellular carcinoma. Its treatment and prognosis vary and depend on the histology and size of tumor, overall health, and how far the tumor has spread. A few of symptoms of hepatocellular carcinoma are loss of appetite, abdominal swelling due to fluid in the abdominal cavity, unintentional weight loss, vomiting, nausea, abdominal pain and tiredness. This book presents the complex subject of hepatocellular carcinoma in the most comprehensible and easy to understand language. It is compiled in such a manner, that it will provide in-depth knowledge about the clinical perspectives of this disease. The book is appropriate for students seeking detailed information in this area as well as for experts.

After months of intensive research and writing, this book is the end result of all who devoted their time and efforts in the initiation and progress of this book. It will surely be a source of reference in enhancing the required knowledge of the new developments in the area. During the course of developing this book, certain measures such as accuracy, authenticity and research focused analytical studies were given preference in order to produce a comprehensive book in the area of study.

This book would not have been possible without the efforts of the authors and the publisher. I extend my sincere thanks to them. Secondly, I express my gratitude to my family and well-wishers. And most importantly, I thank my students for constantly expressing their willingness and curiosity in enhancing their knowledge in the field, which encourages me to take up further research projects for the advancement of the area.

Editor

1

Emerging Targeted Therapies for Treatment of Hepatocellular Carcinoma (HCC)

Sarwat Fatima, Nikki Pui-Yue Lee,
Hiu Yee Kwan and Zhao Xiang Bian

Abstract

Hepatocellular carcinoma (HCC) has dismal diagnosis due to the presence of underlying cirrhosis, late diagnosis, and limited treatment options. Surgery or liver transplantation is restricted to those with small tumours or well-compensated liver diseases. Despite advances in early screening and diagnosis of HCC, survival of patients has not improved greatly. Furthermore, treatment options for advanced HCC are restricted to best supportive care. Currently, sorafenib is the only drug approved for the treatment of advanced HCC patients as well as for those not suitable for transarterial chemoembolization (TACE). Therefore, there is an urgent need to develop new agents for treatment. Hepatocarcinogenesis is a complex multistep process that involves deregulation of various signalling pathways. Thus, there is no dominant molecular mechanism in HCC and understanding of these pathways provides an opportunity for development of potential therapeutic agents in an effort to reverse, prevent or delay tumourigenesis. This review will summarise the significance of these pathways in HCC and discuss the therapeutic benefits or drawbacks of the potential target agents against these pathways especially those that have been part of clinical trials.

Keywords: hepatocellular carcinoma, targeted therapy, sorafenib, signalling pathways, immunotherapeutics

1. Introduction

Hepatocellular carcinoma (HCC) is the most common primary malignancy of liver cancer and is the second biggest cause of cancer-related deaths world-wide. The incidence of HCC is increasing all over the world but the highest rates of HCC are reported in South-East Asia with the leading rate of mortality occurring in China [1]. The risk factors for HCC are well defined, such as hepatitis B virus (HBV) infection, hepatitis C virus (HCV) infection, alcohol consumption, and non-alcoholic steatohepatitis (NASH) [2].

The main reasons for the high rate of mortality are lack of diagnostic methods and limited treatment options for patients with advanced HCC. Surveillance programmes to identify patients with early HCC, such as by ultrasound sound screening and by serum alpha fetoprotein (AFP) levels, are not well implemented. Additionally, AFP levels are also dysregulated in benign liver diseases [3]. Some of the treatment options for HCC patients include surgical resection, liver transplantation (LTx), radiofrequency ablation (RFA), transarterial chemoembolization (TACE) and sorafenib. Surgery has a 5-year survival rate of 70% but unfortunately at the time of diagnosis, only 10–30% of patients are suitable for this option. The biggest risk post-surgery is that of recurrence. The 5-year recurrence rate in patients with early HCC is about 68% after surgery [4]. LTx is suggested to HCC patients with tumours within the Milan criteria (a single lesion ≤5 cm, or up to three lesions ≤3 cm each) and is associated with a 5-year overall survival (OS) rate of 75%. However, the limitation of LTx is shortage of organ donation [5]. RFA is another option for patients with early HCC (<3 cm) and its survival benefits are comparable to those with surgical resection. However, high costs of RFA and complications involving peritoneal bleeding hinder its use [6]. TACE is the standard of care for intermediate HCC with preserved liver function, and with no signs of macrovascular invasion or extrahepatic spread. It has reported a median survival of 34 months and a survival benefit at 1, 3, 5 and 7 year as 82%, 47%, 26% and 16%, respectively. However, TACE is a heterogeneous operating technique with variation in efficacy depending on the choice of chemotherapeutic agents used [7]. For advanced HCC patients, sorafenib is the only drug approved by the

Trial name and no.	**Drug**	**Target**	**Ref**
SHARP, NCT00105443	Sorafenib *versus* placebo	VEGFR, PDGFR, Raf	[8]
Asia Pacific, NCT00492752	Sorafenib *versus* placebo	VEGFR, PDGFR, Raf	[15]
STORM, NCT00692770	Sorafenib *versus* placebo	VEGFR, PDGFR, Raf	[17]
REACH, NCT01140347	Ramucirumab *versus* placebo	VEGFR-2	[23]
--, NCT00699374	Sunitinib *versus* sorafenib	VEGFR, PDGFR	[26]
LIGHT, NCT01009593	Linifanib *versus* sorafenib	VEGFR and PDGFR	[28]
RESOURCE, NCT01774344	Regorafenib *versus* placebo	VEGFR1-3, PDGFR-β, and FGFR-1	[30]
EVOLVE-1, NCT01035229	Everolimus *versus* placebo	mTOR	[39]
SILVER, NCT00355862	Sirolimus *versus* placebo	mTOR	[43]
METIV-HCC, NCT01755767	Tivantinib *versus* placebo	c-MET	[47]
JET-HCC, NCT02029157	Tivantinib *versus* placebo	c-MET	[47]
CELESTIAL, NCT01908426	Cabozantinib *versus* placebo	c-MET and VEGFR, PDGFR	[48]

--: no name assigned; NCT: ClinicalTrials.gov number; VEGFR: vascular endothelial growth factor receptor; PDGFR: platelet-derived growth factor receptor; FGFR: fibroblast growth factor receptor; mTOR: mammalian target of rapamycin.

Table 1. Phase III clinical trials of molecular targets in HCC.

US Food and Drug Administration (FDA) for treatment and although it improves survival compared to placebo in clinical trials it suffers from adverse side-effects and high costs [8]. Unfortunately, with a majority of patients still diagnosed at late stage and with clinical phase III trials failing to improve survival benefits in intermediate and/or advanced HCC, new molecular therapeutics are urgently needed to address the dismal prognosis of HCC. One approach is to identify molecular targets from the several signalling pathways that are dys-regulated in HCC. Several phase III trials have been completed to identify potential molecular targets in HCC (**Table 1**).

2. Vascular endothelial growth factor (VEGF) receptor signalling

Angiogenesis is a critical step for tumour growth and metastasis. With HCC being a highly vascular tumour, controlling tumour-associated angiogenesis offers a promising approach to inhibiting tumour progression.

VEGF is the most well documented growth factor in angiogenesis. It exerts its effect by binding to its receptors, VEGF receptor 1 (VEGF-R1), VEGF-R2, and VEGF-R3, present on endothelial cells. VEGF secreted by tumour cells bind to its receptors and results in activation of signal transduction pathways promoting cell migration, proliferation, and survival of cancer cells leading to angiogenesis. VEGF overexpression is possibly induced by the hypoxic tumour environment, activation by epidermal growth factor (EGF) receptor (EGFR) and cyloonxygenase-2 signalling. Increased levels of VEGF, VEGFRs have been reported in HCC cell lines, tissue and serum of HCC patients. High levels of VEGF in HCC patients has been associated to poor OS and disease-free survival [9], vascular invasion [10] and portal vein emboli [11]. Additionally, Guo et al. [12] and colleagues reported poor prognosis for HCC patients with increased serum VEGF following TACE. VEGF is also more commonly expressed in HCV-associated HCC than in HBV-associated HCC providing clinical implications for different population of HCCs.

Other growth factors stimulating angiogenesis include fibroblast growth factor receptor (FGFR), and platelet-derived growth factor receptor (PDGFR). Overexpression of either of these growth factors has also been associated to poor survival. There are four types of FGFRs (FGFR1, 2, 3, 4) and the PDGFR consist of PDGFRα and PDGFRβ [13, 14].

Sorafenib is currently the only drug approved for treatment of advanced HCC patients who cannot undergo TACE treatment. It is an orally active anti-angiogenic multi-kinase inhibitor. Several clinical studies have reported promising results. In the randomised phase III SHARP trial (ClinicalTrials.gov number NCT00105443), 400 mg of sorafenib twice daily, significantly increased the OS of advanced HCC patients (7.9 months *versus* 10.7 months) and the time to progression (TTP) (2.8 months *versus* 5.5 months) compared to the placebo group [8]. Similarly in another phase III Asia Pacific trial (NCT00492752), sorafenib increased the OS and TTP from 4.2 months to 6.5 months and from 1.4 months to 2.8 months, respectively [15]. The difference in the OS and TTP results in both studies could be due to patient HCC aetiology. The Asia Pacific trail had more HBV-associated HCC compared to the SHARP trial (73% *versus* 12%).

The use of sorafenib as an adjuvant after surgery or TACE remains doubtful. In a small retrospective study with 36 HCC patients, 12 patients received sorafenib post-surgery and the remaining 24 patients had surgery only. The group of patients who received sorafenib post-surgery had a significantly longer OS (37 months *versus* 30 months) and TTP (29 months *versus* 22 months) [16]. However, in the phase III placebo-controlled study (STORM, NCT00692770), which recruited 1602 patients from 28 countries, sorafenib as an adjuvant treatment after surgery/local ablation, did not affect time to recurrence or OS [17]. Similar findings were reported in the SPACE trial (NCT00855218). In this phase II trial Lencioni et al. [18] tested the efficacy of doxorubicin-eluting beads (DEB)-TACE plus sorafenib *versus* sorafenib in patients with intermediate HCC. The authors did not report a significant improvement in TTP following addition of sorafenib to DEB-TACE.

Bevacizumab is an anti-VEGF monoclonal antibody that has demonstrated improved efficacy in patients with unresectable HCC. Treatment with bevacizumab at 5–10 mg/kg produced partial response (PR) in 14% and disease control rates (DCR) in 56% of patients. A phase II trial of bevacizumab with capecitabine and oxaliplatin (chemotherapeutic drugs) also showed encouraging results with a median progression-free survival (PFS) of 6.8 months, and a median OS of 9.8 months. Twenty three patients had stable disease with overall 77.5% disease control rate and eight patients produced (PR) [19]. Hsu et al. [20] investigated the combination of bevacizumab plus capecitabine in a phase II study yielding median PFS and OS of 2.7 and 5.9 months, respectively.

Ramucirumab is another example of monoclonal antibody targeting VEGFR-2. The above mentioned bevacizumab targets the proangiogenic factor VEGF while ramucirumab blocks the receptor. In a phase II study involving advanced HCC patients, ramucirumab monotherapy yielded a disease control rate (DCR) of 50%, PFS of 4.0 months and OS of 12 months [21]. The promising results from this study lead to a phase III trial (REACH, NCT01140347) of ramucirumab monotherapy in advanced HCC patients (post-sorafenib). Although ramucirumab did not improve OS, interestingly in a sub-group of HCC patients with AFP base line levels ≥400 ng/mL, ramucirumab significantly enhanced the OS [22].

Sunitinib is an orally administered multi-kinase inhibitor with activity against various kinases including VEGFR and PDGFR. It has been approved for treatment of renal cell carcinoma (RCC), and imatinib-resistant gastrointestinal stromal tumours (GIST). However, it is not considered for HCC patients due to its high toxicity. In two phase II studies of sunitinib, 50 mg daily of sunitinib orally, 4 weeks on and 2 weeks off, both Barone et al. [23] and Faivre et al. [24] reported high toxicity. Barone et al. [23] observed treatment-related deaths in 18% of patients and with PR in 12% of patients. Median TTP was 2.8 months and median OS was 5.8 months. Faivre et al. [24] reported 10% deaths related to treatment and 80% patients experienced grade 3/4 adverse effects because of which the study could not proceed to the second phase and was terminated [23, 24]. Similarly, a phase III trial (NCT00699374) comparing sunitinib to sorafenib was discontinued. Patients were administered 37.5 mg of sunitinib once daily or 400 mg of sorafenib twice a day but a majority of patients experienced adverse effects such as thrombocytopenia and neutropenia. Additionally, sunitinib did not show a better OS than sorafenib [25].

Linifanib is a multikinase inhibitor targeting VEGFR and PDGFR. In a phase II trial involving 44 HCC patients with unresectable or metastatic HCC, linifanib yielded a median OS of 9.7 months (compared to 10.4 months in patients with Child-Pugh class A hepatic function) [26]. In an open-label phase III trial (LIGHT, NCT01009593), Cainap et al. [27] compared linifanib with sorafenib treatment in advanced HCC. Both drugs had similar OS with 9.1 months for linifanib and 9.8 months for sorafenib. The median TTP was found to be 5.4 months and 4.0 months for linifanib and sorafenib respectively. However, linifanib caused more adverse side effects than sorafenib, implying sorafenib could be more safe than linifanib.

Regorafenib is a novel diphenylurea multikinase inhibiting VEGFR1-3, PDGFR-β, and FGFR-1. It has been approved for treatment of metastatic colorectal cancer after failure of oxaliplatin and irinotecan-based systemic chemotherapy and has also been approved for treatment of metastatic gastrointestinal stroma tumours after failure of imatinib and sunitinib. This year regorafenib was approved by the FDA as a second-line treatment for HCC. HCC patients not responding to sorafenib now have an option of FDA-approved regorafenib as a second line of treatment. This makes regorafenib the first FDA approved drug for treatment of liver cancer in almost a decade. In a small phase II study involving 36 advanced HCC patients who had progressed following sorafenib, regorafenib at 160 mg once daily in cycles of 3 weeks yielded a median TTP of 4.3 months median OS of 13.8 months. The side effects of regorafenib appeared similar to that of sorafenib such as fatigue, diarrhoea, hypertension and, hand–foot skin reaction [28]. A phase III trial of regorafenib (RESOURCE, NCT01774344) involving 573 patients from 21 countries evaluated the efficacy and safety of regorafenib in HCC patients and observed disease progression after systemic first-line treatment with sorafenib. Regorafenib treatment resulted in a survival benefit of 2.8 months compared to placebo (10.6 months *versus* 7.8 months). The median PSF for patients taking regorafenib was 3.1 months compared to 1.5 months for patients taking placebo. The overall response rate was 11% compared to 4% of patients taking placebo [29]. Following these promising results from the RESOURCE trail, regorafenib was approved by the FDA in April 2017 for the treatment of HCC patients who have previously been treated with sorafenib.

3. RAF/MEK/ERK pathway

The mitogen-activated protein kinase (MAPK) cascade consists of serine/threonine kinases, which converts extracellular molecules such as growth factors, hormones, and differentiation factors, into intracellular signals for regulating several cellular processes including proliferation, apoptosis and migration. The four core proteins kinases of this pathway include, Ras, Raf, MEK and ERK. The pathway is activated by binding of ligand to receptor tyrosine kinases (RTK). In the nucleus, phosphorylation of these four protein kinases regulates gene transcription. Around 58% of HCC cases have activated MAPK pathway with Ras, MEK, ERK and MAPK up regulated in 33%, 40%, 50% and 50% of HCC patients, respectively [30]. This pathway has also been shown to be activated by hepatitis virus infections. Dysregulation of this pathway by hepatitis B virus X protein has contributed to loss of function of the tumour suppressor p53 [31]. HCV infection has led to anti-apoptotic effect also following activation by Ras/Raf/Mek/Erk signalling [32].

Selumetinib is an oral MEK inhibitor. In a small phase II study (NCT00604721) involving 19 HCC patients with advanced HCC, selumetinib was given at a dose of 100 mg twice per day but the study was terminated at interim analysis because there was no response and the TTP was only 8 weeks. However western blot of biopsy samples taken pre and post treatment showed phosphorylation of MEK1/2, and ERK1/2, suggesting failure of selumetinib was not due to lack of target inhibition [33]. A recent phase I study (NCT01029418) looked into the safety, maximum tolerated dose (MTD), and tolerability of selumetinib in combination with sorafenib in 27 Asian patients with advanced HCC. The MTD of selumetinib was at 75 mg daily with sorafenib at 400 mg twice daily. Common treatment-related adverse events included diarrhoea, rash, and hypertension, fatigue, anorexia and hand-foot and mouth disease. Seven patients had a PR and stable disease for more than 6 months. The OS was 14.4 months. Due to the acceptable adverse events, this combination of selumetinib and sorafenib deserves further evaluation [34].

Another MEK inhibitor, refametinib, was evaluated in a phase II study (NCT01204177) in combination with sorafenib in 95 patients with unresectable HCC. Patients received twice-daily refametinib at 50 mg plus twice-daily sorafenib at 200 mg (morning)/400 mg (evening), with dose escalation to sorafenib 400 mg twice daily after cycle 2. The TTP was 122 days and OS was 290 days. Interestingly, the best responders to the combination treatment were those harbouring Ras mutation. A recently completed proof of concept phase II trial (NCT01915602) of refametinib in combination with sorafenib in Ras mutant HCC has recently been completed with results expected soon. Given that Ras mutations are only observed in 3–5% of HCC patients, this study raises questions about feasibility and costs of screening large cohort of patients to identify a small sub-group with particular mutations.

4. Mammalian target of rapamycin (mTOR) signalling pathway

This pathway is a critical regulator of numerous physiological processes and also plays a pivotal role in cell proliferation and metastasis of transformed human cancers including HCC. It is upregulated in around 40% of HCC and has been associated to poor prognosis and early recurrence independent of underlying liver aetiology [35]. Two mTOR inhibitors have been studied in clinical trials.

Preclinical studies have shown everolimus (taken orally) to dose-dependently inhibit tumour growth in patient-derived xenograft models of advanced HCC [36]. In a phase I/II study (NCT00516165) in advanced HCC patients, Zhu et al. [37] reported daily dose of 10 mg per day to be well tolerated in 28 patients producing a medium PFS and OS of 3.8 months and 8.4 months respectively. The subsequent phase II study involving 28 patients with prior systemic therapy with daily dose of 10 mg could not be completed as two patients remained progression free for 24 weeks. Although everolimus was well tolerated this study had some limitations including small sample size and lack of randomised control. The efficacy of everolimus was next investigated in advanced HCC patients who did not respond to sorafenib. In a phase III, randomised, double-blind study (EVOLVE-1, NCT01035229) everolimus did not show improvement in OS (7.6 months with everolimus, 7.3 months with placebo). In a separate phase II study (NCT01005199), patients with advanced HCC were compared to those administered sorafenib alone (800 mg) or with everolimus (5 mg) [38]. The results were not encouraging and combination of sorafenib with everolimus did not improve efficacy compared to sorafenib alone with median PFS (6.6 months *versus* 5.7 months), TTP (7.6 months *versus* 6.3 months), and OS (10 months *versus* 12 months) were similar in the Sorafenib alone group *versus* sorafenib + everolimus, respectively. However, loss of tuberous sclerosis complex 2 (TSC2) in HCC has been reported to be predictive of response to everolimus in HCC patients [39]. Immuohistochemical analysis of HCC samples collected in the EVOLVE-1 clinical trial (NCT01035229) had no detection of TSC2 and longer OS than compared to placebo. A larger study is needed to validate the potential of everolimus before it can be used to stratify HCC patients for response to everolimus.

Another mTOR inhibitor, temsirolimus (taken intravenously) has not improved survival either alone or in combination with either sorafenib [40] or bevacizumab [41]. In a recently concluded phase III study (SILVER, NCT00355862), another mTOR inhibitor, sirolimus, did not improve recurrence-free survival (RFS) or OS beyond 5 years in Ltx recipients with HCC but it did improve RFS and OS within 3–5 years. This may suggest the potential use of sirolimus for selection of immunosuppression in LTx recipients with HCC [42].

5. c-MET inhibitors

c-Met is a proto-oncogene that encodes the receptor, MET, for the ligand of hepatocyte growth factor (HGF). MET is a tyrosine kinase receptor regulating metastatic progression. Binding of MET to HGF activates the RAS-MAPK and PI3K-AKT signalling pathways leading to tumour development and metastasis. In HCC, c-MET protein is overexpressed in 70% of HCC and has been associated to poor prognosis [43].

Foretinib was the first c-MET inhibitor of broad spectrum, including c-Met and VEGFR, to be tested in clinical trials. In a phase I/II study (NCT00920192) involving patients with advanced HCC, the median TTP was 4.2 months and the OS was 15.7 months. Its toxicity profile was also acceptable with the most adverse events including hypertension and anorexia. Baseline plasma levels of Interleukin 6 (IL6) and Interleukin 8 (IL8) were identified as independent predictors of OS by multivariate analysis. A larger randomised study is needed to warrant the effects of foretinib [44].

Tivantinib is a selective oral inhibitor of c-MET. In a randomised, placebo controlled phase II study (NCT00988741), advanced HCC patients were administered 240 mg daily resulting in a small improvement in TTP (1.4 months *versus* 1.6 months) compared to the placebo group. Additionally, HCC tumours expressing high levels of c-MET protein, as judged by immunohistochemical analysis, demonstrated an improved OS (7.2 months *versus* 3.8 months) and longer TTP (2.7 months *versus* 1.4 months) compared to placebo. There was no difference in OS and TTP in HCC patients with c-MET protein expression between tivantinib and placebo. These results suggest the potential of c-met protein expression to select HCC patients who may benefit from tivantinib [45]. However, surprisingly, two large randomised double-blind placebo-controlled phase III trials i.e. METIV-HCC (NCT01755767) and JET-HCC (NCT02029157), have both failed to demonstrate improved OS in advanced HCC patients with high c-met protein expression [46].

Cabozantinib is also an oral inhibitor of c-MET, VEGFR and PDGFR. *In vitro* and *in vivo* studies have demonstrated its reduced invasive and migratory properties in HCC. A phase II randomised trial is on-going to investigate the efficacy to cabozantinib in solid tumours. A phase III, randomised, double-blind, controlled trial is underway to evaluate the efficacy of cabozantinib *versus* placebo as a second-line treatment for advanced HCC who have received prior sorafenib (CELESTIAL, NCT01908426) [47].

6. Other potential therapeutic targets in HCC

6.1. Wnt/β-catenin signalling

The Wnt/β-catenin signalling plays a pivotal role in a host of physiological and pathophysiological processes such as embryonic development, cell proliferation, regeneration, angiogenesis and cancer [48]. It is also an important player in maintaining liver health, but it is found to be dysregulated in HCC with mutation in β-catenin observed in about 40–70% of HCC cases, proving to be a potential important target of therapy.

At physiological levels β-catenin is regulated by a destruction complex consisting of adenomatous polyposis coli (APC)/Axin/glycogen synthase kinase 3b (GSK3β), and casein kinase 1 (CK1) which phosphorylates β-catenin at Ser33, Ser37, Thr41, and Ser45 residues located in exon 3. The phosphorylated β-catenin is polyubiquitinated by β-transducin repeat containing protein (β-TrCP) and degraded by the proteasome. However, wnt signalling is activated upon binding of the wnt to one of the frizzled (FZD) family members and to low- density lipoprotein receptor-related protein 5 (LRP5) or LRP6, resulting in the inhibition of β-catenin degradation. The accumulated cytoplasmic β-catenin translocates to the nucleus where it forms a complex with T-cell factor (TCF)/lymphoid, displacing the transcriptional inhibitor Groucho, and the β-catenin-TCF complex enhances transcription of target genes that are implicated in cancer development for example, c-Myc and cyclin D1.

Nuclear β-catenin accumulation has been found to be associated to tumour progression and poor prognosis. Cytoplasmic β-catenin accumulation has been reported in HCCs larger than 5 cm in diameter and with reduced disease-free survival. Dysregulation of the wnt/β-catenin signalling has also shown to regulate angiogenesis and metastasis [49]. Aberrant activation of wnt signalling has also resulted from deregulation of other components of the pathway e.g. up regulation of wnt genes (Wnt3, Wnt4 and Wnt5A) and FZD (FZD3, FZD6 and FZD7) in about 60–90% of HCCs with more than 5% occurring in peritumours, implying that their expression could be an early event in hepatocarcinogenesis [50].

Disruption of β-catenin and TCF association in the nucleus by two fungal-derived compounds, PKF115-584 and CGC049090, has shown dose-dependent cytotoxicity against HCC cells and 10 times reduced toxicity in normal hepatocytes [51]. The disruption reduced expression of wnt/β-catenin target genes (c-Myc, cyclin D1, survivin) and inhibited *in vivo* tumour growth [52]. For reasons yet to be delineated, the presence of EpCAM, hepatic stem cell marker and a direct target of the wnt/β-catenin pathway, sensitised HCC cells to these antagonists [53]. Together these results suggest that EpCAM expression may facilitate HCC prognosis by effective stratification of HCC patients responsive to wnt/β-catenin signalling antagonists.

Recently, two FDA-approved drugs have been identified to antagonise wnt/β-catenin pathway by differing mechanisms. First, pyrvinium was identified in a chemical screen for small molecules. It binds to CK1 potentiating its activity and leading to stabilisation of the destruction complex resulting in degradation of cytoplasmic and nuclear levels of β-catenin [54]. Recently, Pimozide, an antipsychotic drug, has been shown to inhibit cell proliferation and apoptosis in HCC cell lines by reducing EpCAM and β-catenin [55]. The specific role of these inhibitors has yet to be completely elucidated.

Another class of compounds regulate the wnt/β-catenin pathway by inhibiting tankyrases (TNK1 and TNK2). TNKs destabilise Axin leading to β-catenin stabilisation. Thus, inhibition of TNKs prolongs half-life of Axin preventing β-catenin accumulation. These compounds include XAV939 and WXL-8 and also reduce tumourigenicity *in vivo* [56].

Another therapeutic strategy to regulate the wnt/β-catenin signalling is to block the interaction between wnt ligands and FZD receptors. This has been achieved with monoclonal antibodies or using recombinant soluble fragment of FZD (sFZD). A monoclonal antibody, OMP-18R5, developed using the extracellular domain of FZD7, binds to five FZD receptors and blocks wnt signalling. It inhibits *in vivo* tumour growth and acts synergistically with chemotherapeutic drugs including taxol, irinotecan and gemcitabine [57]. OMP-18RS, is the only potential compound targeting the wnt pathway to make it to clinical phase I trials (NCT01345201) for the treatment of solid tumours and myeloid malignancies, suggesting potential use for HCC treatment.

Sorafenib has also been proposed as a potential wnt modulator, decreasing β-catenin and also expression of liver-specific wnt targets (GLUL, LGR5, and TBX3) in several HCC cell lines accompanied by reduced tumour volume *in vivo* using HepG2 xenografts in nude mice [58].

Several studies have also evaluated the significance of combination therapy for targeting the wnt pathway. A small molecular target, FH535 inhibits proliferation of HCC cell lines by inhibiting recruitment of β-catenin coactivators and also suppresses peroxisome proliferator-activated receptor (PPAR) signalling. Galuppo et al. [59] reported FH535 and sorafenib synergistically inhibited HCC cell line and liver cancer stem cells by targeting the RAS/RAF/MAPK and WNT/β-catenin pathways. Western blot demonstrated cleaved increased poly (ADP-ribose) polymerase (PARP) and reduced cyclin D1 and c-Myc.

Identification of pharmacological inhibitors of the wnt/βcatenin pathway is still underway. In the complex network of wnt ligands, receptors and β-catenin, preclinical studies have yielded promising results but wnt inhibitors targeting HCC have not yet reached clinical trials.

6.2. Immunotherapeutics

Immune checkpoints are emerging as promising targets for treatment of HCC. The immune system helps to distinguish body's own cells from foreign cells. To help it achieve this, immune checkpoints which are molecules on certain immune cells, need to be activated or inactivated to start an immune response. Cancer cells find ways to use such checkpoints to escape immune response.

Programed death-1 (PD-1) is a check-point receptor found on $CD8^{+}$T-cells and directs it from attacking other cells in the body. PD-1 binds to PD ligands (PDL)-1 and PDL-2. Cancer cells have high amount of PD-1 and PDL-1 which helps them evade immune response. In HCC, $CD8^{+}$ T-cells that express PD-1 is much higher in both tumour regions and peripheral blood compared to healthy controls [60, 61]. Additionally, several correlative studies have associated PD-1 and PDL-1 in tumours to be significantly associated with HCC recurrence, and poor prognosis [62, 63]. Monoclonal antibodies against PD-1 and PD-L1 have been developed and are under clinical trials in HCC patients.

Cytotoxic T lymphocyte associated antigen 4 (CTLA-4) is another example of an immune check-point, which serves an inhibitory co-receptor that interferes with T cell activation and proliferation. CTLA-4 pathway downregulates an immune response by binding to CD80. Inhibiting the CTLA-4 pathway leads to T-cell activation and proliferation and may help generate memory T cells. Monoclonal antibody against CTLA-4 are also under trial in HCC [64].

Pembrolizumab and nivolumab are monoclonal antibodies targeting PD-1. A phase II study (KEYNOTE-224, NCT02702414) is currently underway to access the toxicity and activity of pembrolizumab in advanced HCC patients who have been treated with sorafenib. The primary objective of this study is to determine the objective response rate (ORR) of pembrolizumab given as monotherapy. Recently, a case study reported a decrease in tumour size and AFP levels in a 75 year old man with metastatic HCC who was treated pembrolizumab after failure to respond to sorafenib [65]. Another single-arm phase II trial of pembrolizumab is underway (Keytruda, NCT02658019) and is recruiting advanced HCC patients with unresectable HCC. The primary end points of this study are PFS, OS, RR, duration of response and toxicity.

A phase I/II study is underway (CheckMate040, NCT01658878) to evaluate the safety and tolerability of nivolumab. HCC patients who were either not responsive to sorafenib or failed sorafenib are also included in the study. Another phase III study (CheckMate-459, NCT02576509) is recruiting HCC patients to compare nivolumab with sorafenib as a first line treatment for advanced HCC patients.

Durvalumab is a monoclonal antibody targeting PDL-1. A phase II study (NCT02519348) is currently recruiting patients with unresectable HCC to evaluate durvalumab and tremelimumab either alone or in combination.

Tremelimumab is an inhibitor of CTLA-4. In a small pilot clinical trial including 21 patients with metastatic HCV-related HCC, tremelimumab induced a significant decrease in viral load and showed promising partial response rate and disease control rate of 17.6% and 76.4%, respectively. The TTP was 6.5 months [66].

6.3. Epigenetic-based therapeutics

Chromatin remodelling is a critical epigenetic mechanism regulating gene expression and plays an important role in cell proliferation, differentiation and DNA repair. Epigenetics alters gene expression without any changes to the DNA sequence and involves the enzymatic covalent modification of histones such as methylation, phosphorylation and acetylation. Histone deacetylases (HDACs) remove the acetyl group from histones, making DNA more compact resulting in gene silencing. There are a total of 18 HDACs identified in mammals. Accumulating evidence suggests the overexpression of HDACs to be correlated advanced tumour stage, recurrence after surgery and poor prognosis in several cancers including HCC [67, 68]. For these reasons HDAC inhibitors may serve as potential therapeutic targets.

Currently 2 HDAC inhibitors have been approved by the FDA i.e. vorinostat and romidepsin, for treatment of cutaneous T cell lymphoma. These inhibitors demonstrate anti-tumour activity by means of histone hyperacetylation reducing DNA-histone affinity and allowing access to transcription factors enhancing gene expression. Currently, a phase I clinical trial (NCT01075113) is underway to evaluate vorinostat in combination with sorafenib in HCC. Romidepsin has not been tested in a clinical setting.

Aberrant up regulation of several HDACs (HDAC1, 2, 3, 4, 5, and 11) and changes in copy number of HDAC3 and HDAC5 have been reported in HCC. Treatment with panobinostat (HDAC inhibitor) demonstrated strong anti-tumour activity *in vitro* and *in vivo* and the effect was enhanced in combination with sorafenib [69]. In a recently completed phase I/II trial (SHELTER, NCT00943449), combination of resminostat (HDAC inhibitor) with sorafenib yielded a progression-free survival-rate of 12.5% for resminostat alone and 62.5% for resminostat plus sorafenib. Median TTP and OS were 1.8 months and 4.1 months for resminostat and 6.5 months and 8.0 months for the combination, respectively [70]. These results support further evaluation of HDAC inhibitors in clinical settings in HCC.

7. Conclusion

New therapeutic options are needed for the treatment of HCC despite the availability of sorafenib, which has limited survival benefits in advanced HCC patients. Several clinical trials are investigating the efficacy and tolerability of combining sorafenib with other agents. Future studies should continue to delineate dysregulated signalling pathways in hepatocarcinogenesis to introduce new molecular targets for therapeutic intervention. Simultaneously it is critical to identify biomarkers and/or aberrant genotypes that would predict clinical efficacy to these targeted agents. Much work also remains to evaluate the role of targeted therapy in adjuvant, neoadjuvant or metastatic settings to determine the most suitable combination of treatment. The battle against HCC is far from over and requires a multidisciplinary approach.

Author details

Sarwat Fatima[1,2*], Nikki Pui-Yue Lee[3], Hiu Yee Kwan[1,2] and Zhao Xiang Bian[1,2]

*Address all correspondence to: sarwat@hkbu.edu.hk

1 Lab of Brain and Gut Research, Centre of Clinical Research for Chinese Medicine, School of Chinese Medicine, Hong Kong Baptist University, Kowloon Tong, Hong Kong SAR, China

2 Centre for Cancer and Inflammation Research, School of Chinese Medicine, Hong Kong Baptist University, Kowloon Tong, Hong Kong SAR, China

3 Department of Surgery, The University of Hong Kong, Pokfulam, Hong Kong SAR, China

References

[1] Torre LA, Bray F, Siegel RL, Ferlay J, Lortet-Tieulent J, Jemal A. Global cancer statistics, 2012. CA: A Cancer Journal for Clinicians. 2015;**65**:87-108. DOI: 10.3322/caac.21262

[2] Ferlay J, Soerjomataram I, Dikshit R, Eser S, Mathers C, Rebelo M, et al. Cancer incidence and mortality worldwide: Sources, methods and major patterns in GLOBOCAN 2012. International Journal of Cancer. 2015;**136**:E359-E386. DOI: 10.1002/ijc.29210

[3] Lui HF. Screening for hepatocellular carcinoma. International Journal of Hepatology. 2011;**2011**:363151. DOI: 10.4061/2011/363151

[4] Gish RG, Finn RS, Marrero JA. Extending survival with the use of targeted therapy in the treatment of hepatocellular carcinoma. Gastroenterology & Hepatology. 2013;**9**:1-24

[5] Mazzaferro V, Bhoori S, Sposito C, Bongini M, Langer M, Miceli R, et al. Milan criteria in liver transplantation for hepatocellular carcinoma: An evidence-based analysis of 15 years of experience. Liver Transplantation: Official Publication of the American Association for the Study of Liver Diseases and the International Liver Transplantation Society. 2011;**17**(Suppl 2):S44-S57. DOI: 10.1002/lt.22365

[6] Chen X, Chen Y, Li Q, Ma D, Shen B, Peng C. Radiofrequency ablation versus surgical resection for intrahepatic hepatocellular carcinoma recurrence: A meta-analysis. The Journal of Surgical Research. 2015;**195**:166-174. DOI: 10.1016/j.jss.2015.01.042

[7] Takayasu K, Arii S, Ikai I, Omata M, Okita K, Ichida T, et al. Prospective cohort study of transarterial chemoembolization for unresectable hepatocellular carcinoma in 8510 patients. Gastroenterology. 2006;**131**:461-469. DOI: 10.1053/j.gastro.2006.05.021

[8] Llovet JM, Ricci S, Mazzaferro V, Hilgard P, Gane E, Blanc JF, et al. Sorafenib in advanced hepatocellular carcinoma. The New England Journal of Medicine. 2008;**359**:378-390. DOI: 10.1056/NEJMoa0708857

[9] Mukozu T, Nagai H, Matsui D, Kanekawa T, Sumino Y. Serum VEGF as a tumor marker in patients with HCV-related liver cirrhosis and hepatocellular carcinoma. Anticancer Research. 2013;**33**:1013-1021

[10] Li XM, Tang ZY, Zhou G, Lui YK, Ye SL. Significance of vascular endothelial growth factor mRNA expression in invasion and metastasis of hepatocellular carcinoma. Journal of Experimental & Clinical Cancer Research: CR. 1998;**17**:13-17

[11] Zhou J, Tang ZY, Fan J, Wu ZQ, Li XM, Liu YK, et al. Expression of platelet-derived endothelial cell growth factor and vascular endothelial growth factor in hepatocellular carcinoma and portal vein tumor thrombus. Journal of Cancer Research and Clinical Oncology. 2000;**126**:57-61

[12] Guo JH, Zhu X, Li XT, Yang RJ. Impact of serum vascular endothelial growth factor on prognosis in patients with unresectable hepatocellular carcinoma after transarterial chemoembolization. Chinese Journal of Cancer Research = Chung-kuo yen cheng yen chiu. 2012;**24**:36-43. DOI: 10.1007/s11670-012-0036-8

[13] Wei T, Zhang LN, Lv Y, Ma XY, Zhi L, Liu C, et al. Overexpression of platelet-derived growth factor receptor alpha promotes tumor progression and indicates poor prognosis in hepatocellular carcinoma. Oncotarget. 2014;**5**:10307-10317. DOI: 10.18632/oncotarget.2537

[14] Zheng N, Wei W, Wang Z. Emerging roles of FGF signaling in hepatocellular carcinoma. Translational Cancer Research. 2016;**5**:1-6

[15] Cheng AL, Kang YK, Chen Z, Tsao CJ, Qin S, Kim JS, et al. Efficacy and safety of sorafenib in patients in the Asia-Pacific region with advanced hepatocellular carcinoma: A phase III randomised, double-blind, placebo-controlled trial. The Lancet Oncology. 2009;**10**:25-34. DOI: 10.1016/s1470-2045(08)70285-7

[16] Li J, Hou Y, Cai XB, Liu B. Sorafenib after resection improves the outcome of BCLC stage C hepatocellular carcinoma. World Journal of Gastroenterology. 2016;**22**:4034-4040. DOI: 10.3748/wjg.v22.i15.4034

[17] Bruix J, Takayama T, Mazzaferro V, Chau GY, Yang J, Kudo M, et al. Adjuvant sorafenib for hepatocellular carcinoma after resection or ablation (STORM): A phase 3, randomised, double-blind, placebo-controlled trial. The Lancet Oncology. 2015;**16**:1344-1354. DOI: 10.1016/s1470-2045(15)00198-9

[18] Lencioni R, Llovet JM, Han G, Tak WY, Yang J, Guglielmi A, et al. Sorafenib or placebo plus TACE with doxorubicin-eluting beads for intermediate stage HCC: The SPACE trial. Journal of Hepatology. 2016;**64**:1090-1098. DOI: 10.1016/j.jhep.2016.01.012

[19] Sun W, Sohal D, Haller DG, Mykulowycz K, Rosen M, Soulen MC, et al. Phase 2 trial of bevacizumab, capecitabine, and oxaliplatin in treatment of advanced hepatocellular carcinoma. Cancer. 2011;**117**:3187-3192. DOI: 10.1002/cncr.25889

[20] Hsu CH, Yang TS, Hsu C, Toh HC, Epstein RJ, Hsiao LT, et al. Efficacy and tolerability of bevacizumab plus capecitabine as first-line therapy in patients with advanced hepatocellular carcinoma. British Journal of Cancer. 2010;**102**(6):981. DOI: 10.1038/sj.bjc.6605580

[21] Zhu AX, Finn RS, Mulcahy M, Gurtler J, Sun W, Schwartz JD, et al. A phase II and biomarker study of ramucirumab, a human monoclonal antibody targeting the VEGF receptor-2, as first-line monotherapy in patients with advanced hepatocellular cancer. Clinical Cancer Research: An Official Journal of the American Association for Cancer Research. 2013;**19**:6614-6623. DOI: 10.1158/1078-0432.ccr-13-1442

[22] Chau I, Peck-Radosavljevic M, Borg C, Malfertheiner P, Seitz JF, Park JO, et al. Ramucirumab as second-line treatment in patients with advanced hepatocellular carcinoma following first-line therapy with sorafenib: Patient-focused outcome results from the randomised phase III REACH study. European Journal of Cancer (Oxford, England: 1990). 2017;**81**:17-25. DOI: 10.1016/j.ejca.2017.05.001

[23] Barone C, Basso M, Biolato M, Pompili M, Rufini V, Miele L, et al. A phase II study of sunitinib in advanced hepatocellular carcinoma. Digestive and Liver Disease: Official Journal of the Italian Society of Gastroenterology and the Italian Association for the Study of the Liver. 2013;**45**:692-698. DOI: 10.1016/j.dld.2013.01.002

[24] Faivre S, Raymond E, Boucher E, Douillard J, Lim HY, Kim JS, et al. Safety and efficacy of sunitinib in patients with advanced hepatocellular carcinoma: An open-label, multicentre, phase II study. The Lancet Oncology. 2009;**10**:794-800. DOI: 10.1016/s1470-2045(09)70171-8

[25] Cheng AL, Kang YK, Lin DY, Park JW, Kudo M, Qin S, et al. Sunitinib versus sorafenib in advanced hepatocellular cancer: Results of a randomized phase III trial. Journal of Clinical Oncology: Official Journal of the American Society of Clinical Oncology. 2013;**31**:4067-4075. DOI: 10.1200/jco.2012.45.8372

[26] Toh HC, Chen PJ, Carr BI, Knox JJ, Gill S, Ansell P, et al. Phase 2 trial of linifanib (ABT-869) in patients with unresectable or metastatic hepatocellular carcinoma. Cancer. 2013;**119**:380-387. DOI: 10.1002/cncr.27758

[27] Cainap C, Qin S, Huang WT, Chung IJ, Pan H, Cheng Y, et al. Linifanib versus Sorafenib in patients with advanced hepatocellular carcinoma: Results of a randomized phase III trial. Journal of Clinical Oncology: Official Journal of the American Society of Clinical Oncology. 2015;**33**:172-179. DOI: 10.1200/jco.2013.54.3298

[28] Bruix J, Tak WY, Gasbarrini A, Santoro A, Colombo M, Lim HY, et al. Regorafenib as second-line therapy for intermediate or advanced hepatocellular carcinoma: Multicentre, open-label, phase II safety study. European Journal of Cancer (Oxford, England: 1990). 2013;**49**:3412-3419. DOI: 10.1016/j.ejca.2013.05.028

[29] Bruix J, Qin S, Merle P, Granito A, Huang YH, Bodoky G, et al. Regorafenib for patients with hepatocellular carcinoma who progressed on sorafenib treatment (RESORCE): A randomised, double-blind, placebo-controlled, phase 3 trial. Lancet (London, England). 2017;**389**:56-66. DOI: 10.1016/s0140-6736(16)32453-9

[30] Hoffmann K, Shibo L, Xiao Z, Longerich T, Buchler MW, Schemmer P. Correlation of gene expression of ATP-binding cassette protein and tyrosine kinase signaling pathway in patients with hepatocellular carcinoma. Anticancer Research. 2011;**31**:3883-3890

[31] Wang XW. Microinjection technique used to study functional interaction between p53 and hepatitis B virus X gene in apoptosis. Molecular Biotechnology. 2001;**18**:169-177. DOI: 10.1385/mb:18:2:169

[32] Schmitz KJ, Wohlschlaeger J, Lang H, Sotiropoulos GC, Malago M, Steveling K, et al. Activation of the ERK and AKT signalling pathway predicts poor prognosis in

hepatocellular carcinoma and ERK activation in cancer tissue is associated with hepatitis C virus infection. Journal of Hepatology. 2008;**48**:83-90. DOI: 10.1016/j.jhep.2007.08.018

[33] O'Neil BH, Goff LW, Kauh JS, Strosberg JR, Bekaii-Saab TS, Lee RM, et al. Phase II study of the mitogen-activated protein kinase 1/2 inhibitor selumetinib in patients with advanced hepatocellular carcinoma. Journal of Clinical Oncology: Official Journal of the American Society of Clinical Oncology. 2011;**29**:2350-2356. DOI: 10.1200/jco.2010.33.9432

[34] Tai WM, Yong WP, Lim C, Low LS, Tham CK, Koh TS, et al. A phase Ib study of selumetinib (AZD6244, ARRY-142886) in combination with sorafenib in advanced hepatocellular carcinoma (HCC). Annals of Oncology: Official Journal of the European Society for Medical Oncology. 2017;**27**:2210-2215. DOI: 10.1093/annonc/mdx060

[35] Villanueva A, Chiang DY, Newell P, Peix J, Thung S, Alsinet C, et al. Pivotal role of mTOR signaling in hepatocellular carcinoma. Gastroenterology. 2008;**135**:1972-1983. DOI: 10.1053/j.gastro.2008.08.008

[36] Huynh H, Chow KH, Soo KC, Toh HC, Choo SP, Foo KF, et al. RAD001 (everolimus) inhibits tumour growth in xenograft models of human hepatocellular carcinoma. Journal of Cellular and Molecular Medicine. 2009;**13**:1371-1380. DOI: 10.1111/j.1582-4934.2008.00364.x

[37] Zhu AX, Abrams TA, Miksad R, Blaszkowsky LS, Meyerhardt JA, Zheng H, et al. Phase 1/2 study of everolimus in advanced hepatocellular carcinoma. Cancer. 2011;**117**:5094-5102. DOI: 10.1002/cncr.26165

[38] Koeberle D, Dufour JF, Demeter G, Li Q, Ribi K, Samaras P, et al. Sorafenib with or without everolimus in patients with advanced hepatocellular carcinoma (HCC): A randomized multicenter, multinational phase II trial (SAKK 77/08 and SASL 29). Annals of Oncology: Official Journal of the European Society for Medical Oncology. 2016;**27**:856-861. DOI: 10.1093/annonc/mdw054

[39] Huynh H, Hao HX, Chan SL, Chen D, Ong R, Soo KC, et al. Loss of tuberous sclerosis complex 2 (TSC2) is frequent in hepatocellular carcinoma and predicts response to mTORC1 inhibitor everolimus. Molecular Cancer Therapeutics. 2015;**14**:1224-1235. DOI: 10.1158/1535-7163.mct-14-0768

[40] Kelley RK, Nimeiri HS, Munster PN, Vergo MT, Huang Y, Li CM, et al. Temsirolimus combined with sorafenib in hepatocellular carcinoma: A phase I dose-finding trial with pharmacokinetic and biomarker correlates. Annals of Oncology: Official Journal of the European Society for Medical Oncology. 2013;**24**:1900-1907. DOI: 10.1093/annonc/mdt109

[41] Knox JJ, Qin R, Strosberg JR, Tan B, Kaubisch A, El-Khoueiry AB, et al. A phase II trial of bevacizumab plus temsirolimus in patients with advanced hepatocellular carcinoma. Investigational New Drugs. 2015;**33**:241-246. DOI: 10.1007/s10637-014-0169-3

[42] Geissler EK, Schnitzbauer AA, Zulke C, Lamby PE, Proneth A, Duvoux C, et al. Sirolimus use in liver transplant recipients with hepatocellular carcinoma: A randomized,

multicenter, open-label phase 3 trial. Transplantation. 2016;**100**:116-125. DOI: 10.1097/tp.0000000000000965

[43] Suzuki K, Hayashi N, Yamada Y, Yoshihara H, Miyamoto Y, Ito Y, et al. Expression of the c-met protooncogene in human hepatocellular carcinoma. Hepatology (Baltimore, Md). 1994;**20**:1231-1236

[44] Yau TCC, Lencioni R, Sukeepaisarnjaroen W, Chao Y, Yen CJ, Lausoontornsiri W, et al. A phase I/II multicenter study of single-agent foretinib as first-line therapy in patients with advanced hepatocellular carcinoma. Clinical Cancer Research: An Official Journal of the American Association for Cancer Research. 2017;**23**:2405-2413. DOI: 10.1158/1078-0432.ccr-16-1789

[45] Santoro A, Rimassa L, Borbath I, Daniele B, Salvagni S, Van Laethem JL, et al. Tivantinib for second-line treatment of advanced hepatocellular carcinoma: A randomised, placebo-controlled phase 2 study. The Lancet Oncology. 2013;**14**:55-63. DOI: 10.1016/s1470-2045(12)70490-4

[46] Pievsky D, Pyrsopoulos N. Profile of tivantinib and its potential in the treatment of hepatocellular carcinoma: The evidence to date. Journal of Hepatocellular Carcinoma. 2016;**3**:69-76. DOI: 10.2147/jhc.s106072

[47] Zhang B, Finn RS. Personalized clinical trials in hepatocellular carcinoma based on biomarker selection. Liver Cancer. 2016;**5**:221-232. DOI: 10.1159/000367763

[48] Klaus A, Birchmeier W. Wnt signalling and its impact on development and cancer. Nature Reviews Cancer. 2008;**8**:387-398. DOI: 10.1038/nrc2389

[49] Qu B, Liu BR, Du YJ, Chen J, Cheng YQ, Xu W, et al. Wnt/beta-catenin signaling pathway may regulate the expression of angiogenic growth factors in hepatocellular carcinoma. Oncology Letters. 2014;**7**:1175-1178. DOI: 10.3892/ol.2014.1828

[50] Bengochea A, de Souza MM, Lefrancois L, Le Roux E, Galy O, Chemin I, et al. Common dysregulation of Wnt/Frizzled receptor elements in human hepatocellular carcinoma. British Journal of Cancer. 2008;**99**:143-150. DOI: 10.1038/sj.bjc.6604422

[51] Lepourcelet M, Chen YN, France DS, Wang H, Crews P, Petersen F, et al. Small-molecule antagonists of the oncogenic Tcf/beta-catenin protein complex. Cancer Cell. 2004;**5**:91-102

[52] Wei W, Chua MS, Grepper S, So S. Small molecule antagonists of Tcf4/beta-catenin complex inhibit the growth of HCC cells in vitro and in vivo. International Journal of Cancer. 2010;**126**:2426-2436. DOI: 10.1002/ijc.24810

[53] Yamashita T, Budhu A, Forgues M, Wang XW. Activation of hepatic stem cell marker EpCAM by Wnt-beta-catenin signaling in hepatocellular carcinoma. Cancer Research. 2007;**67**:10831-10839. DOI: 10.1158/0008-5472.can-07-0908

[54] Thorne CA, Hanson AJ, Schneider J, Tahinci E, Orton D, Cselenyi CS, et al. Small-molecule inhibition of Wnt signaling through activation of casein kinase 1alpha. Nature Chemical Biology. 2010;**6**:829-836. DOI: 10.1038/nchembio.453

[55] Fako V, Yu Z, Henrich CJ, Ransom T, Budhu AS, Wang XW. Inhibition of wnt/beta-catenin signaling in hepatocellular carcinoma by an antipsychotic drug pimozide. International Journal of Biological Sciences. 2016;**12**:768-775. DOI: 10.7150/ijbs.14718

[56] Ma L, Wang X, Jia T, Wei W, Chua MS, So S. Tankyrase inhibitors attenuate WNT/beta-catenin signaling and inhibit growth of hepatocellular carcinoma cells. Oncotarget. 2015;**6**:25390-25401. DOI: 10.18632/oncotarget.4455

[57] Gurney A, Axelrod F, Bond CJ, Cain J, Chartier C, Donigan L, et al. Wnt pathway inhibition via the targeting of Frizzled receptors results in decreased growth and tumorigenicity of human tumors. Proceedings of the National Academy of Sciences of the United States of America. 2012;**109**:11717-11722. DOI: 10.1073/pnas.1120068109

[58] Lachenmayer A, Alsinet C, Savic R, Cabellos L, Toffanin S, Hoshida Y, et al. Wnt-pathway activation in two molecular classes of hepatocellular carcinoma and experimental modulation by sorafenib. Clinical Cancer Research: An Official Journal of the American Association for Cancer Research. 2012;**18**:4997-5007. DOI: 10.1158/1078-0432.ccr-11-2322

[59] Galuppo R, Maynard E, Shah M, Daily MF, Chen C, Spear BT, et al. Synergistic inhibition of HCC and liver cancer stem cell proliferation by targeting RAS/RAF/MAPK and WNT/beta-catenin pathways. Anticancer Research. 2014;**34**:1709-1713

[60] Shi F, Shi M, Zeng Z, Qi RZ, Liu ZW, Zhang JY, et al. PD-1 and PD-L1 upregulation promotes CD8(+) T-cell apoptosis and postoperative recurrence in hepatocellular carcinoma patients. International Journal of Cancer. 2011;**128**:887-896. DOI: 10.1002/ijc.25397

[61] Kuang DM, Zhao Q, Peng C, Xu J, Zhang JP, Wu C, et al. Activated monocytes in peritumoral stroma of hepatocellular carcinoma foster immune privilege and disease progression through PD-L1. The Journal of Experimental Medicine. 2009;**206**:1327-1337. DOI: 10.1084/jem.20082173

[62] Umemoto Y, Okano S, Matsumoto Y, Nakagawara H, Matono R, Yoshiya S, et al. Prognostic impact of programmed cell death 1 ligand 1 expression in human leukocyte antigen class I-positive hepatocellular carcinoma after curative hepatectomy. Journal of Gastroenterology. 2015;**50**:65-75. DOI: 10.1007/s00535-014-0933-3

[63] Gao Q, Wang XY, Qiu SJ, Yamato I, Sho M, Nakajima Y, et al. Overexpression of PD-L1 significantly associates with tumor aggressiveness and postoperative recurrence in human hepatocellular carcinoma. Clinical Cancer Research: An Official Journal of the American Association for Cancer Research. 2009;**15**:971-979. DOI: 10.1158/1078-0432.ccr-08-1608

[64] Kudo M. Immune checkpoint blockade in hepatocellular carcinoma: 2017 update. Liver Cancer. 2016;**6**:1-12. DOI: 10.1159/000449342

[65] Truong P, Rahal A, Kallail KJ. Metastatic hepatocellular carcinoma responsive to pembrolizumab. Cureus. 2016;**8**:e631. DOI: 10.7759/cureus.631

[66] Sangro B, Gomez-Martin C, de la Mata M, Inarrairaegui M, Garralda E, Barrera P, et al. A clinical trial of CTLA-4 blockade with tremelimumab in patients with hepatocellular

carcinoma and chronic hepatitis C. Journal of Hepatology. 2013;**59**:81-88. DOI: 10.1016/j.jhep.2013.02.022

[67] Rikimaru T, Taketomi A, Yamashita Y, Shirabe K, Hamatsu T, Shimada M, et al. Clinical significance of histone deacetylase 1 expression in patients with hepatocellular carcinoma. Oncology. 2007;**72**:69-74. DOI: 10.1159/000111106

[68] Liu C, Liu L, Shan J, Shen J, Xu Y, Zhang Q, et al. Histone deacetylase 3 participates in self-renewal of liver cancer stem cells through histone modification. Cancer Letters. 2013;**339**:60-69. DOI: 10.1016/j.canlet.2013.07.022

[69] Lachenmayer A, Toffanin S, Cabellos L, Alsinet C, Hoshida Y, Villanueva A, et al. Combination therapy for hepatocellular carcinoma: Additive preclinical efficacy of the HDAC inhibitor panobinostat with sorafenib. Journal of Hepatology. 2012;**56**:1343-1350. DOI: 10.1016/j.jhep.2012.01.009

[70] Bitzer M, Horger M, Giannini EG, Ganten TM, Worns MA, Siveke JT, et al. Resminostat plus sorafenib as second-line therapy of advanced hepatocellular carcinoma - The SHELTER study. Journal of Hepatology. 2016;**65**:280-288. DOI: 10.1016/j.jhep.2016.02.043

2

Antiangiogenic Therapy for Hepatocellular Carcinoma

Kosuke Kaji and Hitoshi Yoshiji

Abstract

Angiogenesis plays a pivotal role in many pathological processes, including hepatocellular carcinoma (HCC). This indicates that antiangiogenic agents could be promising candidates for chemoprevention against HCC. Several inhibitors targeting receptor tyrosine kinases (RTKs) for the regulation of tumoral vascularization have been developed and employed in clinical practice, including sorafenib. However, there seem to be several issues for the long-term use of this agent as some patients have experienced adverse effects while taking sorafenib. Therefore, it is desirable for patients with chronic liver diseases to be administered sorafenib as little as possible by combining other safe-to-use antiangiogenic compounds. Various factors, such as renin-angiotensin-aldosterone system (RAAS) and insulin resistance (IR), reciprocally contribute to the promotion of angiogenesis. A blockade of RAAS with an angioten-sin-converting enzyme inhibitor (ACE-I) or angiotensin-II (AT-II) receptor blocker (ARB) markedly attenuates HCC in conjunction with the suppression of angiogenesis. Moreover, the IR status has demonstrated direct acceleration in the progression of HCC via the augmentation of tumoral neovascularization. These findings suggest that a combination therapy involving a lower dose of sorafenib with other clinically used agents [e.g., RAAS blockers, insulin sensitizer agents, and branched-chain amino acids (BCAA)] may reduce the adverse effects of sorafenib without attenuating the inhibitory effect against HCC in comparison to a high-dose administration.

Keywords: hepatocellular carcinoma, fibrosis, renin-angiotensin system

1. Introduction

Angiogenesis is the development of new vasculature from preexisting blood vessels or circulating endothelial cell (EC) stem cells. Emerging evidence indicates that angiogenesis develops in many organs and under multiple pathologic situations, as well as during conditions of tissue growth and regeneration. Abnormal pathological angiogenesis is observed in patients with rheumatoid arthritis, psoriasis, diabetic retinopathy, fibrogenesis, and tumor growth [1]. Although early studies were conducted to determine the molecular processes associated with carcinogenesis and angiogenesis that were performed independently, more recent studies have revealed that both biological phenomena emerge synergistically [2].

Hepatocellular carcinoma (HCC) is the sixth most common cancer and the second leading cause of cancer-related mortality worldwide, accounting for more than 600,000 new cases annually. The greatest risk factors for developing HCC include liver cirrhosis induced by hepatitis B virus (HBV) or hepatitis C virus (HCV) infections, excessive alcohol intake, and metabolic syndrome. Regardless of the etiology, since HCC commonly develops in patients with a chronic liver disease (e.g., liver cirrhosis) only approximately one-third of the patients diagnosed with HCC are eligible for curative treatments (e.g., surgical resection) [3]. Consequently, several alternative therapies have been employed, including percutaneous radiofrequency ablation (RFA) and transarterial chemoembolization (TACE). However, no satisfactory improvement of HCC prognosis has been achieved to date. The notable characteristic of HCC that accounts for its poor prognosis is the risk of high frequency in recurrence attributed to intrahepatic metastasis or the multicentric development. The key feature of HCC progression is also hypervascularity formed by intratumoral angiogenesis as well as the frequent recurrence. Several studies have demonstrated that angiogenesis is implicated in the survival and growth of HCC. It has also been reported that angiogenesis can be induced during the early stages of tumor formation and the various carcinogenic mechanisms have been demonstrated in several different experimental models [4–7]. Therefore, several antiangiogenic agents (i.e., sorafenib) have been developed as novel treatment options for HCC.

In this chapter, mechanistic insights into angiogenesis and its contribution to hepatocarcinogenesis will initially be reviewed. In addition, newly developed antiangiogenic agents will be described in detail.

2. Angiogenesis in HCC

In HCC, tumor angiogenesis leads to a pathologic vascularization pattern, of which intratumoral vascularization is critical for the diagnosis and treatment of HCC, as well as for pathogenesis and patient prognosis [1, 8, 9]. In general, HCC is supplied with blood flow primarily via the hepatic arteries, while noncancerous lesions and the normal liver parenchyma are supplied predominantly by the portal vein. This distinct vascularization is clinically utilized to diagnose HCC radiographically by emphasizing the tumor lesions. Any tumor mass more than 1–2 mm^3 depends entirely on the formation of a vascular network that provides the growing tumor with oxygen and essential nutrients [10].

Of the various proangiogenic factors, vascular endothelial growth factor (VEGF) is one of the most potent and required for both physiological and pathological angiogenesis [11]. VEGF induces EC proliferation, promotes migration and differentiation as well as stimulates permeabilization of blood vessels and vasculogenesis. The several forms of VEGF bind to two tyrosine kinase receptors, *fms*-like tyrosine kinase (flt-1: VEGFR-1) and the kinase insert domain-containing receptor/murine homolog, fetal liver kinase-1 (KDR/Flk-1: VEGFR-2) [11, 12]. Recent reports have demonstrated that upregulated VEGF expression is more frequently observed in the tumor lesions of HCC than noncancerous lesions [13–15]. Moreover, the marked increase of VEGF expression is shown during both hepatocarcinogenesis and HCC growth in accordance with the augmented neovascularization. Our basic studies elucidated that monoclonal antibodies (mAb) against both VEGFR-1 and VEGFR-2 ameliorated the HCC development with antiangiogenic activity in rodents [16]. These findings indicate that a blockade of the VEGF-VEGFR axis contributes to the suppressive effect on HCC development.

In tumor neovascularization, VEGF often coordinates with other angiogenic pathways. The angiopoietins (Ang) bind with receptor tyrosine kinases (RTKs) with immunoglobulin-like and EGF-like domains (Tie1 and Tie2). Increased levels of Ang2 promote tumor angiogenesis, metastasis, and inflammation with augmentation of VEGF activity. VEGF-A is also upregulated by interaction with multiple growth factors, including fibroblast growth factor (FGF), insulin-like growth factor-1 (IGF-1), platelet-derived growth factor (PDGF), and the transforming growth factors (TGF) [17]. Tissue hypoxia also stimulates VEGF-A upregulation via the hypoxia-inducible factors (HIF)-1α and HIF-2α [17].

3. Molecular targeted therapy

Several small-molecule, orally available RTK inhibitors exhibit an antiangiogenic effect of inhibiting VEGF and other kinases. They are expected to have high clinical utility and are currently being tested in clinical trials of varying stages for the treatment of advanced HCC (**Table 1**).

Agent	Target
Sorafenib	A-RAF, B-RAF, C-RAF/Raf-1VEGFR-2, VEGFR-3, PDGFR-β, Flt-3, c-Kit
Sunitinib	VEGFR-1, 2, and 3, PDGFR-α, β, c-Kit, Flt3
Brivanib	VEGFR-1, 2, and 3, FGFR-1, 2, and 3
Lenvatinib	VEGFR-1, 2, and 3, FGFR-1, 2, 3, and 4,PDGFR-α, c-Kit, RET
Cabozantinib	VEGFR-2, MET, RET

Table 1. Molecularly targeted antiangiogenic agents for advanced HCC.

3.1. Sorafenib

Sorafenib (Nexavar®) was developed in 1995 and is the only chemotherapeutic drug that has demonstrated to improve the survival rate in patients with HCC [18, 19]. Sorafenib acts by inhibiting the RAF serine/threonine kinases that play a key role in the transduction of mitogenic and oncogenic pathways through the Raf/mitogen-activated protein kinase (MEK)/

extracellular signal-regulated kinase (ERK)/mitogen-activated protein kinase (MAPK) signaling pathway [20]. Such signaling results in a lower cyclin D1 expression as well as cell cycle arrest. Sorafenib also potently inhibits VEGFR-2, VEGFR-3, PDGFR-β, Flt-3, and c-Kit, which promote angiogenesis [19, 20]. The repression blocks a broad spectrum of different processes involved in proliferation, angiogenesis, or apoptosis, causing a reduction in the blood vessel regions of the tumor and the starving of cancerous cells. Furthermore, sorafenib enhances tumor necrosis factor (TNF)-related apoptosis-inducing ligand (TRAIL)-induced cell death through an SH2 domain, which causes a tyrosine phosphatase (SHP-1)-dependent reduction of signal transducers and activators of transcription type 3 (STAT3) phosphorylation and the related protein myeloid cell leukemia 1 (Mcl-1) (i.e., survivin and cyclin D1) in HCC cells [21]. Sorafenib is also able to repress Mcl-1 activity through an MAPK-independent mechanism, which increases the intrinsic apoptosis pathway in tumor cells. Moreover, recent studies have claimed that the eukaryotic translation initiation factor 4E (eIF4E) might be implicated in sorafenib-dependent Mcl-1 inhibition [22]. Clinically, sorafenib can extend the mean patient survival from 7.9 to 10.7 months [19]. Representative adverse events caused by the treatment of sorafenib consist of diarrhea, weight loss, hand-foot skin reaction, and hypophosphatemia. Currently, sorafenib is the first and only agent to demonstrate a beneficial overall survival (OS) and be approved by regulators globally in patients with advanced HCC [19].

3.2. Sunitinib

Sunitinib (Sutent®) is an oral multi-RTK inhibitor targeting VEGFR-1, 2, and 3, PDGFRs, c-Kit, and other RTKs associated with angiogenesis [23]. Several phase II clinical trials have shown favorable results regarding the antitumor activity of this drug against advanced HCC. In one phase III trial, the median OS was 7.9 and 10.2 in the sunitinib and sorafenib groups, respectively [24]. This indicates that sunitinib had no benefit over sorafenib as a first-line therapy for advanced HCC.

3.3. Brivanib

Brivanib, a dual tyrosine kinase inhibitor, shows potent and selective inhibition of VEGFR and FGFR [25]. Brivanib has exerted an anticancerous effect in xenograft human HCC models expressing FGF receptors [26]. Two phase III trials have been performed: (1) the BRISK-FL study, in which brivanib vs. sorafenib as first-line therapy was evaluated in patients with advanced HCC and (2) the BRISK-PS study, in which brivanib was administered to patients with advanced HCC who were resistant to sorafenib [27, 28]. However, both trials failed to meet the primary endpoint of statistically improving the OS rate.

3.4. Lenvatinib

Lenvatinib (Lenvima®) is an oral multityrosine kinase inhibitor with potent antiangiogenic effects that has recently been approved for use in differentiated thyroid cancer [29]. The drug was established in patient-derived xenograft models that reliably recapitulated the genetic and phenotypic features of HCC [30]. Moreover, in models expressing high levels of FGF receptor

1, lenvatinib exhibited a greater efficacy than sorafenib. Lenvatinib has also shown highly promising data in phase I/II clinical trials involving patients with advanced HCC [31].

3.5. Cabozantinib

Cabozantinib (Cometriq®) was approved in 2012 by the FDA and is a small-molecule RTK inhibitor with potent activity toward VEGFR-2, MET, and RET (rearranged during transfection), leading to the inhibition of tumor angiogenesis [32]. In a phase II study, the observed disease control rate following 12 weeks of treatment with cabozantinib was found to be 68 or 78% of the patients with or without prior sorafenib treatment exhibited tumor regression. A phase III randomized double-blind, controlled trial is ongoing to compare the efficacy of cabozantinib with a placebo as the second-line treatment modality for advanced HCC patients who have previously received sorafenib.

4. Alternative therapy

Sorafenib is the standard therapeutic agent administered for the treatment of advanced stages of HCC and it is likely that other RTK inhibitors will also become commonly utilized drugs. However, chronic liver damage usually lowers the capacity of drug metabolism in patients, and the long-term administration of sorafenib may induce excessive adverse effects. Therefore, to reduce dosage of sorafenib, an alternative approach may be required to identify a clinically available compound targeting tumor angiogenesis. Among the various factors to affect angiogenic activities, many researchers have focused their attention on the mechanisms of angiotensin-II (AT-II) and insulin resistance (IR). These factors have been shown to affect angiogenesis in the liver via close interactions [33]. Moreover, since these factors could also be involved in the HCC, the regulation of these factors might contribute to suppressing the progression of the chronic liver disease.

4.1. RAAS blockers

The renin-angiotensin-aldosterone system (RAAS) is a hormone system that is involved in the regulation of the plasma sodium concentration and arterial blood pressure to maintain body fluid homeostasis [34]. Recent reports have demonstrated that RAAS is locally expressed in a number of tissues, including the kidneys, adrenal glands, heart, vasculature and nervous system, and liver. Actually, RAAS is frequently activated in patients with chronic liver diseases, such as liver cirrhosis [35, 36]. AT-II is an octapeptide derived from its precursor, AT-I, after AT-I converting enzyme (ACE) acts AT-I, proteolytically cleaving the C-terminal dipeptide. During the progression of chronic liver diseases, AT-II is considered to be a potential mediator of portal hypertension. It has been reported that AT-II plasma levels are clinically increased in patients with cirrhosis, and an animal study has shown the elevation of the portal pressure by AT-II administration [37, 38].

AT-II plays a crucial role in the development of several cancers, including HCC. Lever et al. has previously shown the outcome of a retrospective cohort study consisting of 5207 patients with treatment of either an ACE inhibitor (ACE-I) or other antihypertensive agents such as calcium channel blockers, diuretics, and β-blockers with a 10-year follow-up (Glasgow study). Interestingly, in their study, the incidence of cancer and fetal cancer was decreased in the patients with ACE-I treatment as compared with those with other drugs [39]. A recent cohort study has also demonstrated a lower incidence of cancer in patients using ACE-I or an AT-II receptor blocker (ARB) than nonusers [40]. Furthermore, it has been reported that the addition of ACE-I or ARB provided the prolonged survival for the patients with advanced non–small cell lung cancer undergoing platinum-based chemotherapy [41]. Additionally, inhibition of RAAS possibly exerted the beneficial effects on the prognosis of patients with advanced hormone-refractory prostate cancer and pancreatic cancer receiving gemcitabine [42, 43]. In regard to liver cancer, ACE-I showed the suppressive effect on the tumor growth in a murine HCC experimental model [44].

The RAAS, especially AT-II, is potently involved in the regulation of both rarefaction and expansion of the vascular network. Circulating AT-II leads to drive a variety of signaling cascades leading to VEGF, FGF, IGF, and TGF-β expression through mainly binding to the AT1R on ECs [45–47]. AT-II/AT1-R axis plays a key role in the regulation of angiogenic activity in various pathological events, including tumor neovascularization. Actually, inhibition of AT-II by ACE-I and ARB reportedly attenuates **intratumoral neovascularization with down-regulation of** VEGF expression in several cancers [48–50]. These findings indicate that ACE-I and ARB can be candidates for novel antiangiogenic agents against HCC. However, previous report has suggested that monotherapy with only antiangiogenic agent does not exert the sufficient effect on the prognosis in patients with advanced cancer [51]. Therefore, the combination treatment of antiangiogenic agents has been approached to show a synergistic inhibitory effect on cancer progression [51, 52]. For example, the combination of ACE-I and interferon (IFN) suppressed HCC growth more potently than monotherapy with ACE-I [53]. Our report demonstrated that the antitumoral effect of 5-fluorouracil (5-FU) is also enhanced by combination with ACE-I [54].

As well as tumor growth and metastasis, the early stages of carcinogenesis are also regulated by RAAS-mediated angiogenesis [5, 55]. Our animal study has shown that ACE-I significantly suppressed hepatocarcinogenesis at a clinically comparable low dose together with an attenuated neovascularization [56]. Additionally, a combination of ACE-I with supplementation of vitamin K (VK), which is often administered to the patients with osteoporosis, showed a more potent inhibitory effect on rat hepatocarcinogenesis than ACE-I monotherapy [57]. This combination regimen consisting of ACE-I and VK also exhibited the beneficial effect on ameliorating hepatocarcinogenesis in our clinical study [58]. A 48-month follow-up study revealed that a combined ACE-I with VK significantly suppressed the cumulative recurrence of HCC with reduced serum VEGF levels. The serum level of lectin-reactive α-fetoprotein (AFP-L3), known as one of the HCC tumor markers, was also decreased in parallel with VEGF. Accordingly, this combination regimen may represent a new strategy for chemoprevention against HCC.

Aldosterone (Ald), a downstream component of AT-II in RAAS, also affects in the regulation of angiogenesis. **Endocrinologically**, Ald is a mineralocorticoid hormone regulating the plasma sodium (Na^+), the extracellular potassium (K^+) and arterial blood pressure, blood pressure, and electrolyte balance via mineralocorticoid receptors (MR) [59]. Recent data have suggested that Ald plays a key role in endothelial dysfunction, as well as a suggested involvement in the pathogenesis of hypertension [60]. Moreover, the possible involvement of Ald and the MR systems in pathological ocular neovascularization has been reported [61]. Ald was shown to stimulate the proliferation and tubulogenesis of EC, and exacerbated angiogenesis in oxygen-induced retinopathy. In addition, these events could be attenuated by spironolactone. Eplerenone, a selective Ald blocker (SAB), is clinically used as a novel option for the treatment of hypertension. SAB is a selective MR antagonist with higher affinity than spironolactone, contributing to lower side effect by binding the progesterone and androgen receptors. The animal study revealed that murine hepatocarcinogenesis was markedly suppressed by the treatment of SAB with attenuation of VEGF-mediated angiogenesis [62]. These results indicate that SAB is also a viable option for treatment of HCC.

4.2. Regulation of insulin resistance

Recent studies have revealed a close relationship between IR and the progression of liver disease, including HCC [63, 64]. In general, chronic liver diseases impair the metabolic homeostasis of glucose as a result of IR, glucose intolerance, and DM [65]. Several clinical studies have also identified the hyperinsulinemia in patients with chronic hepatitis C (CHC) [66–68]. Experimental evidence with the HCV-transgenic mouse model confirms the contribution of HCV in the development of IR and DM [69]. In this model, the overproduced TNF-α appears to play a pivotal role in the induction of IR and DM. TNF-α is a proinflammatory cytokine, dramatically elevated during inflammation-induced disease pathology. HCV itself induces the phosphorylation of the serine residues associated with the insulin receptor substrate (IRS)-1 and -2 and stimulates the overproduction of suppressor of cytokine-3 (SOC-3), inhibiting the phosphorylation of Akt/PI3K, leading to the blockade of transactivation of GLUT-4, which contributes to inhibit intracellular glucose uptake. Additionally, nonalcoholic fatty liver disease (NAFLD) is a common liver disorder associated with IR and DM [70]. Various factors participate in the progression of NAFLD, such as oxidative stress, endotoxemia, obesity, genetic factors, and IR. Several reports have suggested the association of IR and mitochondrial abnormalities [71].

Recently, a reciprocal relationship between diabetes and HCC has been noticed. A two to threefold increase in the risk of HCC has been observed in the patients with DM, regardless of the etiology of chronic liver diseases [72–74]. A large longitudinal study in the United States demonstrated the twofold higher incidence of HCC in the diabetic patients [74]. Moreover, a recent study has elucidated that the IR status directly facilitated hepatocarcinogenesis [64]. Hyperinsulinemia can generally induce the synthesis and activation of IGF-1, which has a potential to progress a variety of cancer [75]. The altered expression pattern of IGF-1 signaling has been found in human HCC as well as hepatocarcinogenesis in rodent models [76]. Furthermore, IR status may progress hepatocarcinogenesis through the augmentation of hepatic neovascularization and VEGF expression in a rat carcinogenesis model [64].

The diabetic patients with compensated liver diseases initially are treated by a lifestyle change. However, restrictive diets may be liable to aggravate malnutrition in some patients. Thus, the oral antidiabetic drugs are administered to treat the diabetic patients with advanced liver diseases such as cirrhosis [77, 78]. To avoid hyperinsulinemia affecting adversely HCC growth, the drugs exerting insulin-sensitizing effects are preferable such as metformin, pioglitazone, dipeptidyl peptidase 4 inhibitor, or sodium glucose cotransporter inhibitor. Another report has demonstrated that the use of statins, a class of lipid-lowering medications by inhibiting HMG-CoA reductase that plays a central role in the production of cholesterol, significantly lowered the risk of HCC in the patients with DM [79].

The branched-chain amino acid (BCAA), an amino acid having aliphatic side chains with a branch (a central carbon atom bound to three or more carbon atoms), comprises three essential amino acids: leucine, isoleucine, and valine. Several clinical studies have suggested the beneficial effect of the long-term supplementation with BCAA granules on hypoalbuminemia and event-free survival in the patients with cirrhosis [80, 81]. BCAAs have also been shown to induce glucose uptake and improve glucose metabolism in a rat cirrhotic model. Intriguingly, the animal study using obese diabetic rat showed a chemopreventive effect of BCAAs against HCC with the downregulation of VEGF and antiangiogenic activity [82, 83]. Multicenter study in Japan also revealed that BCAAs decreased the incidence of HCC in patients with HCV-related cirrhosis as well as the type 2 DM and obesity [84]. However, a monotherapy with BCAA did not inhibit the recurrence of HCC after curative treatment. Therefore, to utilize BCAAs with sufficient effect against HCC, it is strongly recommended to combine them with other drugs. From previous research, AT-II also plays a key role in the development of IR. Actually, mice genetically lacking ACE exhibited the improvement of glucose tolerance through the reduced fat mass [85]. Moreover, additional administration of ACE-I or ARB to BCAAs is also shown to improve the IR status [33, 86]. Our randomized control trial study demonstrated that the combined BCAAs with ACE-I suppresses the cumulative recurrence of HCC in the patients with IR [87].

Taken together, these findings indicate that the combination of BCAAs supplementation and RAAS blockade may represent a potentially novel therapeutic strategy against HCC in the patients with IR.

5. Conclusions and future perspectives

Angiogenesis plays a crucial role in hepatocarcinogenesis and HCC progression, indicating the requirement of an antiangiogenic therapy as a tool for suppressing HCC. Sorafenib has become a breakthrough drug in the field of HCC, with an improvement in the median survival of almost 3 months. This represents a reduction of greater than 30% for the probability of death during the follow-up period.

However, when using RTK inhibitors, including sorafenib for patients with chronic liver diseases, many patients exhibit adverse effects, and several symptoms are very severe. Since the adverse effects induced by RTK inhibitors emerge in a dose-dependent manner, it is desirable for patients with chronic liver diseases to avoid these drugs as much as possible. Therefore, to lower the dose of such treatments, a clinically available compound to use in combination with RTK inhibitors may be required.

ACE-I, ARB, and SAB are extensively employed as antihypertensive agents in clinical practice without serious adverse effects. Thus, these RAAS blocking agents may provide a novel strategy targeting HCC. However, several reports also suggest that there is a close relationship between AT-II polymorphisms and the progression of chronic liver diseases and cancers. In certain types of cancers, the elevated ACE genetic polymorphisms are significantly involved in their poor prognosis [88, 89]. Additionally, AT-II type I receptor polymorphism reportedly contributes to the occurrence of nonalcoholic steatohepatitis (NASH) [90]. These evidences suggest that the efficacy of RAAS inhibition may vary in each case. Since combination treatment of ACE-I and VK exerted substantially more potent inhibitory effects, a combination treatment involving these agents may be preferable for future clinical applications. Furthermore, under IR conditions, the combination treatment of BCAA and ACE-I would be a promising approach against HCC via the suppression of VEGF-mediated angiogenesis. Since these agents are widely used in clinical practice, the combination of these agents with RTK inhibitors such as sorafenib represents a potential alternative approach against HCC.

Author details

Kosuke Kaji* and Hitoshi Yoshiji

*Address all correspondence to: kajik@naramed-u.ac.jp

Third Department of Internal Medicine, Nara Medical University, Shijo-cho, Kashihara, Nara, Japan

References

[1] Carmeliet P. Angiogenesis in life, disease and medicine. Nature. 2005;438(7070):932–6.

[2] Kalluri R, Sukhatme VP. Fibrosis and angiogenesis. Current Opinion in Nephrology and Hypertension. 2000;9(4):413–8.

[3] Llovet JM, Schwartz M, Mazzaferro V. Resection and liver transplantation for hepatocellular carcinoma. Seminars in Liver Disease. 2005;25(2):181–200.

[4] Li CY, Shan S, Huang Q, Braun RD, Lanzen J, Hu K, et al. Initial stages of tumor cell-induced angiogenesis: evaluation via skin window chambers in rodent models. Journal of the National Cancer Institute. 2000;92(2):143–7.

[5] Bergers G, Benjamin LE. Tumorigenesis and the angiogenic switch. Nature Reviews Cancer. 2003;3(6):401–10.

[6] Bergers G, Javaherian K, Lo KM, Folkman J, Hanahan D. Effects of angiogenesis inhibitors on multistage carcinogenesis in mice. Science. 1999;284(5415):808–12.

[7] Brandvold KA, Neiman P, Ruddell A. Angiogenesis is an early event in the generation of myc-induced lymphomas. Oncogene. 2000;19(23):2780–5.

[8] Carr BI. Hepatocellular carcinoma: current management and future trends. Gastroenterology. 2004;127(5 Suppl 1):S218–24.

[9] Kerbel RS. Tumor angiogenesis. The New England Journal of Medicine. 2008;358(19): 2039–49.

[10] Carmeliet P. VEGF as a key mediator of angiogenesis in cancer. Oncology. 2005;69(Suppl 3):4–10.

[11] Shibuya M. Structure and function of VEGF/VEGF-receptor system involved in angiogenesis. Cell Structure and Function. 2001;26(1):25–35.

[12] Karkkainen MJ, Petrova TV. Vascular endothelial growth factor receptors in the regulation of angiogenesis and lymphangiogenesis. Oncogene. 2000;19(49):5598–605.

[13] Miura H, Miyazaki T, Kuroda M, Oka T, Machinami R, Kodama T, et al. Increased expression of vascular endothelial growth factor in human hepatocellular carcinoma. Journal of Hepatology. 1997;27(5):854–61.

[14] Yamaguchi R, Yano H, Iemura A, Ogasawara S, Haramaki M, Kojiro M. Expression of vascular endothelial growth factor in human hepatocellular carcinoma. Hepatology. 1998;28(1):68–77.

[15] Yamaguchi R, Yano H, Nakashima Y, Ogasawara S, Higaki K, Akiba J, et al. Expression and localization of vascular endothelial growth factor receptors in human hepatocellular carcinoma and non-HCC tissues. Oncology Reports. 2000;7(4):725–9.

[16] Yoshiji H, Kuriyama S, Yoshii J, Ikenaka Y, Noguchi R, Hicklin DJ, et al. Halting the interaction between vascular endothelial growth factor and its receptors attenuates liver carcinogenesis in mice. Hepatology. 2004;39(6):1517–24.

[17] Cook KM, Figg WD. Angiogenesis inhibitors: current strategies and future prospects. CA: Cancer Journal for Clinicians. 2010;60(4):222–43.

[18] Forner A, Llovet JM, Bruix J. Hepatocellular carcinoma. Lancet. 2012;379(9822):1245–55.

[19] Llovet JM, Ricci S, Mazzaferro V, Hilgard P, Gane E, Blanc JF, et al. Sorafenib in advanced hepatocellular carcinoma. The New England Journal of Medicine. 2008;359(4):378–90.

[20] Wilhelm S, Carter C, Lynch M, Lowinger T, Dumas J, Smith RA, et al. Discovery and development of sorafenib: a multikinase inhibitor for treating cancer. Nature Reviews Drug Discovery. 2006;5(10):835–44.

[21] Chen KF, Tai WT, Liu TH, Huang HP, Lin YC, Shiau CW, et al. Sorafenib overcomes TRAIL resistance of hepatocellular carcinoma cells through the inhibition of STAT-Clinical Cancer Research: An Official Journal of the American Association for Cancer Research. 2010;16(21):5189–99.

[22] Rosato RR, Almenara JA, Coe S, Grant S. The multikinase inhibitor sorafenib potentiates TRAIL lethality in human leukemia cells in association with Mcl-1 and cFLIPL down-regulation. Cancer Research. 2007;67(19):9490–500.

[23] Zhu AX, Raymond E. Early development of sunitinib in hepatocellular carcinoma. Expert Review of Anticancer Therapy. 2009;9(1):143–50.

[24] Cheng AL, Kang YK, Lin DY, Park JW, Kudo M, Qin S, et al. Sunitinib versus sorafenib in advanced hepatocellular cancer: results of a randomized phase III trial. Journal of Clinical Oncology: Official Journal of the American Society of Clinical Oncology. 2013;31(32):4067–75.

[25] Bhide RS, Cai ZW, Zhang YZ, Qian L, Wei D, Barbosa S, et al. Discovery and preclinical studies of (R)-1-(4-(4-fluoro-2-methyl-1H-indol-5-yloxy)-5- methylpyrrolo[2,1-f][1,2,4]triazin-6-yloxy)propan-2-ol (BMS-540215), an in vivo active potent VEGFR-2 inhibitor. Journal of Medicinal Chemistry. 2006;49(7):2143–6.

[26] Huynh H, Ngo VC, Fargnoli J, Ayers M, Soo KC, Koong HN, et al. Brivanib alaninate, a dual inhibitor of vascular endothelial growth factor receptor and fibroblast growth factor receptor tyrosine kinases, induces growth inhibition in mouse models of human hepatocellular carcinoma. Clinical Cancer Research: An Official Journal of the American Association for Cancer Research. 2008;14(19):6146–53.

[27] Johnson PJ, Qin S, Park JW, Poon RT, Raoul JL, Philip PA, et al. Brivanib versus sorafenib as first-line therapy in patients with unresectable, advanced hepatocellular carcinoma: results from the randomized phase III BRISK-FL study. Journal of Clinical Oncology: Official Journal of the American Society of Clinical Oncology. 2013;31(28):3517–24.

[28] Llovet JM, Decaens T, Raoul JL, Boucher E, Kudo M, Chang C, et al. Brivanib in patients with advanced hepatocellular carcinoma who were intolerant to sorafenib or for whom sorafenib failed: results from the randomized phase III BRISK-PS study. Journal of Clinical Oncology: Official Journal of the American Society of Clinical Oncology. 2013;31(28):3509–16.

[29] Yeung KT, Cohen EE. Lenvatinib in advanced, radioactive iodine-refractory, differentiated thyroid carcinoma. Clinical Cancer Research: An Official Journal of the American Association for Cancer Research. 2015;21(24):5420–6.

[30] Gu Q, Zhang B, Sun H, Xu Q, Tan Y, Wang G, et al. Genomic characterization of a large panel of patient-derived hepatocellular carcinoma xenograft tumor models for preclinical development. Oncotarget. 2015;6(24):20160–76.

[31] Oikonomopoulos G, Aravind P, Sarker D. Lenvatinib: a potential breakthrough in advanced hepatocellular carcinoma? Future Oncology. 2016;12(4):465–76.

[32] Xiang Q, Chen W, Ren M, Wang J, Zhang H, Deng DY, et al. Cabozantinib suppresses tumor growth and metastasis in hepatocellular carcinoma by a dual blockade of VEGFR2 and MET. Clinical Cancer Research: An Official Journal of the American Association for Cancer Research. 2014;20(11):2959–70.

[33] de Kloet AD, Krause EG, Woods SC. The renin angiotensin system and the metabolic syndrome. Physiology & Behavior. 2010;100(5):525–34.

[34] Ardaillou R. Angiotensin II receptors. Journal of the American Society of Nephrology: JASN. 1999;10(Suppl 11):S30–9.

[35] Helmy A, Jalan R, Newby DE, Hayes PC, Webb DJ. Role of angiotensin II in regulation of basal and sympathetically stimulated vascular tone in early and advanced cirrhosis. Gastroenterology. 2000;118(3):565–72.

[36] Munshi MK, Uddin MN, Glaser SS. The role of the renin-angiotensin system in liver fibrosis. Experimental Biology and Medicine. 2011;236(5):557–66.

[37] Beyazit Y, Ibis M, Purnak T, Turhan T, Kekilli M, Kurt M, et al. Elevated levels of circulating angiotensin converting enzyme in patients with hepatoportal sclerosis. Digestive Diseases and Sciences. 2011;56(7):2160–5.

[38] Lugo-Baruqui A, Munoz-Valle JF, Arevalo-Gallegos S, Armendariz-Borunda J. Role of angiotensin II in liver fibrosis-induced portal hypertension and therapeutic implications. Hepatology Research: the Official Journal of the Japan Society of Hepatology. 2010;40(1):95–104.

[39] Lever AF, Hole DJ, Gillis CR, McCallum IR, McInnes GT, MacKinnon PL, et al. Do inhibitors of angiotensin-I-converting enzyme protect against risk of cancer? Lancet. 1998;352(9123):179–84.

[40] Christian JB, Lapane KL, Hume AL, Eaton CB, Weinstock MA, Trial V. Association of ACE inhibitors and angiotensin receptor blockers with keratinocyte cancer prevention in the randomized VATTC trial. Journal of the National Cancer Institute. 2008;100(17): 1223–32.

[41] Wilop S, von Hobe S, Crysandt M, Esser A, Osieka R, Jost E. Impact of angiotensin I converting enzyme inhibitors and angiotensin II type 1 receptor blockers on survival in patients with advanced non-small-cell lung cancer undergoing first-line platinum-based chemotherapy. Journal of Cancer Research and Clinical Oncology. 2009;135(10): 1429–35.

[42] Uemura H, Hasumi H, Kawahara T, Sugiura S, Miyoshi Y, Nakaigawa N, et al. Pilot study of angiotensin II receptor blocker in advanced hormone-refractory prostate cancer. International Journal of Clinical Oncology. 2005;10(6):405–10.

[43] Nakai Y, Isayama H, Ijichi H, Sasaki T, Sasahira N, Hirano K, et al. Inhibition of renin-angiotensin system affects prognosis of advanced pancreatic cancer receiving gemcitabine. British Journal of Cancer. 2010;103(11):1644–8.

[44] Yoshiji H, Kuriyama S, Kawata M, Yoshii J, Ikenaka Y, Noguchi R, et al. The angiotensin-I-converting enzyme inhibitor perindopril suppresses tumor growth and angiogenesis: possible role of the vascular endothelial growth factor. Clinical cancer Research: An Official Journal of the American Association for Cancer Research. 2001;7(4):1073–8.

[45] Miura S, Saku K. Regulation of angiogenesis and angiogenic factors by cardiovascular medications. Current Pharmaceutical Design. 2007;13(20):2113–7.

[46] Heffelfinger SC. The renin angiotensin system in the regulation of angiogenesis. Current Pharmaceutical Design. 2007;13(12):1215–29.

[47] Greene AS, Amaral SL. Microvascular angiogenesis and the renin-angiotensin system. Current Hypertension Reports. 2002;4(1):56–62.

[48] Huang W, Wu YL, Zhong J, Jiang FX, Tian XL, Yu LF. Angiotensin II type 1 receptor antagonist suppress angiogenesis and growth of gastric cancer xenografts. Digestive Diseases and Sciences. 2008;53(5):1206–10.

[49] Kosaka T, Miyajima A, Takayama E, Kikuchi E, Nakashima J, Ohigashi T, et al. Angiotensin II type 1 receptor antagonist as an angiogenic inhibitor in prostate cancer. The Prostate. 2007;67(1):41–9.

[50] Noguchi R, Yoshiji H, Ikenaka Y, Namisaki T, Kitade M, Kaji K, et al. Synergistic inhibitory effect of gemcitabine and angiotensin type-1 receptor blocker, losartan, on murine pancreatic tumor growth via antiangiogenic activities. Oncology Reports. 2009;22(2):355–60.

[51] Kerbel RS. Clinical trials of antiangiogenic drugs: opportunities, problems, and assessment of initial results. Journal of Clinical Oncology: Official Journal of the American Society of Clinical Oncology. 2001;19(18 Suppl):45S–51S.

[52] Scappaticci FA. Mechanisms and future directions for angiogenesis-based cancer therapies. Journal of Clinical Oncology: Official Journal of the American Society of Clinical Oncology. 2002;20(18):3906–27.

[53] Noguchi R, Yoshiji H, Kuriyama S, Yoshii J, Ikenaka Y, Yanase K, et al. Combination of interferon-beta and the angiotensin-converting enzyme inhibitor, perindopril, attenuates murine hepatocellular carcinoma development and angiogenesis. Clinical Cancer Research: An Official Journal of the American Association for Cancer Research. 2003;9(16 Pt 1):6038–45.

[54] Yanase K, Yoshiji H, Ikenaka Y, Noguchi R, Kitade M, Kaji K, et al. Synergistic inhibition of hepatocellular carcinoma growth and hepatocarcinogenesis by combination of 5-fluorouracil and angiotensin-converting enzyme inhibitor via anti-angiogenic activities. Oncology Reports. 2007;17(2):441–6.

[55] Staton CA, Chetwood AS, Cameron IC, Cross SS, Brown NJ, Reed MW. The angiogenic switch occurs at the adenoma stage of the adenoma carcinoma sequence in colorectal cancer. Gut. 2007;56(10):1426–32.

[56] Yoshiji H, Yoshii J, Ikenaka Y, Noguchi R, Yanase K, Tsujinoue H, et al. Suppression of the renin-angiotensin system attenuates vascular endothelial growth factor-mediated tumor development and angiogenesis in murine hepatocellular carcinoma cells. International Journal of Oncology. 2002;20(6):1227–31.

[57] Yoshiji H, Kuriyama S, Noguchi R, Yoshii J, Ikenaka Y, Yanase K, et al. Combination of vitamin K2 and the angiotensin-converting enzyme inhibitor, perindopril, attenuates the liver enzyme-altered preneoplastic lesions in rats via angiogenesis suppression. Journal of Hepatology. 2005;42(5):687–93.

[58] Yoshiji H, Noguchi R, Toyohara M, Ikenaka Y, Kitade M, Kaji K, et al. Combination of vitamin K2 and angiotensin-converting enzyme inhibitor ameliorates cumulative recurrence of hepatocellular carcinoma. Journal of Hepatology. 2009;51(2):315–21.

[59] Williams GH. Aldosterone biosynthesis, regulation, and classical mechanism of action. Heart Failure Reviews. 2005;10(1):7–13.

[60] Funder JW. Minireview: Aldosterone and mineralocorticoid receptors: past, present, and future. Endocrinology. 2010;151(11):5098–102.

[61] Wilkinson-Berka JL, Tan G, Jaworski K, Miller AG. Identification of a retinal aldosterone system and the protective effects of mineralocorticoid receptor antagonism on retinal vascular pathology. Circulation Research. 2009;104(1):124–33.

[62] Kaji K, Yoshiji H, Kitade M, Ikenaka Y, Noguchi R, Shirai Y, et al. Selective aldosterone blocker, eplerenone, attenuates hepatocellular carcinoma growth and angiogenesis in mice. Hepatology Research: The Official Journal of the Japan Society of Hepatology. 2010;40(5):540–9.

[63] Llovet JM, Bruix J. Novel advancements in the management of hepatocellular carcinoma in Journal of Hepatology. 2008;48 Suppl 1:S20–37.

[64] Kaji K, Yoshiji H, Kitade M, Ikenaka Y, Noguchi R, Yoshii J, et al. Impact of insulin resistance on the progression of chronic liver diseases. International Journal of Molecular Medicine. 2008;22(6):801–8.

[65] Nielsen MF, Caumo A, Aagaard NK, Chandramouli V, Schumann WC, Landau BR, et al. Contribution of defects in glucose uptake to carbohydrate intolerance in liver cirrhosis: assessment during physiological glucose and insulin concentrations. American journal of physiology Gastrointestinal and Liver Physiology. 2005;288(6):G1135–43.

[66] Kawaguchi T, Yoshida T, Harada M, Hisamoto T, Nagao Y, Ide T, et al. Hepatitis C virus down-regulates insulin receptor substrates 1 and 2 through up-regulation of suppressor of cytokine signaling The American Journal of Pathology. 2004;165(5):1499–508.

[67] Hui JM, Sud A, Farrell GC, Bandara P, Byth K, Kench JG, et al. Insulin resistance is associated with chronic hepatitis C virus infection and fibrosis progression [corrected]. Gastroenterology. 2003;125(6):1695–704.

[68] Petit JM, Bour JB, Galland-Jos C, Minello A, Verges B, Guiguet M, et al. Risk factors for diabetes mellitus and early insulin resistance in chronic hepatitis C. Journal of Hepatology. 2001;35(2):279–83.

[69] Shintani Y, Fujie H, Miyoshi H, Tsutsumi T, Tsukamoto K, Kimura S, et al. Hepatitis C virus infection and diabetes: direct involvement of the virus in the development of insulin resistance. Gastroenterology. 2004;126(3):840–8.

[70] Bugianesi E, McCullough AJ, Marchesini G. Insulin resistance: a metabolic pathway to chronic liver disease. Hepatology. 2005;42(5):987–1000.

[71] Sanyal AJ, Campbell-Sargent C, Mirshahi F, Rizzo WB, Contos MJ, Sterling RK, et al. Nonalcoholic steatohepatitis: association of insulin resistance and mitochondrial abnormalities. Gastroenterology. 2001;120(5):1183–92.

[72] Davila JA, Morgan RO, Shaib Y, McGlynn KA, El-Serag HB. Diabetes increases the risk of hepatocellular carcinoma in the United States: a population based case control study. Gut. 2005;54(4):533–9.

[73] El-Serag HB, Tran T, Everhart JE. Diabetes increases the risk of chronic liver disease and hepatocellular carcinoma. Gastroenterology. 2004;126(2):460–8.

[74] El-Serag HB, Richardson PA, Everhart JE. The role of diabetes in hepatocellular carcinoma: a case-control study among United States Veterans. The American Journal of Gastroenterology. 2001;96(8):2462–7.

[75] Siddique A, Kowdley KV. Insulin resistance and other metabolic risk factors in the pathogenesis of hepatocellular carcinoma. Clinics in Liver Disease. 2011;15(2):281–96, vii-x.

[76] Alexia C, Fallot G, Lasfer M, Schweizer-Groyer G, Groyer A. An evaluation of the role of insulin-like growth factors (IGF) and of type-I IGF receptor signalling in hepatocarcinogenesis and in the resistance of hepatocarcinoma cells against drug-induced apoptosis. Biochemical Pharmacology. 2004;68(6):1003–15.

[77] Donadon V, Balbi M, Mas MD, Casarin P, Zanette G. Metformin and reduced risk of hepatocellular carcinoma in diabetic patients with chronic liver disease. Liver International: Official Journal of the International Association for the Study of the Liver. 2010;30(5):750–8.

[78] Khattab M, Emad M, Abdelaleem A, Eslam M, Atef R, Shaker Y, et al. Pioglitazone improves virological response to peginterferon alpha-2b/ribavirin combination therapy in hepatitis C genotype 4 patients with insulin resistance. Liver International: Official Journal of the International Association for the Study of the Liver. 2010;30(3): 447–54.

[79] El-Serag HB, Johnson ML, Hachem C, Morgana RO. Statins are associated with a reduced risk of hepatocellular carcinoma in a large cohort of patients with diabetes. Gastroenterology. 2009;136(5):1601–8.

[80] Marchesini G, Bianchi G, Merli M, Amodio P, Panella C, Loguercio C, et al. Nutritional supplementation with branched-chain amino acids in advanced cirrhosis: a double-blind, randomized trial. Gastroenterology. 2003;124(7):1792–801.

[81] Muto Y, Sato S, Watanabe A, Moriwaki H, Suzuki K, Kato A, et al. Effects of oral branched-chain amino acid granules on event-free survival in patients with liver cirrhosis. Clinical Gastroenterology and Hepatology: The Official Clinical Practice Journal of the American Gastroenterological Association. 2005;3(7):705–13.

[82] Yoshiji H, Noguchi R, Kaji K, Ikenaka Y, Shirai Y, Namisaki T, et al. Attenuation of insulin-resistance-based hepatocarcinogenesis and angiogenesis by combined treatment with branched-chain amino acids and angiotensin-converting enzyme inhibitor in obese diabetic rats. Journal of Gastroenterology. 2010;45(4):443–50.

[83] Yoshiji H, Noguchi R, Kitade M, Kaji K, Ikenaka Y, Namisaki T, et al. Branched-chain amino acids suppress insulin-resistance-based hepatocarcinogenesis in obese diabetic rats. Journal of Gastroenterology. 2009;44(5):483–91.

[84] Muto Y, Sato S, Watanabe A, Moriwaki H, Suzuki K, Kato A, et al. Overweight and obesity increase the risk for liver cancer in patients with liver cirrhosis and long-term oral supplementation with branched-chain amino acid granules inhibits liver carcinogenesis in heavier patients with liver cirrhosis. Hepatology Research: The Official Journal of the Japan Society of Hepatology. 2006;35(3):204–14.

[85] Jayasooriya AP, Mathai ML, Walker LL, Begg DP, Denton DA, Cameron-Smith D, et al. Mice lacking angiotensin-converting enzyme have increased energy expenditure, with reduced fat mass and improved glucose clearance. Proceedings of the National Academy of Sciences of the United States of America. 2008;105(18):6531–6.

[86] Manrique C, Lastra G, Gardner M, Sowers JR. The renin angiotensin aldosterone system in hypertension: roles of insulin resistance and oxidative stress. The Medical Clinics of North America. 2009;93(3):569–82.

[87] Yoshiji H, Noguchi R, Ikenaka Y, Kaji K, Aihara Y, Yamazaki M, et al. Combination of branched-chain amino acids and angiotensin-converting enzyme inhibitor suppresses the cumulative recurrence of hepatocellular carcinoma: a randomized control trial. Oncology Reports. 2011;26(6):1547–53.

[88] Fabris C, Smirne C, Fangazio S, Toniutto P, Burlone M, Minisini R, et al. Influence of angiotensin-converting enzyme I/D gene polymorphism on clinical and histological correlates of chronic hepatitis C. Hepatology Research: The Official Journal of the Japan Society of Hepatology. 2009;39(8):795–804.

[89] Medeiros R, Vasconcelos A, Costa S, Pinto D, Lobo F, Morais A, et al. Linkage of angiotensin I-converting enzyme gene insertion/deletion polymorphism to the progression of human prostate cancer. The Journal of Pathology. 2004;202(3):330–5.

[90] Yoneda M, Hotta K, Nozaki Y, Endo H, Uchiyama T, Mawatari H, et al. Association between angiotensin II type 1 receptor polymorphisms and the occurrence of nonalcoholic fatty liver disease. Liver International: Official Journal of the International Association for the Study of the Liver. 2009;29(7):1078–85.

3

Molecular Mechanisms of Hepatocellular Carcinoma Related to Aflatoxins: An Update

Xi-Dai Long, Yan Deng, Xiao-Ying Huang, Jin-Guang Yao, Qun-Ying Su, Xue-Min Wu, Juan Wang, Qun-Qing Xu, Xiao-Ying Zhu, Chao Wang, Bing-Chen Huang and Qiang Xia

Abstract

Hepatocellular carcinoma (hepatocarcinoma) is a major type of primary liver cancer and one of the most frequent human malignant neoplasms. Aflatoxins are I-type chemical carcinogen for hepatocarcinoma. Increasing evidence has shown that hepatocarcinoma induced by aflatoxins is the result of interaction between aflatoxins and hereditary factor. Aflatoxins can induce DNA damage including DNA strand break, adducts formation, oxidative DNA damage, and gene mutation and determine which susceptible individuals feature cancer. Inheritance such as alterations may result in the activation of proto-oncogenes and the inactivation of tumor suppressor genes and determine individual susceptibility to cancer. Interaction between aflatoxins and genetic susceptible factors commonly involve in almost all pathologic sequence of hepatocarcinoma: chronic liver injury, cirrhosis, atypical hyperplastic nodules, and hepatocarcinoma of early stages. In this review, we discuss the biogenesis, toxification, and epidemiology of aflatoxins and signal pathways of aflatoxin-induced hepatocarcinoma. We also discuss the roles of some important genes related to cell apoptosis, DNA repair, drug metabolism, and tumor metastasis in hepatocarcinogenesis related to aflatoxins.

Keywords: hepatocellular carcinoma, molecular mechanism, aflatoxin

1. Introduction

Hepatocellular carcinoma (also called hepatocarcinoma or liver carcinoma) is a major type of primary liver cancer and one of the most frequent human malignant neoplasms. This malignancy has been proved to correlate with aflatoxins, especially aflatoxin B1 (AFB1) [1–3].

Increasing evidence has exhibited that several mechanisms, including the toxic production from metabolism, the accumulation of DNA damage and genic mutation–induced aflatoxins, the decreasing DNA repair capacity, and dysregulation of signal pathways may play a central role in the tumorigenesis of aflatoxin-induced hepatocarcinoma [4–6]. In this review, we discuss the biogenesis, metabolism, and genic toxification of aflatoxins. We also discuss the molecular mechanisms of aflatoxin-induced hepatocarcinoma, involving in aflatoxin toxification, abnormal change of tumor relative genes, the interaction of aflatoxins and genetic factors, and signal pathway for tumorigenesis. The roles of some important genes related to cell apoptosis, DNA repair, drug metabolism, and tumor metastasis in hepatocarcinogenesis related to aflatoxins are further emphasized.

2. Aflatoxin biosynthesis, metabolism, and toxification

2.1. Aflatoxin biosynthesis

The biosynthesis of aflatoxins has been fully summarized in several previous reviews [7, 8]. In brief, aflatoxins are an important type of mycotoxins, which were the most early identified in the *Aspergillus flavus* (*A. flavus*) and regarded as causative agents of "turkey X" disease in the late 1950s and early 1960s. Thus, these toxins were named as "aflatoxins (namely *A. flavus* toxins)" according to their origin fungus [9]. Until now, 17 related aflatoxin isoforms and aflatoxin metabolites have been identified, and 4 of them often contaminated a number of agricultural commodities [10]. According to the amounts and fluorescent reactions, four aflatoxins primarily identified in foodstuffs are named as AFB1, aflatoxin B2 (AFB2), aflatoxin G1 (AFG1), and aflatoxin G2 (AFG2). Among these four known aflatoxins, AFB1 and AFB2 are named as B-type aflatoxins because they are attached to a pentanone and can produce blue-color fluorescent under UV light, whereas AFG1 and AFG2 are termed as G-type aflatoxins because of their attachment to a 6-membered lactone and producing green fluorescent color feature. These aflatoxins are mainly produced by *A. flavus*, *Aspergillus parasiticus* (*A. parasiticus*), *Aspergillus nidulans* (*A. nidulans*), *Aspergillus pseudotamarii* (*A. pseudotamarii*), and *Aspergillus bombycis* (*A. bombycis*) [7, 8].

Toxigenic strains of *A. flavus* produce only B-type aflatoxins, but do not synthesize G-type aflatoxins due to the deletion of an unstable microsome enzyme and a-220 kDa cytosolic protein. The other aflatoxigenic species including *A. parasiticus*, *A. nidulans*, *A. pseudotamarii*, and *A. bombycis* can produce all four aflatoxins [8].

Numeral synthetical genes, such as aflatoxin regulatory protein gene (aflR), are required for aflatoxin biosynthesis and act as a huge neighbor gene cluster consisting of about 60–70 kb in original fungi (**Figure 1**) [8–10]. All corresponding gene-encoding enzymes and transcription factors produce aflatoxin production and regulate biosynthesis. Increasing evidence has proved that aflatoxin biosynthesis involves in at least 3 stages and 18 enzyme steps (**Figures 2–4**). The first stage, including the first (R01) to eighth reaction (R08) of biosynthesis, refers from acetyl CoA to hydroxyversicolorone. The primary product hydroxyversicolorone will be formed and regulated by transcription factors aflR and aflJ (**Figure 2**) [8, 10]. The second (biosynthesis

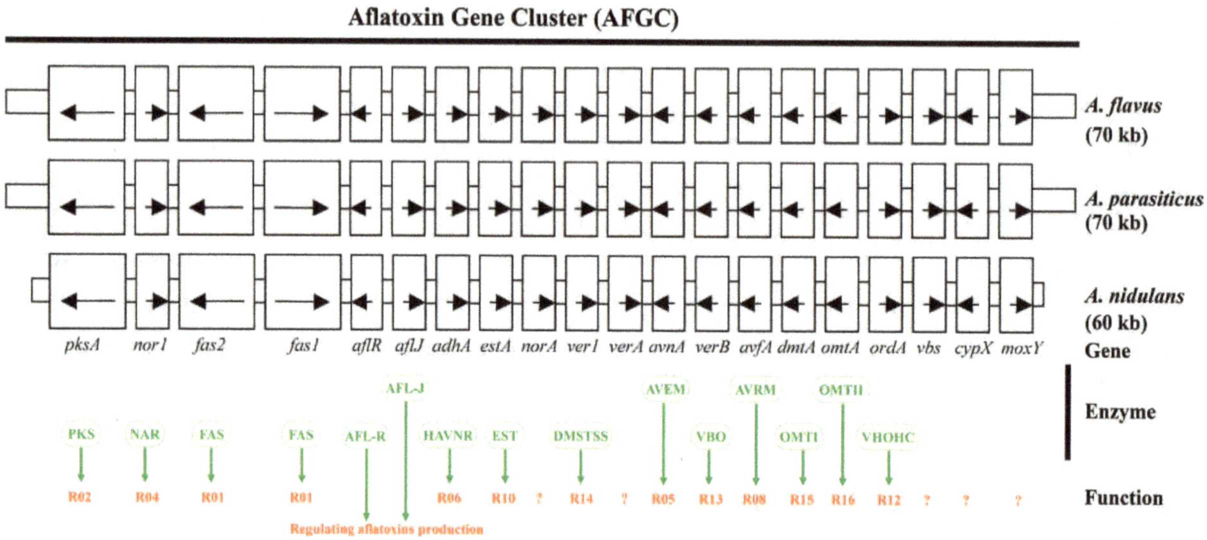

Figure 1. The aflatoxin gene cluster and their expression productions and functions. In the fungus-producing aflatoxins including *A. nidulans, A. parasiticus,* and *A. flavus,* genes encoding the enzymes and the transcription factors involving in aflatoxin biosynthesis commonly locate within a huge gene cluster of about 60–70 kb in the genomes. These genes, except for aflR and aflJ, involve in the 18 enzyme reaction steps (R01–R18) of aflatoxin biosynthesis, whereas aflR and aflJ expressing proteins are two important transcription factors and can regulate enzyme-related gene expression. "?" shows that the function of the corresponding gene is unknown (Note: adapted from Yabe and Nakajima [7]). *Abbreviations.* MCA, malonyl CoA; HAS, hexanoate synthase (also termed fatty acid synthase); PKS, polyketide synthase; NAS, Norsolorinic acid (NA) synthase; NAR, norsolorinic acid (NA) reductase; AVN, averantin; AVNM, averantin (AVN) monooxygenase; HAVN, 5′-hydroxyaverantin; HAVNR, 5′-hydroxyaverantin reductase; OVENC, 5′-oxoaverantin (OAVN) cyclase; AVRM, averufin (AVR) monooxygenase; VHAS, versiconal hemiacetal acetate (VHA) synthase; VHOHC, versiconal (VHOH) cyclase (also called versicolorin B synthase); VHAR, versiconal hemiacetal acetate (VHA) reductase; VBD, versicolorin B (VB) desaturase; DMSTSS, demethylsterigmatocystin (DMST) synthase system; OMTI, *O*-methyltransferase I; OMTII, *O*-methyltransferase II; OAE, OrdA enzyme.

reaction: R09–R12) (**Figure 3**) and third stages (biosynthesis reaction: R13–R18) (**Figure 4**) refer from hydroxyversicolorone to versicolorin B and from versicolorin B (VB) to the formation of ultimate products, respectively. These two stages involve in the formation of hydroxy- and non–hydroxy-versicolorone, and toxins. During the aflatoxin synthesis, more than 10 nicotinamide-adenine dinucleotide phosphate reduced form (NAPDH), one nicotinamide-adenine dinucleotide (NAD), and 2*S*-adenosylmethionine (SAM) are required. These cofactors may play a critical role in the control of aflatoxin biosynthesis [7–10].

2.2. The metabolism of aflatoxins in liver

Aflatoxins synthesized in the mycelia are finally excreted into such mediums as cereals (maize, wheat, sorghum, rice, and millet), nuts (peanuts, pistachios, walnuts, Brazil nut, and coconut), spices (chili, turmeric, paprika, black pepper, and ginger), and seeds. Epidemiological studies have exhibited that AFB1 is the most common in contaminated human foods [8, 10]. Once this aflatoxin in the mediums is taken into body, it is metabolized via two-stage reactions in the liver. The first-stage metabolisms include reduction reaction (ketoreduction to aflatoxicol), oxidative reaction (O-dealkylation to aflatoxin P1), and hydrolytic reactions (hydroxylation to aflatoxin M1, aflatoxin Q1, and aflatoxin B2). This stage reaction involves numerous enzymes such as cytochromes P450 (CYP450), monooxygenases, amino-oxidases, alcohol dehydrogenases, epoxide-hydrolases, aldehyde-reductases, and ketone-reductases. The second-stage reaction mainly comprises covalent binding reaction (toxic produces) and conjugation reaction (excretion and detoxification). Through these metabolites, aflatoxins ultimately transform into nontoxic secretions and toxic products [10, 11].

2.3. The toxification of aflatoxins in liver

Toxification of aflatoxins in liver is mainly divided into acute and chronic toxic effects. Data from epidemiological, experimental, and clinical studies have shown that above 6000 mg exposure of aflatoxin through digestion will cause acute severe liver damage and subsequent

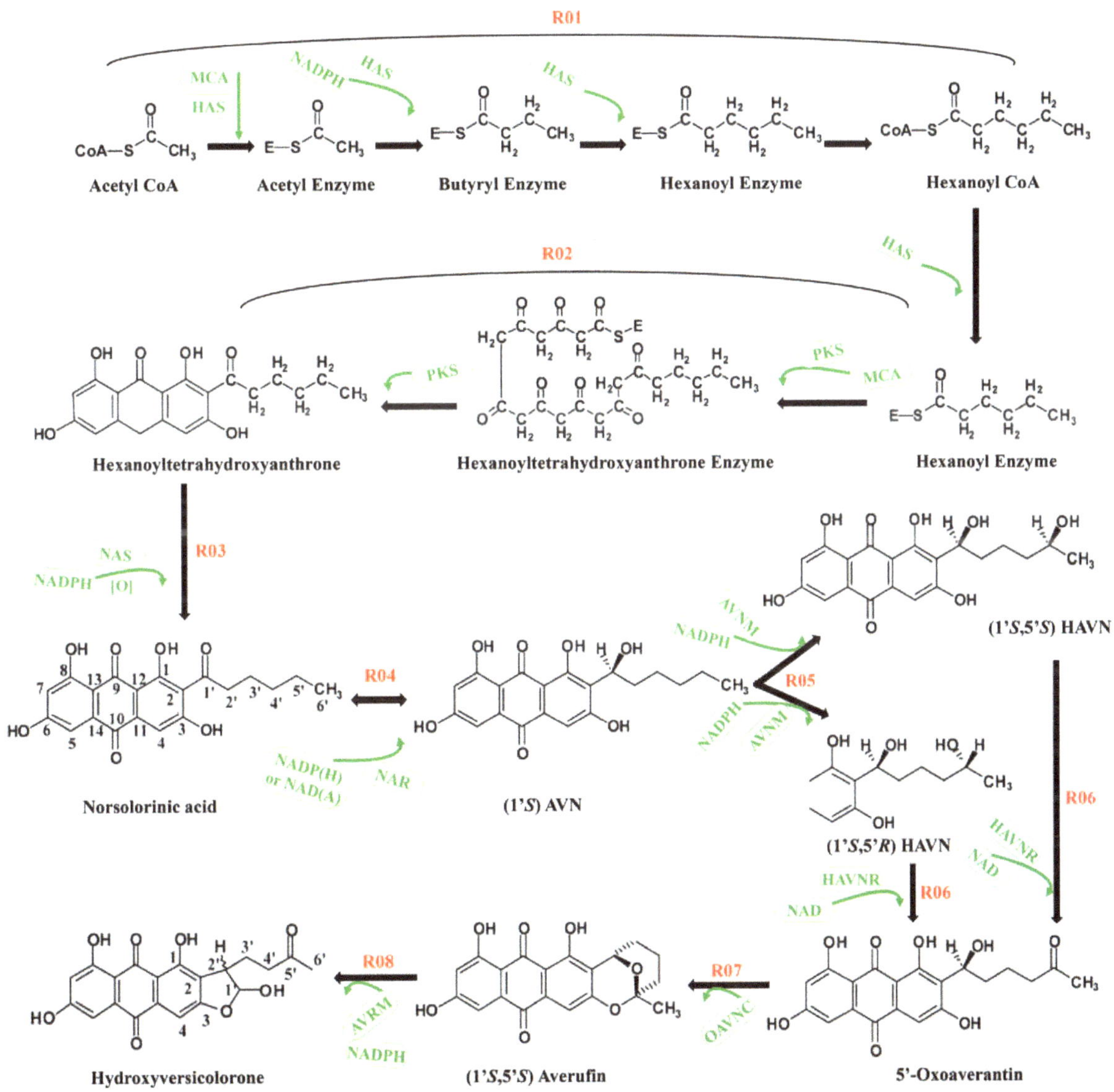

Figure 2. The first stage of aflatoxin biosynthesis. The first stage of aflatoxin biosynthesis, including the first (R01) to eighth reaction (R08) of biosynthesis, refers from acetyl CoA to hydroxyversicolorone. *Abbreviations.* MCA, malonyl CoA; HAS, hexanoate synthase (also termed fatty acid synthase); PKS, polyketide synthase; NAS, norsolorinic acid (NA) synthase; NAR, norsolorinic acid (NA) reductase; AVN, averantin; AVNM, averantin (AVN) monooxygenase; HAVN, 5'-hydroxyaverantin; HAVNR, 5'-hydroxyaverantin reductase; OVENC, 5'-oxoaverantin (OAVN) cyclase; AVRM, averufin (AVR) monooxygenase; NADP, nicotinamide adenine dinucleotide phosphate; NADPH, nicotinamide-adenine dinucleotide phosphate (reduced form); CoA, coenzyme A. *Noted:* adapted from Yabe and Nakajima [7].

illness or death. This kind of acute effect is mainly associated with malfunction of the liver induced by toxic metabolic products. For chronic toxic effects, chronic exposure of aflatoxins can induce DNA damage and produce genotoxicity and carcinogenicity. In the past decades, increasing evidence has proved that AFB1 as aflatoxins often induce genic mutations such as TP53 and are among the most carcinogenic substances known and the major cancerous hepatocarcinoma risk factor.

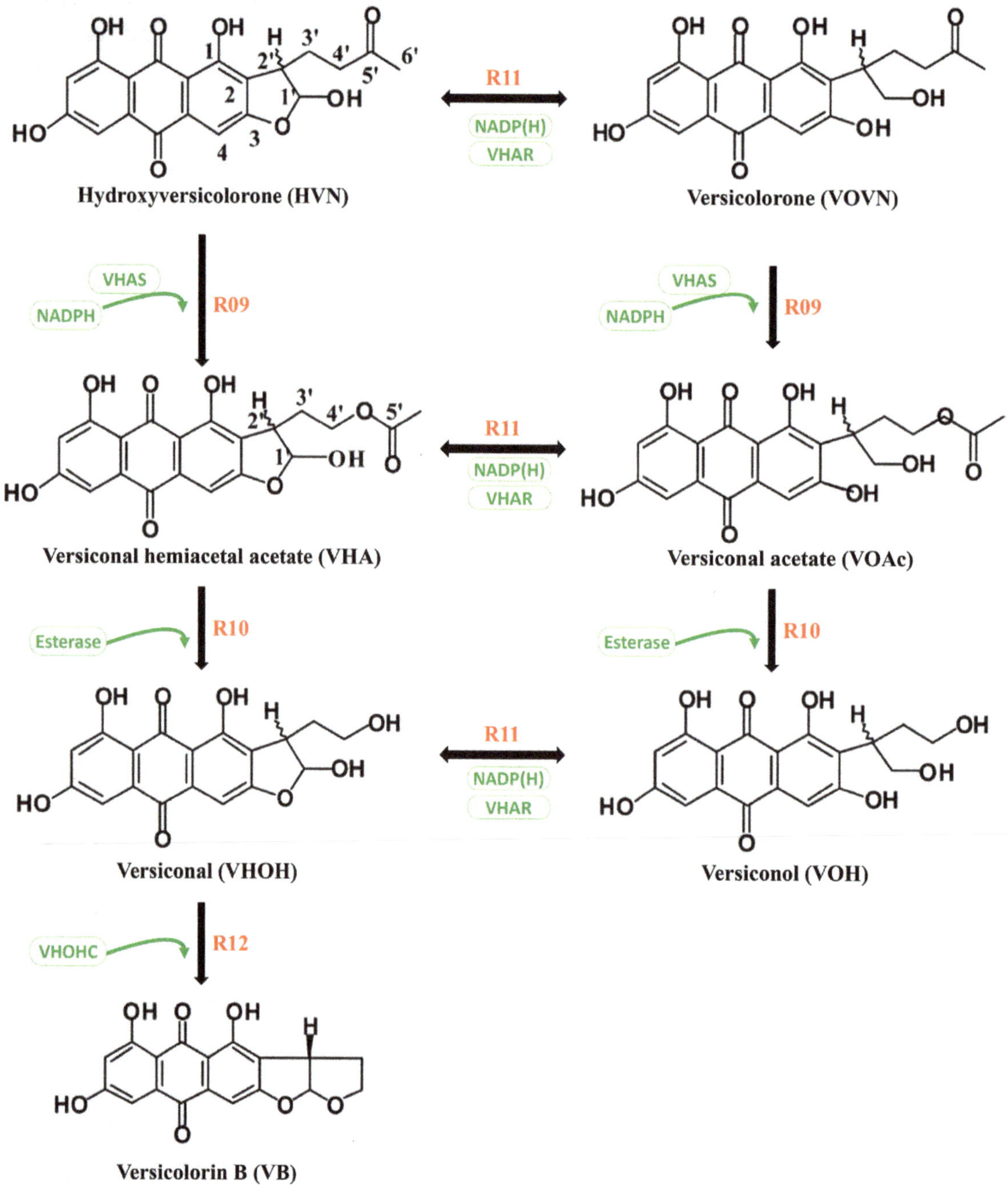

Figure 3. The second stage of aflatoxin biosynthesis. The second stage of aflatoxin biosynthesis, including the ninth (R09) to twelfth reaction (R12) of biosynthesis, refers from hydroxyversicolorone to versicolorin B (VB). *Abbreviations.* VHAS, versiconal hemiacetal acetate (VHA) synthase; VHOHC, versiconal (VHOH) cyclase (also called versicolorin B synthase); VHAR, versiconal hemiacetal acetate (VHA) reductase; NADP, nicotinamide adenine dinucleotide phosphate; NADPH, nicotinamide-adenine dinucleotide phosphate (reduced form). *Noted:* adapted from Yabe and Nakajima [7].

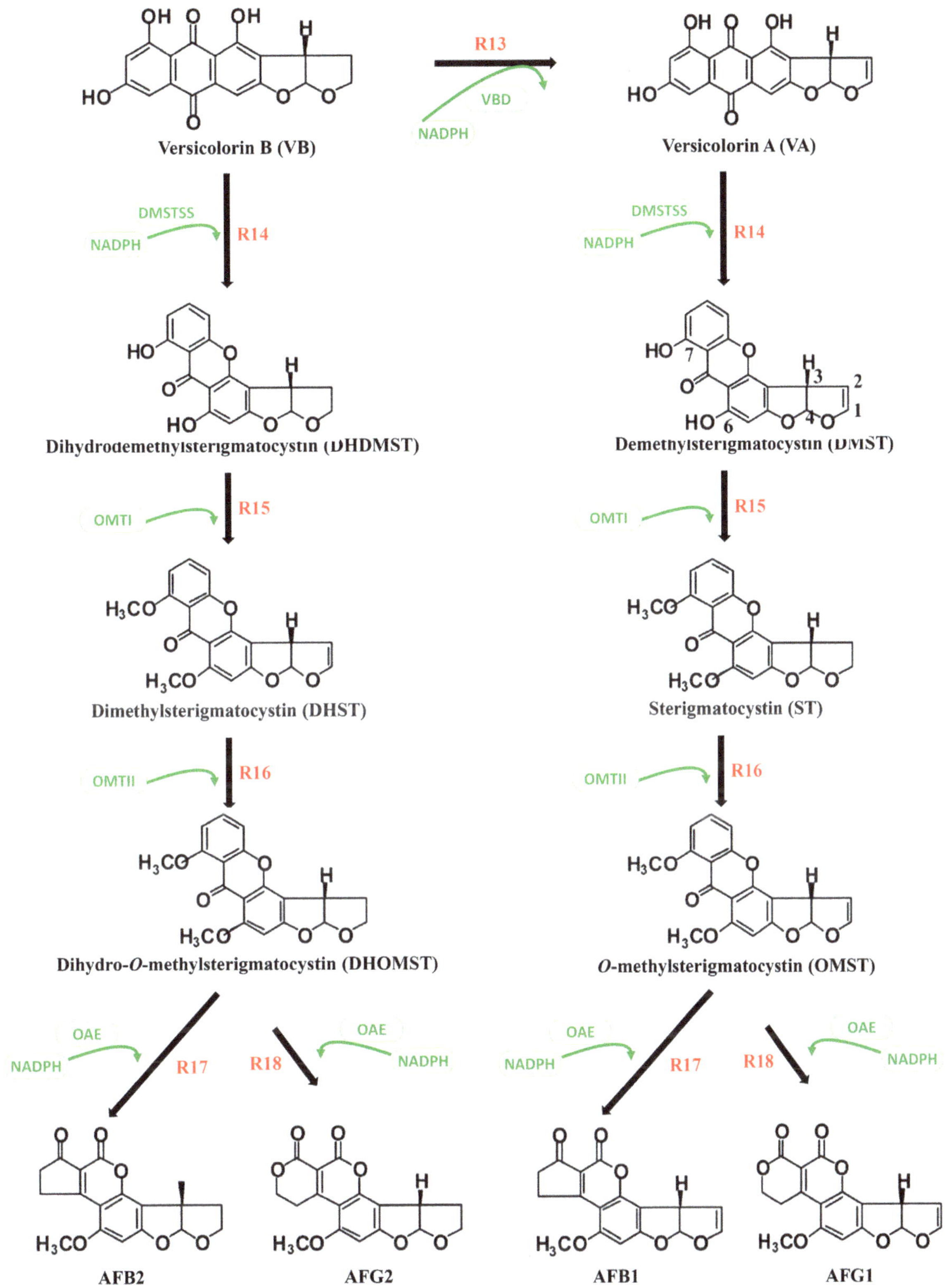

Figure 4. The third stage of aflatoxin biosynthesis. The third stage of aflatoxin biosynthesis, including the 13th (R13) to 18th reaction (R18) of biosynthesis, refers from versicolorin B (VB) to the formation of aflatoxin B1 (AFB1), aflatoxin B2 (AFB2), aflatoxin G1 (AFG1), and aflatoxin G2 (AFG2). *Abbreviations.* VBD, versicolorin B (VB) desaturase; DMSTSS, demethylsterigmatocystin (DMST) synthase system; OMTI, *O*-methyltransferase I; OMTII, *O*-methyltransferase II; OAE, OrdA enzyme; NADP, nicotinamide adenine dinucleotide phosphate; NADPH, nicotinamide-adenine dinucleotide phosphate (reduced form). *Noted:* adapted from Yabe and Nakajima [7].

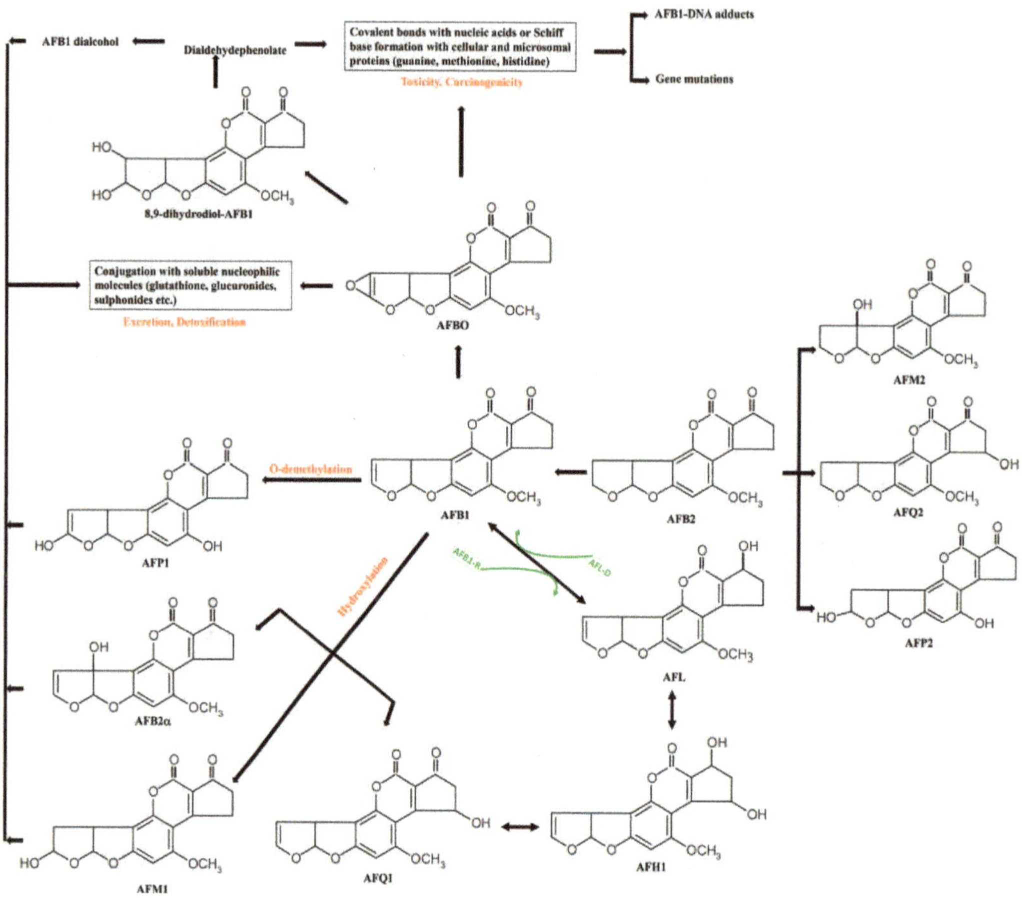

Figure 5. The metabolite of aflatoxins in the liver. Aflatoxins are metabolized via four metabolic pathways: O-dealkylation to aflatoxin P1 (AFP1), ketoreduction to aflatoxicol (AFL), epoxidation to AFB1-8,9-epoxide (AFBO, highly toxic, mutagenic, and carcinogenic), and hydroxylation to aflatoxin M1 (AFM1, highly toxic), AFP1, aflatoxin Q1 (AFQ1), or aflatoxin B2a (AFB2a). *Abbreviations.* AFM2, aflatoxin M2; AFP2, aflatoxin P2; AFQ2, aflatoxin Q2; AFL-D, aflatoxicol dehydrogenase; AFB1-R, aflatoxin B1 reductase. *Noted:* adapted from Wu and Jezkova [10].

3. The molecular mechanisms of aflatoxin-induced hepatocarcinoma

As described earlier, the main chronic toxification of aflatoxins is chronic liver damage and induced tumorigenesis of hepatocarcinoma. AFB1 has been proved as an I-type chemical carcinogen. Mechanisms of AFB1-induced hepatocarcinoma mainly involve in DNA damage and repair, the inactivation of tumor suppressor genes and the activation of oncogenes from genic mutations, abnormal immunoreaction, and inheritance alterations.

3.1. Aflatoxin-induced DNA damage

Increasing evidence has shown that the carcinogenicity of aflatoxins results from aflatoxin-induced DNA damage, including the formation of DNA adducts, DNA single strand breaks (SSBs) or double strand breaks (DSBs), chromosomal aberration damage (CAD), unscheduled DNA synthesis (USDS), abnormal chromatid exchange (ACE), the formation of micronuclei and macronuclei, and oxidation DNA damage. Of these DNA damages, AFB1-DNA adducts are the most common damage types and consist of 8,9-dihydro-8-(N^7-guanyl)-9-hydroxy–AFB1 adduct (AFB1-GA) and ring-opened formamidopyrimidine AFB1 adduct (AFB1-FAPYA). The formation of AFB1-GA begins from AFB1 covalent binding to DNA and its product 8,9-epoxide-AFB1 (AFBE) by CYP450 [12, 13]. This adduct can automatically not only give rise to AFB1-FAYPA, which is accumulated using a time-dependence and nonenzyme pathway, but also be transferred into AFP1, AFM1, AFQ1, and other products by metabolic enzymes.

Additionally, AFB1 also induces oxidation DNA damage such as 8-oxodeoxyguanosine (8-_{oxyG}). These damages induced by aflatoxins, if not timely repaired, can cause subsequent repair-resistant adducts and depurination or lead to error-prone DNA repair resulting in DSBs, SSBs, USDs, CAD, ACE, and frame shift mutations. Interestingly, the accumulation of DNA damages is positively associated with the time and the levels of aflatoxin exposure and modifies the risk of hepatocarcinoma through regulating the expression of some genes such as a disintegrin and metalloproteinase with thrombospondin motifs 5 (ADAMTS5) [14], X-ray repair complementing 4 (XRCC4) [15], microRNA-4651 [16], and so on (**Table 1**). For example, Huang et al. [14] investigated the association between AFB1-DNA adducts via a hospital-based case control study and found increasing AFB1-DNA adducts negatively correlated with ADAMTS5 expression. It is known that ADAMTS5 may act as a tumor suppressor gene via decreasing vascular endothelial growth factor (VEGF) expression and inhibiting tumor angiogenesis and metastasis [17]. The downregulation of XRCC4 by increasing AFB1-DNA adducts decreases repair capacity for SSBs and DSBs and increases risk of tumor suppressor gene TP53 mutation and tumors [15, 18–22]. These genes progress the tumorigenesis and progression of hepatocarcinoma via regulating DNA repair capacity and angiogenesis. Although AFB1-DNA adducts are mainly produced in liver cells, they are also found in the immune cells and may regulate the immune function. Thus, DNA damage may be an important molecular event and may play a crucial role in the carcinogenesis of hepatocarcinoma caused by aflatoxins.

3.2. The mutagenesis of aflatoxins

Aflatoxin-induced DNA adducts can produce depurination, DSBs, the substitution of DNA bases, and frame shift mutations. In the past decades, the *in vivo* and *in vitro* studies have shown that the mutagenesis of aflatoxins can induce the mutation from GC to TA. As previously shown, mispairing of the aflatoxin-DNA adducts can cause both transition and transversion mutations [25–27]. In an *in vitro* non-sense analysis, Foster et al. found that the action form of AFB1 (namely AFBE) can induce more than 90% of GC to TA mutation [28]. This

Gene	Expression change	Role of change in the hepatocarcinoma carcinogenesis	Ref
ADAMTS5	Down	Angiogenesis, metastasis, prognosis	[14]
XRCC4	Down	Low DNA repair capacity, gene mutation	[15]
MicroRNA-4651	Up	Angiogenesis, metastasis, prognosis	[16]
MicroRNA-24	Up	Angiogenesis, metastasis, prognosis	[23]
MicroRNA-429	Up	Angiogenesis, metastasis, prognosis	[24]

Table 1. The change of gene expression related to DNA damage induced by aflatoxins.

mutation was further proved to locate in the GC-rich regions via the plasmid system identifying mutational target enzyme and named as hot-spot regions for aflatoxin-induced mutations [29–31]. Results from quantitative analyses based on the *in vitro* cell model, which was transfected by pS189 (a shuttle vector having mutative targets), also showed that more than 90% of mutative spectra caused by aflatoxins was GC to TA (about 50% of mutations) and GG to TC transversion (about 30% of mutations) [32]. It has been proved that the accumulation of these transversions will result in the mutations of some important genes such as TP53 and Ras and promote hepatocarcinogenesis [31, 33].

3.3. The abnormality of tumor suppressor genes induced by aflatoxins

Studies *in vivo* and *in vitro* have examined the abnormality of tumor suppressor genes by aflatoxin exposure (**Table 2**). Among these known genes, the abnormality of TP53 induced by aflatoxins has been proved to be an important molecule change [34, 35]. In high aflatoxin-exposure areas, the mutations of TP53 gene, especially hot-spot mutation at codon 249, are present among more than 40% of patients with AFB1-related hepatocarcinoma, whereas this kind of mutation is very rare among cases with null or low AFB1 exposure [14, 36, 37]. Therefore, the mutation at codon 249 of TP53 gene has been defined as a molecular symbol for hepatocarcinoma caused by AFB1 exposure. Results from clinical sample and experimental studies further display that consistent exposure of aflatoxins may result in the accumulation of TP53 mutant protein and abnormal DNA damage repair, apoptosis, and immunoreaction [38]. Other genes such as bcl2, p27, p16, and p21 are found to produce different expression or abnormal structural change under the conditions of aflatoxin expression (**Table 2**). Taken together, inactivation of tumor suppressor genes from mutation and increasing mutant expression may be a crucial step of malignant transformation for liver cells.

3.4. The abnormality of oncogenes induced by aflatoxins

In the past decades, the abnormality of oncogenes induced by aflatoxins has mainly been focused on c-myc and ras genes, involving in the activation, expression, and mutation of proto-oncogenes (**Table 3**). For example, Tashiro et al. investigated the effects of AFB1 exposure on oncogenes based on rat model with AFB1-induced hepatomas and found that the expression of both c-myc and c-Ha-ras was upregulated in all the tumors [65]. They also observed c-Ha-ras amplification and rearrangement [65]. In Fischer rat models with AFB1- and AFG1-induced liver tumors, Sinha et al. observed that aflatoxins can induce activation of N-ras and spot mutation of G to A at codon 12 of Ki-ras [66]. This type of activation and mutation will increase in the tissues with liver cancer than those with noncancers [66–69]. Results from *in vitro* studies have further proved that aflatoxins can induce gene mutations of oncogenes [70]. Together, these data suggest that aflatoxins may activate proto-oncogenes by inducing gene mutations and promote the carcinogenesis of hepatocarcinoma.

3.5. The interaction of aflatoxins and hepatitis B virus promoting hepatocarcinogenesis

The interaction of aflatoxins and hepatitis B virus (HBV) has been proved in the carcinogenesis of hepatocarcinoma by molecular epidemiological and clinicopathological studies and sys-

Gene	Study design	Change	Significance	Ref
TP53	Mice model with HNP	Expression ↑	DNA damage ↑	[39]
bcl2	Mice model with HNP	Expression ↓	DNA damage ↑	[39]
p27	Hepatocytes *in vitro*	Expression ↓	DNA damage ↑	[40]
p21	Hepatocytes *in vitro*	Expression ↓	DNA damage ↑	[40]
TP53	HCCs (n = 223)	Expression ↑, multiplot mutation	Carcinogenesis	[41]
TP53	HCCs (n = 124)	Mutation at codon 249: 60%	Carcinogenesis	[42]
H2AX	HCC cells *in vitro*	Phosphorylation	Carcinogenesis	[43]
BP1	HCC cells *in vitro*	Phosphorylation	Carcinogenesis	[43]
TP53	HCCs (n = 52)	Mutation at codon 249: 50%	Carcinogenesis	[44]
p16	HCCs (n = 40)	Methylation	Carcinogenesis	[45]
p53	HCCs (n = 40)	Multiplot mutation	Carcinogenesis	[45]
p53	AFB1-induced mutation *in vitro*	Multiplot mutation at CpG	Carcinogenesis	[46]
TP53	HCCs (n = 64) plus a meta-analysis	Mutation at codon 249: 36%, protein accumulation: 50%	Carcinogenesis	[47]
TP53	Mice model with HNP	Multiplot mutation	Carcinogenesis	[48]
TP53	HCC cells *in vitro*	AFB1-induced mutation at codon 249 promoting IGF-II expression	Carcinogenesis	[49]
TP53	Atcc-Ccl13 *in vitro*	Mutation at codon 249	Carcinogenesis	[50]
TP53	HCCs (n = 36)	Mutation at codon 249	Carcinogenesis	[51]
TP53	Mice model	Mutation at codon 249 and 346, mutant protein increasing	Carcinogenesis	[52–57]
TP53	HCCs (n = 60)	Mutation at codon 249: 69%	Carcinogenesis	[58, 59]
TP53	Hepatocytes *in vitro*	Multiplot mutation	Carcinogenesis	[60]
TP53	HCCs (n = 110)	Mutation at codon 249: 69%	DNA damage, carcinogenesis	[61]
TP53	HCCs (n = 15)	Mutation at codon 249 and 254	Carcinogenesis	[62]
TP53	HCC cells *in vitro*	AFB1-induced Mutation at codon 249	Carcinogenesis	[63]
TP53	HCCs (n = 18)	Mutation at codon 249: 53%	Carcinogenesis	[64]

Abbreviations. HNP, hepatic neoplasms; HCC, hepatocarcinoma.

Table 2. The change information of tumor suppressor genes induced by aflatoxins in hepatic cells and hepatocarcinoma cells.

Gene	Study design	Change	Significance	Ref
N-ras	HCCs (n = 36)	Mutation at codon 61	Carcinogenesis	[51]
c-myc	Mice model with HNP	Expression ↑, amplification, rearrangement	Carcinogenesis	[65]
c-Ha-ras	Mice model with HNP	Expression ↑, amplification, rearrangement	Carcinogenesis	[65]
Ki-ras	Mice model with HNP	Activation	Carcinogenesis	[69]
N-ras	Mice model with HNP	Activation	Carcinogenesis	[66]
Ki-ras	Mice model with HNP	Mutation at codon 12	Carcinogenesis	[66]
N-ras	Mice model with HCC	Activation	Carcinogenesis	[67]
Ki-ras	Mice model with HCC	Activation	Carcinogenesis	[67]
c-Ha-ras	Mice model with HNP	Mutation at codon 61: 40–60%	Carcinogenesis	[71, 72]

Abbreviations. HNP, hepatic neoplasms; HCC, hepatocarcinoma.

Table 3. The change information of oncogenes induced by aflatoxins.

tematically reviewed by several studies [73–75]. In brief, the first clinicopathological evidence of aflatoxins interacting with HBV was provided by Yeh et al. [76]. Through a case-control study design conducted in Guangxi Area, they found that these HBV-positive individuals with high AFB1 exposure consumption featured 10-times the mortality rate compared with those with low exposure consumption. Results from multivariable interactive analyses have further convinced that AFB1 multiplicatively interacted with HBV status for promoting hepatocarcinoma risk [77–80]. For example, Williams et al. reported that the risk of developing hepatocarcinoma was 6.37 for aflatoxin exposure, 11.3 for HBV infection, and 73.0 for the combination of aflatoxin and HBV [77]. The following several molecular epidemiological studies with large-size samples from areas with high aflatoxin exposure and high HBV infection in China showed remarkably multiplicative effect for hepatocarcinoma risk (multiplicative interaction: $63.2_{\text{(both positive)}} > 1.9_{\text{(AFB1 positive)}} \times 9.5_{\text{(HBV positive)}}$ [78–80].

This interaction of two hepatocarcinogenic causes has been proved in the transgenic mice models with overexpressing HBV large envelope polypeptide [81]. Results from this study exhibited that animals will produce more rapid and extensive hepatic dysplasia and hepatocarcinoma under the conditions with aflatoxin consumption [81]. Similar findings have also shown in the studies based on woodchuck and duck models [82–84].

The aflatoxins interacting with HBV infection promoting hepatocarcinoma development mechanically involve in the following aspects. First, HBV infection directly or indirectly increases the sensitivity of hepatocytes on the toxification of aflatoxins. Evidence from observation studies have displayed that HBV-positive carriers have more amount of aflatoxin adducts than those with negative HBV status, although they are from the same high aflatoxin exposure area [85, 86]. The active product of aflatoxin AFBE is found to significantly increase the risk of viral DNA integrating into damaged DNA strand [87]. This promotes malignant transformation of damaged hepatocytes by aflatoxins. Second, HBV infection increases the mutation frequency at codon 249 of TP53 gene and coordinates with aflatoxins for abrogating the normal functions of TP53 (such as the control of cell cycle, DNA damage repair, and cell apoptosis), which contributes to multisteps of hepatic carcinogenesis [64, 88]. Third, the HBV X gene–expressing protein inhibits base excision repair potential and results in an increasing accumulation of aflatoxin-DNA adducts [89]. Finally, HBV infections can cause hepatocytic necrosis, inflammatory proliferation, and oxygen/nitrogen active products, which may increase the likelihood of aflatoxin-induced mutations and the cellular clonal expansion containing mutations [90–92].

3.6. The interaction of aflatoxins and inheritance alterations promoting hepatocarcinogenesis

Increasing evidence has exhibited that the genetic alterations in DNA repair genes increase the amount of AFB1-DNA adducts and the frequency of hot-spot mutation at codon 249 of TP53 gene and may promote hepatic toxification of aflatoxins [1, 19, 20, 22, 37, 93–98]. Joint analyses based on meta-analyses further showed this kind of toxic effects (**Table 4**) [1, 22]. The genetic variants in other genes, such as CYP450, glutathione *S*-transferase T1 (GSTT1), glutathione *S*-transferase M1 (GSTM1), and microsomal epoxide hydrolase (HEHY), also display similar modificative effects on aflatoxin-induced hepatocarcinoma [98–101]. Interestingly, the multiplicatively interactive effects between aflatoxins and genetic alterations in these genes have been identified in the risk elucidation of hepatocarcinoma related to aflatoxins [22]. Taken together, genetic deficiency in the DNA repair and detoxification capacity may play a vital role in the carcinogenetic process of aflatoxin-induced hepatocarcinoma.

3.7. The aflatoxin-caused immunosuppression promoting hepatocarcinogenesis

Increasing evidence from *in vitro* and *in vivo* studies has proved that the immunosuppression induced by aflatoxins plays an important role in the carcinogenesis of hepatocarcinoma. Several known mechanisms may involve in this progression step. First, aflatoxins can significantly suppress the functions of macrophages via affecting the expression and secretions of cytokines such as tumor necrosis factor (TNF)-α, interleukin (IL)-1, IL-2, IL-3, IL-6, and reactive intermediates (including nitric oxide, hydrogen peroxide, and superoxide anion) [102, 103]. The suppression of macrophages by aflatoxins may be also correlated with the arrest in the G1/G0 phase [104] and altered expression of CD14 (a cell surface protein functionally regulating immunoreaction) [105]. This suppression may result in the dysregulation of the immune response and homeostasis, which contributes to the accumulation of abnormal cells with DNA damage and altered genome induced by aflatoxins, and ultimately progresses tumorigenesis. Second, aflatoxin exposure can decrease the secretion of antibody such as IgA [106]. For example, Turner et al. investigated effects of aflatoxin exposure on antibody production based on a large molecular epidemiological study [106]. In their study, they tested the levels of saliva secretory IgA (sIgA) in Gambian children (n = 472) with different degree exposure of aflatoxins and found that these individuals with high aflatoxin exposure featured lower level of sIgA in their saliva compared to those without high exposure (50.4 vs. 70.2 μg/mg protein). Finally, aflatoxins may alter T-cell functions (including decreased T-cell populations and suppressed CD4+ T-cell function) and increase individuals' susceptibility to other carcinogens [77, 107].

Gene	RS#	Genotype	TP53M			DNA adducts	
			%	Risk	*P*	Mean	*P*
XRCC1	rs25487	CC	46.51	Reference		3.276	
		CT	45.25	2.419	3.371×10^{-11}	3.264	0.899
		TT	8.24	5.028	6.651×10^{-6}	3.640	0.026
XRCC3	rs861539	GG	32.17	Reference		2.990	
		GA	43.55	1.380	0.018	3.216	0.025
		AA	24.28	1.524	0.011	3.897	4.962×10^{-14}
XRCC7	rs7003908	AA	21.24	Reference		2.879	
		AC	46.06	1.883	1.372×10^{-5}	3.347	1.663×10^{-5}
		CC	32.71	2.089	4.368×10^{-6}	3.550	1.751×10^{-8}
XRCC4	rs28383151	GG	67.03	Reference		3.308	
		GA	21.68	1.688	0.001	3.405	0.069
		AA	11.29	3.829	7.387×10^{-6}	3.721	2.867×10^{-4}
XRCC4	rs3734091	GG	72.31	Reference		3.229	
		GT	17.56	2.799	9.191×10^{-7}	3.439	0.095
		TT	10.13	5.104	3.826×10^{-6}	3.654	0.005
XPD	rs13181	TT	34.41	Reference		2.926	
		TG	41.85	1.458	0.005	3.253	0.011
		GG	23.75	1.744	0.001	4.062	4.265×10^{-6}
XPC	rs2228001	TT	34.05	Reference		3.083	
		TG	48.30	1.500	0.002	3.332	0.001
		GG	17.65	1.818	0.001	3.666	3.404×10^{-22}

Noted: Adapted from Refs. [13] and [84]. *Abbreviations.* TP53M, hot-spot mutation at codon 249 of TP53 gene; RS#, the number of polymorphism.

Table 4. Polymorphisms in DNA repair genes and HCC risk.

Altogether, the data available to date make it clear that aflatoxins can exert an immunosuppressive effect via different pathways. However, more detailed mechanisms by which this effect is mediated remain unknown.

4. Limitation and further direction

In the past decades, the advance in pathological mechanisms of aflatoxin-related hepatocarcinoma held great promise. However, we are still far from a comprehensive view of this kind of potentials. First, the detailed metabolic step and corresponding enzymes, especially the first-stage reaction and toxicity mechanisms, have not been elucidated. Second, although the activation of aflatoxins is found to act as a crucial step, it is unclear how the tumorigenesis of hepatocarcinoma is triggered by aflatoxins. Third, the vast literature for aflatoxin-induced hepatocarcinoma mainly focuses on the studies on AFB1, and some important information may have been lost. Fourth, in spite of some evidence of AFB1 inducing abnormal immunoreaction and interacting with hepatitis virus and genetic factors, they are at the primary stage and still far from elucidation. Therefore, the detailed toxicity mechanisms of aflatoxins and corresponding carcinogenesis mechanism will greatly benefit our understanding of aflatoxin-related hepatocarcinoma.

5. Summary

It has been shown that increasing exposure of aflatoxins may promote the carcinogenesis of hepatocarcinoma. Molecular mechanisms of aflatoxin-induced hepatocarcinoma involve in DNA damage, gene mutations, the inactivation of such tumor suppressor gene as TP53, the activation of proto-oncogenes, abnormal immunoreaction, and the interaction between aflatoxins and other carcinogens such as HBV. However, an understanding of aflatoxin-induced hepatocarcinoma is far from complete, and further research in this field is looked forward to elucidating more detailed mechanisms responsible for hepatocarcinoma related to aflatoxins in the future.

Conflicts of interest and source of funding

The authors declare no competing financial interests. This study was supported in part by the National Natural Science Foundation of China (Nos. 81760502, 81572353, 81372639, 81472243, 81660495, and 81460423), the Innovation Program of Guangxi Municipal Education Department (Nos. 201204LX674 and 201204LX324), Innovation Program of Guangxi Health Department (No. Z2013781), the Natural Science Foundation of Guangxi (Nos. 2017GXNSFGA198002, 2017JJF10001, 2017GXNSFAA198002, 2016GXNSFDA380003, 2015GXNSFAA139223, 2013GXNSFAA019251, 2014GXNSFDA118021, and 2014GXNSFAA118144), Research Program of Guangxi "Zhouyue Scholar" (No. 2017-38), Research Program of Guangxi Specially-invited Expert (No. 2017-6th), Research Program of Guangxi Clinic Research Center of Hepatobiliary Diseases (No. AD17129025), and Open Research Program from Molecular Immunity Study Room Involving in Acute & Severe Diseases in Guangxi Colleges and Universities (Nos. kfkt20160062 and kfkt20160063).

Abbreviations

AFB1	aflatoxin B1
AFB2	aflatoxin B2
AFG1	aflatoxin G1

AFG2	aflatoxin G2
AFP	α-fetoprotein
A. flavus	*Aspergillus flavus*
A. parasiticus	*Aspergillus parasiticus*
A. nidulans	*Aspergillus nidulans*
A. pseudotamarii	*Aspergillus pseudotamarii*
A. bombycis	*Aspergillus bombycis*
HBV	hepatitis virus B
HCV	hepatitis virus C
Hepatocarcinoma	hepatocellular carcinoma
NAPDH	nicotinamide-adenine dinucleotide phosphate reduced form
NAD	one nicotinamide-adenine dinucleotide
SAM	*S*-adenosylmethionine
CYP450	cytochromes P450

Author details

Xi-Dai Long[1,2,3*†], Yan Deng[4†], Xiao-Ying Huang[1†], Jin-Guang Yao[1†], Qun-Ying Su[1†], Xue-Min Wu[1†], Juan Wang[1†], Qun-Qing Xu[3], Xiao-Ying Zhu[3], Chao Wang[5], Bing-Chen Huang[1] and Qiang Xia[2]

*Address all correspondence to: sjtulongxd@263.net

1 Department of Pathology, the Affiliated Hospital of Youjiang Medical University for Nationalities, Baise, China

2 Department of Liver Surgery, Ren Ji Hospital, School of Medicine, Shanghai Jiao Tong University, Shanghai, China

3 Guangxi Clinic Research Center of Hepatobiliary Diseases, Baise, China

4 Department of Epidemiology, Youjiang Medical University for Nationalities, Baise, China

5 Department of Medicine, the Affiliated Hospital of Youjiang Medical University for Nationalities, Baise, China

† These authors contributed equally to this work.

References

[1] Long XD, Yao JD, Yang Q, Huang CH, Liao P, Nong LG, Tang YJ, Huang XY, Wang C, Wu XM, Huang BC, Ban FZ, Zeng LX, Ma Y, Zhai B, Zhang JQ, Xue F, Lu CX, Xia Q. Polymorphisms of DNA repair genes and toxicological effects of aflatoxin B1 exposure. In: Faulkner AG, editor. Aflatoxins: Food Sources, Occurrence and Toxicological Effects. 1st ed. New York: Nova Science Publishers; 2014. pp. 107-124. DOI: 978-1-63117-298-4

[2] Siegel RL, Miller KD, Jemal A. Cancer statistics, 2017. CA: A Cancer Journal for Clinicians. 2017;**67**:7-30. DOI: 10.3322/caac.21387

[3] Chen W, Zheng R, Baade PD, Zhang S, Zeng H, Bray F, Jemal A, Yu XQ, He J. Cancer statistics in China, 2015. CA: A Cancer Journal for Clinicians. 2016;**66**:115-132. DOI: 10.3322/caac.21338

[4] Umesha S, Manukumar HM, Chandrasekhar B, Shivakumara P, Shiva Kumar J, Raghava S, Avinash P, Shirin M, Bharathi TR, Rajini SB, Nandhini M, Vinaya Rani GG, Shobha M, Prakash HS. Aflatoxins and food pathogens: Impact of biologically active aflatoxins and their control strategies. Journal of the Science of Food and Agriculture. 2017;**97**:1698-1707. DOI: 10.1002/jsfa.8144

[5] Sarma UP, Bhetaria PJ, Devi P, Varma A. Aflatoxins: Implications on health. Indian Journal of Clinical Biochemistry. 2017;**32**:124-133. DOI: 10.1007/s12291-017-0649-2

[6] Kowalska A, Walkiewicz K, Koziel P, Muc-Wierzgon M. Aflatoxins: characteristics and impact on human health. Postepy Higieny i Medycyny Doświadczalnej (Online). 2017;**71**:315-327. DOI: 10.5604/01.3001.0010.3816

[7] Yabe K, Nakajima H. Enzyme reactions and genes in aflatoxin biosynthesis. Applied Microbiology and Biotechnology. 2004;**64**:745-755. DOI: 10.1007/s00253-004-1566-x

[8] Abrar M, Anjum FM, Butt MS, Pasha I, Randhawa MA, Saeed F, Waqas K. Aflatoxins: Biosynthesis, occurrence, toxicity, and remedies. Critical Reviews in Food Science and Nutrition. 2013;**53**:862-874. DOI: 10.1080/10408398.2011.563154

[9] Kensler TW, Roebuck BD, Wogan GN, Groopman JD. Aflatoxin: A 50-year odyssey of mechanistic and translational toxicology. Toxicological Sciences. 2011;**120**(Suppl 1):S28-S48. DOI: 10.1093/toxsci/kfq283

[10] Wu Q, Jezkova A, Yuan Z, Pavlikova L, Dohnal V, Kuca K. Biological degradation of aflatoxins. Drug Metabolism Reviews. 2009;**41**:1-7. DOI: 10.1080/03602530802563850

[11] Woloshuk CP, Shim WB. Aflatoxins, fumonisins, and trichothecenes: A convergence of knowledge. FEMS Microbiology Reviews. 2013;**37**:94-109. DOI: 10.1111/1574-6976.12009

[12] Essigmann JM, Croy RG, Nadzan AM, Busby WF Jr, Reinhold VN, Buchi G, Wogan GN. Structural identification of the major DNA adduct formed by aflatoxin B1 in vitro. Proceedings of the National Academy of Sciences of the United States of America. 1977;**74**:1870-1874. DOI: 10.1073/pnas.PMC431033

[13] Croy RG, Essigmann JM, Reinhold VN, Wogan GN. Identification of the principal aflatoxin B1-DNA adduct formed in vivo in rat liver. Proceedings of the National Academy of Sciences of the United States of America. 1978;**75**:1745-1749. DOI: 10.1073/pnas.PMC392416

[14] Huang XY, Yao JG, Huang BC, Ma Y, Xia Q, Long XD. Polymorphisms of a disintegrin and metalloproteinase with thrombospondin motifs 5 and aflatoxin B1-related hepatocellular carcinoma. Cancer Epidemiology, Biomarkers & Prevention. 2016;**25**:334-343. DOI: 10.1158/1055-9965.EPI-15-0774

[15] Lu J, Wang XZ, Zhang TQ, Huang XY, Yao JG, Wang C, Wei ZH, Ma Y, Wu XM, Luo CY, Xia Q, Long XD. Prognostic significance of XRCC4 expression in hepatocellular carcinoma. Oncotarget. 2017;**8**:87955-87970. DOI: 10.18632/oncotarget.21360

[16] Wu XM, Xi ZF, Liao P, Huang HD, Huang XY, Wang C, Ma Y, Xia Q, Yao JG, Long XD. Diagnostic and prognostic potential of serum microRNA-4651 for patients with hepatocellular carcinoma related to aflatoxin B1. Oncotarget. 2017;**8**:81235-81249. DOI: 10.18632/oncotarget.16027

[17] Li C, Xiong Y, Yang X, Wang L, Zhang S, Dai N, Li M, Ren T, Yang Y, Zhou SF, Gan L, Wang D. Lost expression of ADAMTS5 protein associates with progression and poor prognosis of hepatocellular carcinoma. Drug Design, Development and Therapy. 2015;**9**:1773-1783. DOI: 10.2147/DDDT.S77069

[18] Long XD, Ma Y, Huang YZ, Yi Y, Liang QX, Ma AM, Zeng LP, Fu GH. Genetic polymorphisms in DNA repair genes XPC, XPD, and XRCC4, and susceptibility to helicobacter pylori infection-related gastric antrum adenocarcinoma in Guangxi population. China Molecular Carcinogenesis. 2010;**49**:611-618. DOI: 10.1002/mc.20630

[19] Long XD, Yao JG, Zeng Z, Ma Y, Huang XY, Wei ZH, Liu M, Zhang JJ, Xue F, Zhai B, Xia Q. Polymorphisms in the coding region of X-ray repair complementing group 4 and aflatoxin B1-related hepatocellular carcinoma. Hepatology. 2013;**58**:171-181. DOI: 10.1002/hep.26311

[20] Long XD, Zhao D, Wang C, Huang XY, Yao JG, Ma Y, Wei ZH, Liu M, Zeng LX, Mo XQ, Zhang JJ, Xue F, Zhai B, Xia Q. Genetic polymorphisms in DNA repair genes XRCC4 and XRCC5 and aflatoxin B1-related hepatocellular carcinoma. Epidemiology. 2013;**24**:671-681. DOI: 10.1097/EDE.0b013e31829d2744

[21] Lin ZH, Chen JC, Wang YS, Huang TJ, Wang J, Long XD. DNA repair gene XRCC4 codon 247 polymorphism modified diffusely infiltrating astrocytoma risk and prognosis. International Journal of Molecular Sciences. 2014;**15**:250-260. DOI: 10.3390/ijms15010250

[22] Yao JG, Huang XY, Long XD. Interaction of DNA repair gene polymorphisms and aflatoxin B1 in the risk of hepatocellular carcinoma. International Journal of Clinical and Experimental Pathology. 2014;**7**:6231-6244. DOI: 10.2016/1936-2625.25337275

[23] Liu YX, Long XD, Xi ZF, Ma Y, Huang XY, Yao JG, Wang C, Xing TY, Xia Q. MicroRNA-24 modulates aflatoxin B1-related hepatocellular carcinoma prognosis and tumorigenesis. BioMed Research International. 2014;**2014**:482926. DOI: 10.1155/2014/482926

[24] Huang XY, Yao JG, Huang HD, Wang C, Ma Y, Xia Q, Long XD. MicroRNA-429 modulates hepatocellular carcinoma prognosis and tumorigenesis. Gastroenterology Research and Practice. 2013;**2013**:804128. DOI: 10.1155/2013/804128

[25] Hagiwara N, Mechanic LE, Trivers GE, Cawley HL, Taga M, Bowman ED, Kumamoto K, He P, Bernard M, Doja S, Miyashita M, Tajiri T, Sasajima K, Nomura T, Makino H, Takahashi K, Hussain SP, Harris CC. Quantitative detection of p53 mutations in plasma DNA from tobacco smokers. Cancer Research. 2006;**66**:8309-8317. DOI: 10.1158/0008-5472. CAN-06-0991

[26] Harris LC, Remack JS, Houghton PJ, Brent TP. Wild-type p53 suppresses transcription of the human O6-methylguanine-DNA methyltransferase gene. Cancer Research. 1996; **56**:2029-2032

[27] Harris CC. Tumour suppressor genes, multistage carcinogenesis and molecular epidemiology. IARC Scientific Publications. 1992:67-85 DOI: PMID1428103

[28] Foster PL, Eisenstadt E, Miller JH. Base substitution mutations induced by metabolically activated aflatoxin B1. Proceedings of the National Academy of Sciences of the U S A. 1983;**80**:2695-2698. DOI: PMC393894

[29] Qi LN, Bai T, Chen ZS, Wu FX, Chen YY, De Xiang B, Peng T, Han ZG, Li LQ. The p53 mutation spectrum in hepatocellular carcinoma from Guangxi, China: Role of chronic hepatitis B virus infection and aflatoxin B1 exposure. Liver International. 2014. DOI: 10.1111/liv.12460

[30] Golli-Bennour EE, Kouidhi B, Bouslimi A, Abid-Essefi S, Hassen W, Bacha H. Cytotoxicity and genotoxicity induced by aflatoxin B1, ochratoxin A, and their combination in cultured Vero cells. Journal of Biochemical and Molecular Toxicology. 2010;**24**:42-50. DOI: 10.1002/jbt.20310

[31] Paget V, Sichel F, Garon D, Lechevrel M. Aflatoxin B1-induced TP53 mutational pattern in normal human cells using the FASAY (functional analysis of separated alleles in yeast). Mutation Research. 2008;**656**:55-61. DOI: 10.1016/j.mrgentox.2008.07.009

[32] Levy DD, Groopman JD, Lim SE, Seidman MM, Kraemer KH. Sequence specificity of aflatoxin B1-induced mutations in a plasmid replicated in xeroderma pigmentosum and DNA repair proficient human cells. Cancer Research 1992;**52**:5668-5673. DOI: 10.1158/0008-5472. CAN-Published-October-1992

[33] Wang JS, Groopman JD. DNA damage by mycotoxins. Mutation Research. 1999;**424**:167-181. DOI: 10.1016/S0027-5107(99)00017-2

[34] Long XD, Yao JG, Zeng Z, Huang CH, Huang ZS, Huang YZ, Ban FZ, Huang XY, Yao LM, Fan LD, Fu GH. DNA repair capacity-related to genetic polymorphisms of DNA repair genes and aflatoxin B1-related hepatocellular carcinoma among Chinese population. In: Kruman I, editor. DNA Repair. Rijeka: InTech; 2011. pp. 505-524. DOI: 10.5772/20792

[35] Xia Q, Huang XY, Xue F, Zhang JJ, Zhai B, Kong DC, Wang C, Huang ZQ, Long XD. Genetic polymorphisms of DNA repair genes and DNA repair capacity related to aflatoxin

b1 (AFB1)-induced DNA damages. In: Chen C, editor. New Research Directions in DNA Repair. 1st ed. Rijeka: InTech; 2013. pp. 377-412. DOI: 10.5772/53967

[36] Chen BP, Long XD, Fu GH. Meta-analysis of XRCC1 codon 399 polymorphism and susceptibility of hepatocellular carcinoma. Journal of Shanghai Jiao Tong University (Medical Science). 2011;**31**:1588-1602. DOI: 10.3969/j.issn.1674-8115.2011.11.018

[37] Long XD, Huang HD, Huang XY, Yao JG, Xia Q. XPC codon 939 polymorphism is associated with susceptibility to DNA damage induced by aflatoxin B1 exposure. International Journal of Clinical and Experimental Medicine. 2015;**8**:1197-1204. DOI: PMC4358568

[38] Shen HM, Ong CN. Mutations of the p53 tumor suppressor gene and ras oncogenes in aflatoxin hepatocarcinogenesis. Mutation Research. 1996;**366**:23-44. DOI: 10.1016/S0165-1110(96)90005-6

[39] Alm-Eldeen AA, Basyony MA, Elfiky NK, Ghalwash MM. Effect of the Egyptian propolis on the hepatic antioxidant defense and pro-apoptotic p53 and anti-apoptotic bcl2 expressions in aflatoxin B1 treated male mice. Biomedicine & Pharmacotherapy. 2017;**87**:247-255. DOI: 10.1016/j.biopha.2016.12.084

[40] Ranchal I, Gonzalez R, Bello RI, Ferrin G, Hidalgo AB, Linares CI, Aguilar-Melero P, Gonzalez-Rubio S, Barrera P, Marchal T, Nakayama KI, de la Mata M, Muntane J. The reduction of cell death and proliferation by p27(Kip1) minimizes DNA damage in an experimental model of genotoxicity. International Journal of Cancer. 2009;**125**:2270-2280. DOI: 10.1002/ijc.24621

[41] Qi LN, Bai T, Chen ZS, Wu FX, Chen YY, De Xiang B, Peng T, Han ZG, Li LQ. The p53 mutation spectrum in hepatocellular carcinoma from Guangxi, China: Role of chronic hepatitis B virus infection and aflatoxin B1 exposure. Liver International. 2015;**35**:999-1009. DOI: 10.1111/liv.12460

[42] Chittmittrapap S, Chieochansin T, Chaiteerakij R, Treeprasertsuk S, Klaikaew N, Tangkijvanich P, Komolmit P, Poovorawan Y. Prevalence of aflatoxin induced p53 mutation at codon 249 (R249s) in hepatocellular carcinoma patients with and without hepatitis B surface antigen (HBsAg). Asian Pacific Journal of Cancer Prevention. 2013;**14**:7675-7679. DOI: PMID24460352

[43] Gursoy-Yuzugullu O, Yuzugullu H, Yilmaz M, Ozturk M. Aflatoxin genotoxicity is associated with a defective DNA damage response bypassing p53 activation. Liver International. 2011;**31**:561-571. DOI: 10.1111/j.1478-3231.2011.02474.x

[44] Pineau P, Marchio A, Battiston C, Cordina E, Russo A, Terris B, Qin LX, Turlin B, Tang ZY, Mazzaferro V, Dejean A. Chromosome instability in human hepatocellular carcinoma depends on p53 status and aflatoxin exposure. Mutation Research. 2008;**653**:6-13. DOI: 10.1016/j.mrgentox.2008.01.012

[45] Zhang YJ, Rossner P Jr, Chen Y, Agrawal M, Wang Q, Wang L, Ahsan H, Yu MW, Lee PH, Santella RM. Aflatoxin B1 and polycyclic aromatic hydrocarbon adducts, p53 mutations and p16 methylation in liver tissue and plasma of hepatocellular carcinoma patients. International Journal of Cancer. 2006;**119**:985-991. DOI: 10.1002/ijc.21699

[46] Chan KT, Hsieh DP, Lung ML. In vitro aflatoxin B1-induced p53 mutations. Cancer Letters. 2003;**199**:1-7. DOI: 10.1016/S0304-3835(03)00337-9

[47] Stern MC, Umbach DM, Yu MC, London SJ, Zhang ZQ, Taylor JA. Hepatitis B, aflatoxin B(1), and p53 codon 249 mutation in hepatocellular carcinomas from Guangxi, People's Republic of China, and a meta-analysis of existing studies. Cancer Epidemiology Biomarkers & Prevention. 2001;**10**:617-625. DOI: PMID11401911

[48] Park US, Su JJ, Ban KC, Qin L, Lee EH, Lee YI. Mutations in the p53 tumor suppressor gene in tree shrew hepatocellular carcinoma associated with hepatitis B virus infection and intake of aflatoxin B1. Gene. 2000;**251**:73-80. DOI: 10.1016/S0378-1119(00)00183-9

[49] Lee YI, Lee S, Das GC, Park US, Park SM, Lee YI. Activation of the insulin-like growth factor II transcription by aflatoxin B1 induced p53 mutant 249 is caused by activation of transcription complexes; implications for a gain-of-function during the formation of hepatocellular carcinoma. Oncogene. 2000;**19**:3717-3726. DOI: 10.1038/sj.onc.1203694

[50] Uwaifo O. P53 gene of chang-liver cells (Atcc-Ccl13) exposed to aflatoxin B1 (Afb): The effect of lysine on mutation at codon 249 of exon 7. African Journal of Medicine and Medical Sciences. 1999;**28**:71-75. DOI: PMID12953991

[51] Chao HK, Tsai TF, Lin CS, Su TS. Evidence that mutational activation of the ras genes may not be involved in aflatoxin B(1)-induced human hepatocarcinogenesis, based on sequence analysis of the ras and p53 genes. Molecular Carcinogenesis. 1999;**26**:69-73. DOI: 10.1002/(SICI)1098-2744(199910)26:2<69::AID-MC1>3.0.CO;2-A

[52] Ghebranious N, Sell S. The mouse equivalent of the human p53ser249 mutation p53ser246 enhances aflatoxin hepatocarcinogenesis in hepatitis B surface antigen transgenic and p53 heterozygous null mice. Hepatology. 1998;**27**:967-973. DOI: 10.1002/hep.510270411

[53] Ghebranious N, Sell S. Hepatitis B injury, male gender, aflatoxin, and p53 expression each contribute to hepatocarcinogenesis in transgenic mice. Hepatology. 1998;**27**:383-391. DOI: 10.1002/hep.510270211

[54] Liu YP, Lin Y, Ng ML. Immunochemical and genetic analysis of the p53 gene in liver preneoplastic nodules from aflatoxin-induced rats in one year. Annals of the Academy of Medicine of Singapore. 1996;**25**:31-36

[55] Hulla JE, Chen ZY, Eaton DL. Aflatoxin B1-induced rat hepatic hyperplastic nodules do not exhibit a site-specific mutation within the p53 gene. Cancer Research. 1993;**53**:9-11. DOI: PMID8380129

[56] Lilleberg SL, Cabonce MA, Raju NR, Wagner LM, Kier LD. Alterations in the structural gene and the expression of p53 in rat liver tumors induced by aflatoxin B1. Molecular Carcinogenesis. 1992;**6**:159-172. DOI: 10.1002/mc.2940060211

[57] Lilleberg SL, Cabonce MA, Raju NR, Wagner LM, Kier LD. Alterations in the p53 tumor suppressor gene in rat liver tumors induced by aflatoxin B1. Progress in Clinical and Biological Research. 1992;**376**:203-222

[58] Deng ZL, Ma Y. Aflatoxin sufferer and p53 gene mutation in hepatocellular carcinoma. World Journal of Gastroenterology. 1998;**4**:28-29. DOI: 10.3748/wjg.v4.i1.28

[59] Deng Z, Pan L, Ma Y. Sequence alterations in p53 gene of hepatocellular carcinoma from high aflatoxin risk area in Guangxi. Zhonghua Zhong Liu Za Zhi. 1997;**19**:18-21. DOI: PMID10743047

[60] Mace K, Aguilar F, Wang JS, Vautravers P, Gomez-Lechon M, Gonzalez FJ, Groopman J, Harris CC, Pfeifer AM. Aflatoxin B1-induced DNA adduct formation and p53 mutations in CYP450-expressing human liver cell lines. Carcinogenesis. 1997;**18**:1291-1297. DOI: PMID9230270

[61] Lunn RM, Zhang YJ, Wang LY, Chen CJ, Lee PH, Lee CS, Tsai WY, Santella RM. p53 mutations, chronic hepatitis B virus infection, and aflatoxin exposure in hepatocellular carcinoma in Taiwan. Cancer Reserch. 1997;**57**:3471-3477. DOI: PMID9270015

[62] Hollstein MC, Wild CP, Bleicher F, Chutimataewin S, Harris CC, Srivatanakul P, Montesano R. p53 mutations and aflatoxin B1 exposure in hepatocellular carcinoma patients from Thailand. International Journal of Cancer. 1993;**53**:51-55. DOI: 10.1002/ijc.2910530111

[63] Aguilar F, Hussain SP, Cerutti P. Aflatoxin B1 induces the transversion of G-->T in codon 249 of the p53 tumor suppressor gene in human hepatocytes. Proceedings of the National Academy of Sciences U S A. 1993;**90**:8586-8590. DOI: PMC47402

[64] Ozturk M. p53 mutation in hepatocellular carcinoma after aflatoxin exposure. Lancet. 1991;**338**:1356-1359. DOI: 10.1016/0140-6736(91)92236-U

[65] Tashiro F, Morimura S, Hayashi K, Makino R, Kawamura H, Horikoshi N, Nemoto K, Ohtsubo K, Sugimura T, Ueno Y. Expression of the c-Ha-ras and c-myc genes in aflatoxin B1-induced hepatocellular carcinomas. Biochemical and Biophysical Research Communications. 1986;**138**:858-864. DOI: 10.1016/S0006-291X(86)80575-7

[66] Sinha S, Webber C, Marshall CJ, Knowles MA, Proctor A, Barrass NC, Neal GE. Activation of ras oncogene in aflatoxin-induced rat liver carcinogenesis. Proceedings of the National Academy of Sciences U S A. 1988;**85**:3673-3677. DOI: PMC280280

[67] Soman NR, Wogan GN. Activation of the c-Ki-ras oncogene in aflatoxin B1-induced hepatocellular carcinoma and adenoma in the rat: Detection by denaturing gradient gel electrophoresis. Proceedings of the National Academy of Sciences U S A. 1993;**90**:2045-2049. DOI: PMC46017

[68] McMahon G, Hanson L, Lee JJ, Wogan GN. Identification of an activated c-Ki-ras oncogene in rat liver tumors induced by aflatoxin B1. Proceedings of the National Academy of Sciences U S A. 1986;**83**:9418-9422. DOI: PMC387149

[69] McMahon G, Davis EF, Huber LJ, Kim Y, Wogan GN. Characterization of c-Ki-ras and N-ras oncogenes in aflatoxin B1-induced rat liver tumors. Proceedings of the National Academy of Sciences U S A. 1990;**87**:1104-1108. DOI: PMC53419

[70] Riley J, Mandel HG, Sinha S, Judah DJ, Neal GE. In vitro activation of the human Harvey-ras proto-oncogene by aflatoxin B1. Carcinogenesis. 1997;**18**:905-910. DOI: PMID9163674

[71] Bauer-Hofmann R, Buchmann A, Wright AS, Schwarz M. Mutations in the Ha-ras proto-oncogene in spontaneous and chemically induced liver tumours of the CF1 mouse. Carcinogenesis. 1990;**11**:1875-1877. DOI: PMID2119910

[72] Wiseman RW, Stowers SJ, Miller EC, Anderson MW, Miller JA. Activating mutations of the c-Ha-ras protooncogene in chemically induced hepatomas of the male B6C3 F1 mouse. Proceedings of the National Academy of Sciences U S A. 1986;**83**:5825-5829. DOI: PMC386388

[73] Kew MC. Synergistic interaction between aflatoxin B1 and hepatitis B virus in hepatocarcinogenesis. Liver International. 2003;**23**:405-409. DOI: 10.1111/j.1478-3231.2003.00869.x

[74] Kew MC. Aflatoxins as a cause of hepatocellular carcinoma. Journal of Gastrointestinal and Liver Diseases. 2013;**22**:305-310. DOI: PMID24078988

[75] Moudgil V, Redhu D, Dhanda S, Singh JA. Review of molecular mechanisms in the development of hepatocellular carcinoma by aflatoxin and hepatitis B and C viruses. Journal of Environmental Pathology, Toxicology and Oncology. 2013;**32**:165-175. DOI: 10.1615/JEnvironPatholToxicolOncol.2013007166

[76] Yeh FS, Mo CC, Yen RC. Risk factors for hepatocellular carcinoma in Guangxi, People's Republic of China. National Cancer Institute Monograph. 1985;**69**:47-48. DOI: PMID3010122

[77] Williams JH, Phillips TD, Jolly PE, Stiles JK, Jolly CM, Aggarwal D. Human aflatoxicosis in developing countries: A review of toxicology, exposure, potential health consequences, and interventions. The American Journal of Clinical Nutrition. 2004;**80**:1106-1122. DOI: PMID15531656

[78] Qian GS, Ross RK, Yu MC, Yuan JM, Gao YT, Henderson BE, Wogan GN, Groopman JD. A follow-up study of urinary markers of aflatoxin exposure and liver cancer risk in Shanghai, People's Republic of China. Cancer Epidemiology, Biomarkers & Prevention. 1994;**3**:3-10. DOI: PMID8118382

[79] Wang JS, Qian GS, Zarba A, He X, Zhu YR, Zhang BC, Jacobson L, Gange SJ, Munoz A, Kensler TW, et al. Temporal patterns of aflatoxin-albumin adducts in hepatitis B surface antigen-positive and antigen-negative residents of Daxin, Qidong County, People's Republic of China. Cancer Epidemiology, Biomarkers & Prevention: A publication of the American Association for Cancer Research, Cosponsored by the American Society of Preventive Oncology. 1996;**5**:253-261. DOI: PMID8722216

[80] Ross RK, Yuan JM, MC Y, Wogan GN, Qian GS, JT T, Groopman JD, Gao YT, Henderson BE. Urinary aflatoxin biomarkers and risk of hepatocellular carcinoma. Lancet. 1992;**339**:943-946. DOI: 10.1016/0140-6736(92)91528-G

[81] Sell S, Hunt JM, Dunsford HA, Chisari FV. Synergy between hepatitis B virus expression and chemical hepatocarcinogens in transgenic mice. Cancer Reserch. 1991;**51**:1278-1285. DOI: PMID1847661

[82] Bannasch P, Khoshkhou NI, Hacker HJ, Radaeva S, Mrozek M, Zillmann U, Kopp-Schneider A, Haberkorn U, Elgas M, Tolle T, et al. Synergistic hepatocarcinogenic effect of hepadnaviral infection and dietary aflatoxin B1 in woodchucks. Cancer Reserch. 1995;**55**:3318-3330. DOI: PMID7614467

[83] Li Y, Su JJ, Qin LL, Yang C, Ban KC, Yan RQ. Synergistic effect of hepatitis B virus and aflatoxin B1 in hepatocarcinogenesis in tree shrews. Annals of the Academy of Medicine Singapore. 1999;**28**:67-71. DOI: PMID10374028

[84] Cova L, Wild CP, Mehrotra R, Turusov V, Shirai T, Lambert V, Jacquet C, Tomatis L, Trepo C, Montesano R. Contribution of aflatoxin B1 and hepatitis B virus infection in the induction of liver tumors in ducks. Cancer Reserch. 1990;**50**:2156-2163. DOI: PMID2107970

[85] Allen SJ, Wild CP, Wheeler JG, Riley EM, Montesano R, Bennett S, Whittle HC, Hall AJ, Greenwood BM. Aflatoxin exposure, malaria and hepatitis B infection in rural Gambian children. Transactions of the Royal Society of Tropical Medicine and Hygiene. 1992;**86**: 426-430. DOI: PMID1440826

[86] Turner PC, Mendy M, Whittle H, Fortuin M, Hall AJ, Wild CP, Hepatitis B. Infection and aflatoxin biomarker levels in Gambian children. Tropical Medicine & International Health. 2000;**5**:837-841. DOI: 10.1046/j.1365-3156.2000.00664.x

[87] Groopman JD, Wang JS, Scholl P. Molecular biomarkers for aflatoxins: From adducts to gene mutations to human liver cancer. Canadian Journal of Physiology and Pharmacology. 1996;**74**:203-209. DOI: PMID8723033

[88] Coursaget P, Depril N, Chabaud M, Nandi R, Mayelo V, LeCann P, Yvonnet B. High prevalence of mutations at codon 249 of the p53 gene in hepatocellular carcinomas from Senegal. British Journal of Cancer. 1993;**67**:1395-1397. DOI: PMC1968506

[89] Kew MC, Hepatitis B. Virus x protein in the pathogenesis of hepatitis B virus-induced hepatocellular carcinoma. Journal of Gastroenterology and Hepatology. 2011;**26**(Suppl 1): 144-152. DOI: 10.1111/j.1440-1746.2010.06546.x

[90] Gomez-Moreno A, Garaigorta U, Hepatitis B. Virus and DNA damage response: Interactions and consequences for the infection. Virus. 2017;**9**. DOI: 10.3390/v9100304

[91] Castelli G, Pelosi E, Testa U. Liver cancer: Molecular characterization, clonal evolution and cancer stem cells. Cancers (Basel). 2017;**9**. DOI: 10.3390/cancers9090127

[92] Ghouri YA, Mian I, Rowe JH. Review of hepatocellular carcinoma: Epidemiology, etiology, and carcinogenesis. Journal of Carcinogenesis. 2017;**16**:1. DOI: 10.4103/jcar.JCar_9_16

[93] Long XD, Huang HD, Xia Q. The polymorphism of XRCC3 codon 241 and the hotspot mutation in the TP53 gene in hepatocellular carcinoma induced by aflatoxin B1. Journal of Tumor. 2014;**2**:272-277. DOI: 10.6051/j.issn.1819-6187.2014.02.57

[94] Long XD, Yao JG, Huang YZ, Huang XY, Ban FZ, Yao LM, Fan LDDNA. Repair gene XRCC7 polymorphisms (rs#7003908 and rs#10109984) and hepatocellular carcinoma related to AFB1 exposure among Guangxi population, China. Hepatology Research. 2011;**41**:1085-1093. DOI: 10.1111/j.1872-034X.2011.00866.x

[95] Long XD, Ma Y, Zhou YF, Ma AM, Fu GH. Polymorphism in xeroderma pigmentosum complementation group C codon 939 and aflatoxin B1-related hepatocellular carcinoma in the Guangxi population. Hepatology. 2010;**52**:1301-1309. DOI: 10.1002/hep.23807

[96] Long XD, Ma Y, Zhou YF, Yao JG, Ban FZ, Huang YZ, Huang BC. XPD Codon 312 and 751 polymorphisms, and AFB1 exposure, and hepatocellular carcinoma risk. BMC Cancer. 2009;**9**:400. DOI: 10.1186/1471-2407-9-400

[97] Long XD, Ma Y, Huang HD, Yao JG, Qu de Y, Lu YL. Polymorphism of XRCC1 and the frequency of mutation in codon 249 of the p53 gene in hepatocellular carcinoma among Guangxi population, China. Molecular Carcinogenesis 2008;**47**:295-300. doi: 10.1002/mc.20384

[98] Long XD, Ma Y, Wei YP, Deng ZL. The polymorphisms of GSTM1, GSTT1, HYL1*2, and XRCC1, and aflatoxin B1-related hepatocellular carcinoma in Guangxi population, China. Hepatology Research. 2006;**36**:48-55. DOI: 10.1016/j.hepres.2006.06.004

[99] Long XD, Ma Y, Deng ZL. GSTM1 and XRCC3 polymorphisms: Effects on levels of aflatoxin B1-DNA adducts. Chinese Journal of Cancer Research. 2009;**21**:177-184. DOI: 10.1007/s11670-009-0177-6

[100] Long XD, Ma Y, Wei YP, Deng ZL. A study about the association of detoxication gene GSTM1 polymorphism and the susceptibility to aflatoxin B1-related hepatocellular carcinoma. Zhonghua Gan Zang Bing Za Zhi. 2005;**13**:668-670. DOI: PMID16174455

[101] Long XD, Ma Y, Wei YP, Deng ZL. Study on the detoxication gene gstM1-gstT1-null and susceptibility to aflatoxin B1 related hepatocellular carcinoma in Guangxi. Zhonghua Liu Xing Bing Xue Za Zhi. 2005;**26**:777-781. DOI: PMID16536303

[102] Moon EY, Rhee DK, Pyo S. In vitro suppressive effect of aflatoxin B1 on murine peritoneal macrophage functions. Toxicology. 1999;**133**:171-179. DOI: PMID10378483

[103] Moon EY, Rhee DK, Pyo S. Inhibition of various functions in murine peritoneal macrophages by aflatoxin B1 exposure in vivo. International Journal of Immunopharmacology. 1999;**21**:47-58. DOI: 10.1016/S0192-0561(98)00069-1

[104] Bianco G, Russo R, Marzocco S, Velotto S, Autore G, Severino L. Modulation of macrophage activity by aflatoxins B1 and B2 and their metabolites aflatoxins M1 and M2. Toxicon. 2012;**59**:644-650. DOI: 10.1016/j.toxicon.2012.02.010

[105] Bruneau JC, Stack E, O'Kennedy R, Loscher CE. Aflatoxins B(1), B(2) and G(1) modulate cytokine secretion and cell surface marker expression in J774A.1 murine macrophages. Toxicology In Vitro. 2012;**26**:686-693. DOI: 10.1016/j.tiv.2012.03.003

[106] Turner PC, Moore SE, Hall AJ, Prentice AM, Wild CP. Modification of immune function through exposure to dietary aflatoxin in Gambian children. Environmental Health Perspectives. 2003;**111**:217-220. DOI: PMC1241353

[107] Oswald IP, Marin DE, Bouhet S, Pinton P, Taranu I, Accensi F. Immunotoxicological risk of mycotoxins for domestic animals. Food Additives and Contaminants. 2005;**22**:354-360. DOI: 10.1080/02652030500058320

4

Innovative Blood Tests for Hepatocellular Carcinoma: Liquid Biopsy and Evaluation of Systemic Inflammatory Reaction

Ilze Strumfa, Dzeina Mezale, Boriss Strumfs,
Andrejs Vanags, Arturs Kalva, Dainis Balodis,
Ilze Fridrihsone, Arnis Abolins and Janis Gardovskis

Abstract

Hepatocellular carcinoma (HCC) is an aggressive tumour associated with dismal prognosis. To improve the outcome, early diagnostics is important. At present, classical HCC diagnostics is based on evaluation of risk factors, surveillance in cirrhotic patients, preference for non-invasive diagnosis by computed tomography or magnetic resonance imaging and biopsy confirmation in controversial cases. However, ambiguous radiological presentation, biopsy-related complications or insufficient representation of the pathology in the tissue core are well-known problems. Panel assessment of microRNAs has diagnostic and prognostic value; thus, in future, microRNA-based liquid biopsy could partially reduce the need for core biopsies. Systemic inflammatory reaction (SIR), characterised mainly by neutrophil-to-lymphocyte ratio, platelet-to-lymphocyte ratio and Glasgow prognostic score, may have prognostic value and can be incorporated in criteria for certain treatment approaches, e.g., becoming an adjunct to Milan criteria. Thus, innovations in HCC diagnostics are expected in the field of miRNA-based liquid biopsy for diagnosis/prognosis and SIR for prognosis/selection of treatment.

Keywords: hepatocellular carcinoma, HCC, liquid biopsy, miRNA, systemic inflammatory response, neutrophil-to-lymphocyte ratio, platelet-to-lymphocyte ratio, Glasgow prognostic score, prognosis

1. Introduction

Hepatocellular carcinoma is one of the most aggressive human cancers. The total oncological mortality is decreasing in many developed countries, e.g., it has been reduced by 23% since 1991 in the United States of America (USA). In contrast, death rate of HCC is increasing, along with the incidence of this tumour [1, 2]. Positive changes are expected due to risk factor eradication by vaccination against hepatitis B and improved treatment of chronic hepatitis C. The treatment of HCC has also developed significantly, including radiofrequency ablation, transarterial chemoembolisation, liver resection and transplantation as well as molecular targeted treatment by sorafenib. However, SEER-based analysis has revealed that survival has improved in early but not in advanced cases [2]. Thus, timely diagnostics remain an important goal.

Most of the hepatocellular carcinoma cases develop on the background of liver cirrhosis or chronic inflammatory liver disease in precirrhotic stage, e.g. chronic viral hepatitis B or C, alcohol-induced or autoimmune liver disease or non-alcoholic steatohepatitis (NASH). This might facilitate the diagnostics by screening of the risk population. Nowadays, screening by ultrasonography and non-invasive radiological diagnosis by the means of computed tomography or magnetic resonance imaging is the mainstay of HCC diagnostics. However, the radiological findings in early cases can be difficult to interpret. Biopsy is indicated in such controversial cases.

However, the biological course of HCC can result in diagnostic difficulties even in biopsy. HCC frequently develops in a dysplastic cirrhotic nodule. Such early HCC is typically well differentiated. Over time, it progresses to advanced dedifferentiated HCC. The resulting heterogeneity can lead to diagnostic problems and failures in biopsy due to sampling errors. For instance, if a small nodule seemed suspicious but not overtly malignant by radiological imaging, leading to biopsy, the differential diagnosis between dysplastic nodule and HCC will frequently imply the necessity to distinguish between premalignant process and well-differentiated tumour, usually lacking marked cell atypia or clear-cut invasion. In addition, both processes can be adjacent in the tissues. Consequently, early diagnostics of HCC is not straightforward even in biopsy.

In addition, biopsy can cause complications, including arterial hypotension, bleeding, pneumothorax, haemothorax, haemobilia, acute pancreatitis, visceral perforation, biliary fistulas, sepsis and needle breakage. Arterial hypotension is seen frequently (1.1–4.0%), mostly due to vasovagal reaction. In few cases, falling arterial blood pressure might indicate bleeding, if it is unusually severe. Bleeding can develop in the liver tissues or in the peritoneal cavity. It is seen in 4.5% of patients and is more frequent if INR is elevated: frequency of bleeding was 3.3% in patients having INR 1.3–1.5 and 7.1% among those who had INR > 1.5. Pneumothorax and haemothorax have been reported in 0.35 and 0.18% of patients, if the needle has accidentally passed through lung or diaphragmatic and intercostal blood vessels. Haemobilia has been described in 0.1% of patients and can induce acute pancreatitis via biliary obstruction. The frequency of visceral perforation, biliary fistulas, sepsis and needle breakage is 0.01% each. In addition, biopsy can result in pain, experienced in up to 84% of patients. In 40% of cases, pain lasts for 24 hours. It is attributable to skin and liver capsule damage, viscerosomatic irradiation (to shoulder) or complications that lead to peritoneal irritation (bleeding, bile accumulation in the peritoneum perforation of the internal organs). Few death cases have been reported after liver biopsy: 0.01–0.1% of patients [3].

Non-invasive means of HCC diagnostics would be beneficial. Two promising pathways include so-called liquid biopsy by microRNA analysis in blood and assessment of tumour-induced systemic inflammatory reaction (SIR). MicroRNA spectrum might have diagnostic and prognostic value. Regarding SIR, prognostic aspects have been studied and appear as promising adjunct how to select patients for treatment.

2. miRNAs in the diagnostics of hepatocellular carcinoma

MicroRNAs (miRNAs) are small, double-stranded, non-coding RNA molecules consisting of approximately 22 nucleotides. MiRNAs regulate gene expression at the post-transcriptional level [4, 5] acting as large-scale molecular switches. MiRNAs are found not only in cells but also in body fluids. Due to the stable and relatively simple structure, these molecules are good biomarkers for diagnostic and prognostic evaluation complying with the idea of so-called liquid biopsy—a patient-friendly blood test bringing the same information as a biopsy. In order to increase the diagnostic value of such tests, panels of miRNAs have been advocated. However, the biological course of HCC cause a possible pitfall in the elaboration of such diagnostic tests: as HCC mainly arise on the background of liver cirrhosis, inflammatory or metabolic liver diseases, these preceding pathologies can also alter the levels of miRNAs.

MiRNA-122 is attractive for its wide expression in liver tissues suggesting significant role in liver functions. MiRNA-122 is upregulated in serum of HCC patients and downregulated in HCC tissues suggesting specific excretion of miRNA-122 in blood by HCC. Although miRNA-122 shows high specificity and sensitivity for HCC in comparison with healthy controls (83.3 and 81.6%, respectively), levels of miRNA-122 change in other liver pathologies as well, limiting the diagnostic application [6].

Comparing HCC patients with those having hepatitis B or liver cirrhosis, serum levels of exosomal miRNA-18a, miRNA-221, miRNA-222 and miRNA-224 were increased, while miRNA-101, miRNA-106b, miRNA-122 and miRNA-195 were decreased. MiRNA-16 was decreased in HCC, and the levels significantly differed from those found in hepatitis C virus (HCV) infection because chronic viral hepatitis C and non-alcoholic fatty liver disease are characterised by the contrary changes—increase in miRNA-16. MiRNA-21 is characterised by positive characteristics in meta-analysis showing specificity and sensitivity for HCC diagnosis of 84.8 and 81.2%, respectively. The changes of miRNA-21 serum levels in HCC patients significantly differ from cases of chronic hepatitis; however, other malignant tumours can also yield higher serum concentration of miRNA-21 [7].

Several panels of miRNAs have been recommended. Exploring nine serum miRNAs (miRNA-21, miRNA-30c, miRNA-93, miRNA-122, miRNA-125b, miRNA-126, miRNA-130a, miRNA-193b and miRNA-222) in HCC and chronic viral hepatitis C patients, nine markers were decreased in chronic hepatitis C *versus* healthy controls, while seven markers (miRNA-21, miRNA-30c, miRNA-93, miRNA-122, miRNA-125b, miRNA-130a and miRNA-222) were significantly ($p < 0.05$) decreased in HCC *versus* chronic viral hepatitis C patients and four (miRNA-93, miRNA-122, miRNA-125b and miRNA-130a) in HCC *versus* non-HCC patients [8]. Panel of three miRNAs (upregulated miRNA-92a-3p, downregulated miRNA-3126-5p and upregulated miRNA-107) could discriminate HCC from healthy controls [9] Evaluating serum levels of 13 miRNAs in HCV-associated chronic hepatitis, liver cirrhosis and HCC *versus* healthy controls, panel of three miRNAs (miRNA-122, miRNA-885-5p and miRNA-29b) in association with serum alpha-fetoprotein (AFP) level could identify HCC *versus* healthy persons, while four miRNAs (miRNA-122, miRNA-885-5p, miRNA-221 and miRNA-22) and AFP were recommended for HCC diagnostics in liver cirrhosis and two (miRNA-22, miRNA-199a-3p) along with AFP—in chronic hepatitis [10]. In another study of HCV-infected patients including cases of HCV-related chronic hepatitis, liver cirrhosis and HCC, serum levels of miRNA-126, miRNA-129, miRNA-155, miRNA-203 and miRNA-223 were significantly decreased in HCC *versus* non-HCC patients [11]. Panel of eight miRNAs was assessed in hepatitis B virus-infected patients diagnosed with HCC or liver cirrhosis as well as in healthy controls. The levels of hsa-miRNA-206, hsa-miRNA-141-3p, hsa-miRNA-433-3p and hsa-miRNA-1228-5p were significantly increased in HCC *versus* control group comprising both healthy and cirrhosis patients, while hsa-miRNA-199a-5p, hsa-miRNA-122-5p, hsa-miRNA-192-5p and hsa-miRNA-26a-5p were downregulated [4].

In addition to the diagnostic role, miRNAs have been evaluated in the prognostic aspect. The influence of miRNAs upon HCC stem cells has been exploited. It has also been suggested that miRNAs could become treatment targets [12].

3. Systemic inflammatory response

Many tumours, including hepatocellular carcinoma, evoke systemic inflammatory reaction (SIR). In the recent years, cancer-induced SIR has become an attractive research area as changes in blood cell counts or ratios or blood levels of certain proteins are associated with the biological potential, course and treatment response in many malignant tumours. Although complex pathogenesis lies behind these changes, SIR can be evaluated by simple, widely available and economically feasible blood tests.

SIR in cancer patients develops through local and central mechanisms. Locally, the invasive growth of malignant tumour injures surrounding parenchyma, connective tissues and endothelium. The tissue damage leads to inflammation necessitating supply of inflammatory cells from the bone marrow through the circulation. The production of acute phase proteins becomes upregulated as well. Endothelial injury activates platelets; indeed, the association between hypercoagulation and advanced cancers is classical. Tumour necrosis and hypoxia are additional causes of local inflammatory response. Cancer can also evoke immune response manifesting by local cellular reactions. In turn, the inflammation can have both tumour-enhancing and tumour-suppressing outcomes. The released cytokines and transcription factors can upregulate the proliferation of malignant cells. Release of metalloproteinases and other enzymes can promote tissue degradation facilitating invasion. Angiogenesis can be upregulated as well. The immune system, in turn, can limit growth of the tumour.

The systemic effects of cancer include alterations in bone marrow function, especially myelopoiesis. Besides the increased production and release of leukocytes, immature myeloid cells, including the precursors of granulocytes and monocytes, are retained in early stages of differentiation. Immature myeloid cells can act as immune suppressors and generate pre-metastatic niches, among other pathogenetic processes [13]. Thus, it has even been stated that cancer is an inflammatory disease [14]. Further, neutrophils can form neutrophil extracellular traps developed from externalised DNA network. These nets are bidirectionally associated with platelet activation and can contribute to cancer progression via several mechanisms; therefore, neutrophil extracellular traps also represent an attractive treatment target [15].

Cancer-related SIR involves cells of innate and adaptive immunity as well as soluble factors. Macrophages are recruited in tumour by hypoxia and tumour-released molecular agents including growth factors and cytokines [16]. Macrophage phenotype switch from tumour-suppressing classical M1 to tumour-promoting M2 subtype promotes angiogenesis and immunosuppression. Platelet activation contributes to cancer progression and patient mortality [15]. Neutrophils are locally recruited in the cancer via chemokine signalling. Neutrophil activation can contribute to angiogenesis and increased blood vessel permeability locally and metastatic spread systemically. In addition, immature myeloid cells and neutrophil extracellular traps might have tumour-promoting activity. These molecular events also highlight the association between infection or surgery-induced inflammation [17] and cancer relapse or metastatic spread. Thus, innate immunity is generally thought to act as tumour enhancers. In contrast, lymphocytes representing the adaptive immunity are considered to have tumour-suppressing effects [16], although contrary effects have been ascribed to certain subpopulations [18].

HCC can be considered a classical inflammation-induced cancer, as its most common risk factors are hepatitis B and hepatitis C virus infections. Inflammation is also present in liver tissues in patients affected by alcohol-induced hepatitis or NASH. Thus, SIR is not expected to have diagnostic value. Indeed, SIR parameters change before the tumour develops, e.g., increased NLR has been observed in chronic viral hepatitis C [19]. NLR is an independent prognostic factor in liver cirrhosis [20].

Wide variety of inflammation-based markers could be used as indicators of HCC prognosis, tumour recurrence and response to specific treatment. In particular, neutrophil, lymphocyte and platelet counts as well as C-reactive protein and albumin and their combinations, neutrophil-to-lymphocyte ratio (NLR), platelet-to-lymphocyte ratio (PLR) and Glasgow prognostic score (GPS) have prognostic value.

3.1. Neutrophil-to-lymphocyte ratio in HCC

Neutrophil-to-lymphocyte ratio is the most extensively evaluated parameter of SIR in HCC. NLR, calculated as the ratio between count of neutrophils and lymphocytes in blood, seems to reflect the intensity of systemic pro- and anti-tumour reaction. NLR has shown prognostic importance in surgically treated HCC cases, including early stage tumours; in liver transplantation; sorafenib treatment and different ablation techniques.

Several meta-analyses have been devoted to NLR in HCC patients. Thus, baseline NLR was associated with overall survival and recurrence-free survival, while post-treatment NLR was significantly associated with overall survival [21]. In meta-analysis of NLR in HCC patients treated by liver transplantation, significant association with overall and recurrence-free survival was found [22]. In an early study, NLR was already confirmed as a prognostic factor in HCC. NLR was associated with overall and disease-free survival both generally and after different treatment approaches [23].

3.2. Neutrophil-to-lymphocyte ratio in surgically treated HCC

In HCC patients subjected to curative resection, several research groups have identified high NLR as an independent, significant predictive factor, associated with worse overall survival [24–27], shorter recurrence-free survival [24, 25, 28] and higher frequency of recurrence [29].

The studies show some variability in design, group size and cut-off level. However, the reported differences in survival are not only statistically significant but also biologically important. In 672 HCC patients treated by surgical resection, the recurrence rate within 1, 3 and 5 years was 77.4, 55.2 and 44.8% in those having low NLR ($\leq$2.5), while the corresponding recurrence rates were 64.1, 45.2 and 35.5% ($p = 0.016$) in high NLR group [29]. In 303 patients who underwent surgical liver resection for HCC, high NLR (>2.0, based on ROC-detected cut-off) was significantly associated both with shorter recurrence-free and overall survival (both $p < 0.001$), but multivariate analysis confirmed it as an independent prognostic factor only for overall survival (hazard ratio (HR) 1.724; 95% confidence interval (CI): 1.241–2.394; $p = 0.001$). Huang et al. evaluated 1659 HCC patients, stratifying them by NLR quartiles. The 5-year overall survival rate was 60% in the lowest quartile contrasting with 27% in the highest quartile. NLR was associated by HR of mortality 1.031; 95% CI: 1.002–1.060; $p = 0.033$ [30]. In a large Japanese study, enrolling 958 patients who underwent hepatectomy, the 5-year survival rate was 72.9% in low NLR (<2.81) group *versus* 51.5% in patients with high NLR [24]. In another 256 Japanese patients, NLR was confirmed by multivariate analysis as an independent prognostic factor both for overall and recurrence-free interval. The respective hazard ratios were 2.59; 95% CI: 1.56–4.31; $p < 0.001$ and 2.11; 95% CI = 1.44–3.11; $p < 0.001$ [25]. In a smaller study of 113 patients, the recurrence-free survival was 42.4 months in patients having NLR < 3 but 7.9 months in those having NLR $\geq$ 3.0. The respective HR was 2.58; $p = 0.002$ [28].

The findings in Western patients have been less positive. In the largest Western series comprising 370 patients, treated in Memorial Sloan Kettering Cancer Center in New York, USA, PLR, but not NLR, was independently associated with worse recurrence-free survival and overall survival [31].

NLR retains prognostic value in several subgroups of surgically treated patients, including early cases. By multivariate analysis, preoperative NLR (at cut-off 2.8) was the strongest independent prognostic factor for overall survival after liver resection with curative intent for TNM stage I HCC. The HR was 2.69; 95% CI: 1.57–4.59; $p < 0.001$. The 5-year survival in high *versus* low NLR group was 45.0 *versus* 76.4%; $p < 0.001$. Interestingly, the association with survival in stage II or III was not significant, reflected by $p = 0.283$ and $p = 0.155$. In stage I patients, high NLR predicted more frequent extrahepatic recurrence ($p = 0.006$). As growth of HCC is associated with grade progression, these results suggest that NLR reflects the biological potential of HCC [32]. In Chinese cohort of 222 patients, preoperative NLR, using cut-off at

2.1, predicted overall survival in solitary small (≤5 cm) HCC after surgical resection and could discriminate outcome in patients having AFP levels not exceeding 400 ng/mL [33]. Further, in a large study of 963 HCC patients treated by potentially curative surgical resection, high NLR (>2.81) was an independent risk factor for overall and recurrence-free survival (both $p < 0.001$) in the general group as well as in early or intermediate stage HCC: Barcelona Clinic Liver Cancer (BCLC) stages 0/A or B (both $p < 0.05$) while no association was found in stage C [34]. NLR was also not associated with early (<1 year) mortality from cancer recurrence after liver resection for huge (at least 10 cm in diameter) HCC in 166 patients [35]. NLR was an independent factor that predicted ($p = 0.029$) early recurrence after curative resection of HCC presenting as a single focus in 193 Japanese patients [36]. However, contrary results have been reported as well, e.g., NLR had no prognostic significance in early HCC (BCLC stage 0/A) treated by surgical resection in 324 patients [37].

Somewhat contrasting data are reported regarding NLR in surgically treated patients with more advanced HCC. Although limited significance of NLR was previously noted in high-stage or large HCC, some authors have found significant role of NLR in advanced cases. Thus, in 81 hepatectomy-treated HCC patients with portal or hepatic vein tumour thrombosis, high NLR (defined as >2.9) was an independent prognostic factor for worse overall survival, characterised by HR 1.866; 95% CI: 1.048–3.322; $p = 0.034$. Significant association with recurrence-free interval was found as well. The overall survival in high *versus* low NLR groups was 6.2 months *versus* 15.7 months; $p = 0.007$, while the recurrence-free survival was 2.2 *versus* 3.7 months; $p = 0.039$ [38].

Not only baseline NLR but also the dynamic changes of NLR were found to be important. In 189 patients treated by curative resection for small HCC, the temporal change of NLR was an independent prognostic factor for overall (HR 2.637; 95% CI: 1.356–5.128; $p = 0.004$) and recurrence-free (HR 2.372; 95% CI: 1.563–3.601; $p < 0.001$) survival. The 1-, 3- and 5-year survival was 92.7, 70.0 and 53.0% in patients experiencing NLR increase *versus* 96.2, 87.5 and 75.9% in those with decreasing NLR ($p = 0.003$). High preoperative or postoperative NLR had lower prognostic value in this study [39]. Paralleling observations have been reported by Hung et al., studying patients with HCC recurrence after liver resection. The 5-year post recurrence survival was better (45.9%) in those continuously having NLR ≤ 2.5. Patients who had low NLR (≤2.5) at resection but high level (>2.5) at recurrence had 5-year survival of only 24.6%; the difference was significant as reflected by $p = 0.013$ [29].

3.3. Neutrophil-to-lymphocyte ratio in patients receiving transplantation for HCC

Different aspects of NLR have been evaluated in HCC patients subjected to liver transplantation, including transplantation from living donor. The prognostic value of NLR was revealed already in the early studies. Thus, NLR (applying the cut-off level at 5.0) was an independent predictor of overall and recurrence-free survival in 219 Italian patients after liver transplantation for HCC [40].

By univariate analysis, preoperative NLR was significantly associated by disease-free survival and overall survival in HCC patients after liver transplantation. The 1-, 3- and 5-year overall survival rate in high *versus* low NLR group was 81.3, 56.7 and 51.0 *versus* 90.9, 74.2 and 66.8% ($p = 0.041$). Similarly, the 1-, 3- and 5-year recurrence-free survival rate in high *versus* low NLR group was 65.3, 48.5 and 39.4 *versus* 80.0, 68.0 and 65.2%. The difference was also significant as reflected by $p = 0.013$ [41]. Further, NLR was an independent prognostic factor for overall and recurrence-free survival after liver transplantation for HCC as was shown by multivariate analysis of 160 Western patients [42]. NLR was proved to be an independent risk factor for overall survival ($p < 0.001$) and recurrence-free survival ($p = 0.003$) in 248 male patients treated by liver transplantation [43]. Harimoto et al. reported on 213 patients receiving living donor liver transplantation for HCC. High preoperative NLR ≥ 2.66 was an independent predictor of recurrence [44].

NLR can be used in prognostic models to identify patients who exceed Milan criteria but still have good overall and tumour-free survival. In study reported by Wang et al., male patients were enrolled and thus the proposed models were verified in males only [43]. Combination of NLR and Hangzhou criteria has been suggested to identify patients who can be successfully treated by liver transplantation [45]. NLR has been included in the MORAL scores to predict recurrence after liver transplantation, and these scores were superior to Milan criteria [46]. Complex evaluation of NLR along with fibrinogen increases the prognostic accuracy in order to predict disease-free survival and overall survival in HCC patients treated by liver transplantation [41]. Pretransplantation NLR along with levels of C-reactive protein has been combined with Milan criteria to develop new selection criteria for living donor liver transplantation beyond Milan criteria [47].

However, contrasting findings have been published as well. Thus, NLR did not predict post-transplantation recurrence or worse overall survival in 150 patients within Milan criteria [48]. Limited prognostic impact of NLR was found in 124 patients who underwent living donor liver transplantation [49]. In Western patients, NLR was not predictive of treatment success regarding liver transplantation or other tested approaches (hepatectomy, transarterial chemo-embolisation). Although the group was quite small (75), Child-Pugh and Model for End Stage Liver Disease (MELD) scores were informative [50].

3.4. Neutrophil-to-lymphocyte ratio in sorafenib-treated HCC patients

In patients with unresectable HCC, treated by multikinase inhibitor sorafenib, high NLR (>3.1) was a significant independent prognostic factor, associated with worse overall survival. Better treatment response was observed in patients with low NLR [51]. The findings were confirmed by another study, reporting on 442 sorafenib-treated patients (Japan, Italy and United Kingdom) with advanced HCC. High NLR again was an independent prognostic factor, predicting shorter survival with HR 1.218; 95% CI: 1.108–1.322; $p < 0.0001$ [52].

Regarding combined approach, high pre-treatment NLR (>3.0) was an independent predictor of worse overall survival in 40 patients with unresectable HCC treated by transcatheter arterial embolisation and sorafenib. The median survival in high *versus* low NLR group was 14 months (95% CI = 10.1–17.9) *versus* 26 months (95% CI = 17.4–34.6). The difference was significant ($p = 0.001$) and biologically remarkable [53]. Other researchers have also confirmed that NLR was independent predictor of overall survival in patients with advanced HCC treated by sorafenib [54].

3.5. Neutrophil-to-lymphocyte ratio in HCC patients undergoing tumour ablation

NLR has been investigated in regard to different embolisation and ablation techniques. High NLR (>3) predicted significantly worse treatment results ($p = 0.014$) and early disease progression ($p < 0.0001$) in 86 treatment-naive patients subjected to arterial chemoembolisation or radioembolisation [55]. Elevated pre-treatment NLR (>1.85) was associated with overall survival and disease-free survival in 178 HCC patients subjected to transcatheter arterial chemoembolisation (TACE). The median survival in high *versus* low NLR group was 8 *versus* 17.5 months. The 1-, 3- and 5-year overall survival rates in these groups were 42.1, 19.6 and 9.5 *versus* 57.3, 44.1 and 27.2%, respectively ($p < 0.001$). Differences in disease-free survival were significant as well ($p < 0.001$). Multivariate analysis confirmed NLR as a significant ($p = 0.04$), independent prognostic factor for survival after TACE [56].

In patients with advanced HCC treated by hepatic arterial infusion chemotherapy, high NLR was a significant predictor of lower response rate, worse progression-free and overall survival [57]. Baseline NLR was a significant predictor of treatment response and progression-free survival after hepatic arterial infusion chemotherapy for advanced HCC [58]. In patients receiving hepatic arterial infusion chemotherapy by cisplatin and fluorouracil, response rate and overall survival were associated with NLR [59].

Dynamic changes of NLR had independent prognostic significance ($p = 0.035$) in HCC with portal vein tumour thrombosis treated by microwave ablation after transarterial chemoembolisation [60]. In 506 patients treated by thermal ablation of recurrent HCC, high pre-treatment NLR (≥2.14) was a prognostic factor for recurrence-free survival, confirmed by Cox multiple regression analysis. The 1- and 3-year recurrence rates in high *versus* low NLR groups were 57.9 and 82.5 *versus* 20.7 and 31.6%. The difference was statistically significant, confirmed by $p < 0.001$ [61].

Pre-treatment NLR was associated with worse overall survival in early HCC after radiofrequency ablation. Post-treatment NLR was associated both with worse overall survival and recurrence in early HCC after radiofrequency ablation [62]. Similarly, NLR dynamics, but not pre-treatment NLR, was an independent prognostic factor for overall survival and recurrence-free survival in patients with small HCC treated by radiofrequency ablation [63]. In patients treated by radiofrequency ablation for HCC, post-treatment NLR was associated with recurrence and survival. Pre-treatment NLR was associated with recurrence only in patients who had HBV infection and HCC but not in those who developed HCC in association with HCV infection [64]. In unresectable HCC treated by radioembolisation, elevated NLR was an independent predictor of worse survival [65].

3.6. Neutrophil-to-lymphocyte ratio and tumour characteristics

NLR has been mostly assessed in correlation with survival or treatment response. However, some observations are reported on the association between systemic inflammatory response and tumour morphology in gross and microscopic level. Thus, high NLR is observed in patients having larger tumours, multiple HCC foci, higher grade of HCC and vascular invasion [29]. In few studies, the infiltration of neutrophils and macrophages in liver tumours has been assessed. Peritumoural tissues are characterised by higher ratio between neutrophils and T lymphocytes, and higher ratio also correlates with lower overall survival. The combination of these findings suggests that neutrophils might facilitate tumour progression. They suppress adaptive immunity by death ligand expression [66]. Correlation between NLR and PD-L1 expression in the centre of tumour but not peritumoural tissues has been described [67]. High NLR was associated with CD163-positive tumour-associated macrophages [24]. High NLR was associated with higher peritumoural but not intratumoural CD163 and IL-17-expressing cells [68].

3.7. Platelet-to-lymphocyte ratio in HCC patients

Platelet-to-lymphocyte ratio (PLR) is another frequently assessed estimate of SIR, although fewer publications have been devoted to PLR than to NLR. Nevertheless, prognostic role of PLR has been evaluated in different aspects of HCC patient treatment, including surgery [31, 69, 70], transplantation, sorafenib treatment, TACE and ablation techniques.

In the largest Western series enrolling 370 HCC patients, treated by surgical resection, higher preoperative PLR was identified as an independent risk factor of worse overall survival and recurrence-free survival [31]. Other research groups have confirmed the association between PLR and prognosis. Higher preoperative PLR is an independent predictor of worse overall survival in HCC patients undergoing curative liver resection [69, 70] as was shown in two large Eastern cohorts comprising 778 [70] and 1804 [69] patients, respectively. The significant association with overall survival ($p < 0.001$) was retained in specific subgroups, e.g., patients having cirrhosis or being positive for HbsAg [70]. In some studies, the associations between PLR and prognosis were statistically significant but not independent. Thus, PLR was significantly associated with disease-free and overall survival in 332 HCC patients after hepatectomy [71]. The association between higher PLR and shorter recurrence-free survival in HCC patients undergoing curative liver resection was statistically significant but not independent [70]. Finally, no association has been found in some studies. Hence, in 113 HCC patients undergoing curative resection, PLR was not confirmed as a significant prognostic factor for recurrence-free survival. NLR was found to be superior in this study [28].

PLR has been analysed in the context of liver transplantation. Already in early studies, statistically significant association was found between pretransplantation PLR and cancer recurrence after liver transplantation. In 146 patients, the recurrence-free survival was 80.7 *versus* 91.6%; the difference was statistically significant as confirmed by $p = 0.02$ [72].

In 122 Chinese patients undergoing transarterial chemoembolisation (TACE) for HBV-related HCC, high pre-treatment PLR (≥96.13) was an independent, statistically significant ($p = 0.001$) factor that predicted worse survival [73].

In 414 patients affected by recurrent HCC and treated by thermal ablation, high pre-treatment PLR (≥87.87) was associated with higher risk of recurrence and worse recurrence-free survival. The 1- and 3-year recurrence rates in high *versus* low PLR groups were 56.0 and 79.5 *versus* 39.9 and 54.8%; $p < 0.05$ [74].

Regarding sorafenib-treated cases, PLR has not shown prognostic value in patients receiving sorafenib for advanced HCC. Although the negative result could be attributed to the small group size (16 patients), significant association with NLR was still confirmed [75].

Several meta-analyses have recently been carried out to evaluate PLR in hepatocellular carcinoma. Significant association between higher PLR and increased risk of death was reported by Hu and Yu, reporting odds ratio for death 1.59; 95% CI: 1.15–2.20 on the basis of meta-analysis of six studies with 1446 HCC patients [76]. The association between high PLR and worse overall survival was confirmed by Ma et al., Song et al., and Zhao et al. [77–79]. In a meta-analysis of nine studies including 2017 patients, high PLR was associated with poor overall survival (HR 1.63; 95% CI: 1.42–1.88; $p < 0.001$) as reported by Ma et al. [77]. Evaluating 2507 patients in 11 studies, high PLR was significantly associated with worse overall survival, as reflected by hazard ratio HR = 1.78; 95% CI: 1.36–2.34; $p < 0.001$ [78]. In a meta-analysis of 10 studies including 2315 patients, high PLR was associated with the HR for worse overall survival of 1.60; 95% CI: 1.23–2.08; $p = 0.0005$ [79].

Controversial findings are reported regarding PLR and recurrence-free survival. The association has been confirmed by some research groups [77, 78] but denied by others. In a meta-analysis of nine studies including 2017 patients, high PLR was significantly ($p < 0.001$) associated with poor recurrence-free survival: HR = 1.32; 95% CI: 1.15–1.52. In a meta-analysis of 11 studies comprising 2507 patients, elevated PLR was significantly associated with worse recurrence-free survival, as reflected by hazard ratio HR = 1.82; 95% CI: 1.56–2.13; $p < 0.001$. In contrast, by meta-analysis of 2315 patients in 10 studies, high PLR was not significantly associated with worse recurrence-free survival as the HR was 1.21; 95% CI: 0.87–1.67; $p = 0.26$ [79].

High PLR also showed correlation with high tumour size exceeding 3 cm, TNM stage, lymph node metastases and distant metastases [78]. The findings regarding vascular invasion are controversial again, as the association is confirmed in some studies [78] but not others [77]. No association between PLR and tumour multifocality and higher grade has been confirmed [77].

3.8. Glasgow prognostic score in hepatocellular carcinoma

The prognosis and treatment options of HCC patients depend not only on tumour progression but also on the extent of liver dysfunction. As a consequence, several staging systems have been proposed to predict prognosis for HCC, including Glasgow prognostic score (GPS), based on the levels of C-reactive protein and albumin (**Table 1**). GPS in HCC patients with hepatocellular carcinoma is an independent prognostic predictor after hepatic resection, with higher score indicating worse prognosis [80]. Thus, among 144 patients who underwent surgical resection for HCC, GPS 2 was associated with worse disease-free (HR = 2.527; 95% CI: 1.163–5.490; $p = 0.019$) and overall (HR = 8.012; 95% CI: 2.818–22.784; $p < 0.001$) survival, but GPS 1 with shorter overall (HR = 2.277; 95% CI: 1.029–5.039; $p = 0.042$) survival than seen in patients preoperatively presenting with GPS 0 [80]. The independent prognostic role of GPS for overall survival was confirmed by other research teams [81] and meta-analysis [82]. Modified GPS score and dynamics of GPS score have also shown prognostic value. Thus, elevated modified GPS was associated with overall survival (HR = 2.21; 95% CI: 1.73–2.82; $p < 0.05$) in a meta-analysis of 2047 HCC patients [83]. Dynamics of GPS (assessed in association with hepatitis B infection status) was an independent predictor of overall survival in 247 patients treated by liver resection [84]. In addition, GPS was related to blood transfusion requirement and postoperative pulmonary complications after liver resection for HCC [85]. In patients undergoing liver transplantation for HCC, elevated GPS, reaching 1 or 2, was

Score	Definition
Glasgow prognostic score	
0	C-reactive protein (CRP) < 10 mg/L AND albumin ≥35 g/L
1	One high-risk finding: CRP ≥ 10 mg/L OR albumin <35 g/L
2	Both high-risk findings: CRP ≥ 10 mg/L AND albumin <35 g/L
Modified Glasgow prognostic score	
0	CRP ≤ 10 mg/L irrespective of albumin level
1	Increased CRP on the background of normal albumin level: CRP > 10 mg/L AND albumin ≥35 g/L
2	Increased CRP and hypoalbuminaemia: CRP > 10 mg/L AND albumin <35 g/L

Table 1. Glasgow prognostic score and its modifications [30].

significantly associated with poor overall ($p = 0.018$) and recurrence-free ($p = 0.030$) survival. Complex scoring system has been created on the basis of Milan criteria and GPS [86].

Regarding advanced HCC, GPS retained independent prognostic value for survival (HR = 1.410; 95% CI = 1.060–1.874; $p = 0.018$). In addition to the statistical significance of results, the biological survival differences by GPS were also remarkable, e.g., median survival was 480 days in patients presenting with GPS 0 and 154 days in those having GPS 1 or 2 [87]. GPS was an independent prognostic factor (HR = 5.483; 95% CI: 2.563–11.729; $p < 0.001$) for overall survival in patients undergoing sorafenib treatment: the median survival in those having GPS 0 *versus* elevated GPS 1 or 2 was 18.1 *versus* 5.2 months; $p < 0.001$ [88].

In HCC patients undergoing transarterial chemoembolisation, GPS was an independent prognostic factor for overall survival (HR = 1.697; 95% CI: 1.325–2.174; $p < 0.001$). It was also found to be superior to other inflammation scores as NLR, PLR or modified GPS. Based on these findings, the authors proposed a new complex score that included Child-Pugh stage, number of tumour nodules and proportion of affected liver, AFP, presence or absence of portal vein thrombosis and GPS. The new score was also a significant predictor of survival as the HR was 1.724; 95% CI: 1.347–2.285; $p < 0.001$ [89].

4. Conclusions

HCC is a frequent and aggressive malignant tumour. Longer survival can be reached in early diagnosed and properly treated cases. In the future, diagnosis of HCC might be based on combination of radiological features and miRNA profile representing liquid biopsy. MiRNA profile can have both diagnostic and prognostic value. Thus, further lowering of the needs for core biopsy might be expected, leading to patient-friendly examination and avoiding the rare but still possible complications. After the diagnosis of HCC has been confirmed, SIR assessment by NLR and PLR represents innovative means of prognostic evaluation.

Acknowledgements

BS was financially supported by post-doctoral research project 1.1.1.2./VIAA/1/16/242.

Author details

Ilze Strumfa[1*], Dzeina Mezale[1], Boriss Strumfs[2], Andrejs Vanags[3], Arturs Kalva[1], Dainis Balodis[1], Ilze Fridrihsone[1], Arnis Abolins[1] and Janis Gardovskis[3]

*Address all correspondence to: ilze.strumfa@rsu.lv

1 Department of Pathology, Riga Stradins University, Riga, Latvia

2 Latvian Institute of Organic Synthesis, Riga, Latvia

3 Department of Surgery, Riga Stradins University, Riga, Latvia

References

[1] Siegel RL, Miller KD, Jemal A. Cancer statistics, 2016. CA: A Cancer Journal for Clinicians. 2016;**66**(1):7-30

[2] Shah C, Mramba LK, Bishnoi R, Bejjanki H, Chhatrala HS, Chandana SR. Survival differences among patients with hepatocellular carcinoma based on the stage of disease and therapy received: Pre and post sorafenib era. Journal of Gastrointestinal Oncology. 2017;**8**(5):789-798

[3] Filingeri V, Francioso S, Sforza D, Santopaolo F, Oddi FM, Tisone G. A retrospective analysis of 1.011 percutaneous liver biopsies performed in patients with liver transplantation or liver diseases: Ultrasonography can reduce complications? European Review for Medical and Pharmacological Sciences. 2016;**20**(17):3609-3617

[4] Tan Y, Ge G, Pan T, Wen D, Chen L, Yu X, Zhou X, Gan J. A serum microRNA panel as potential biomarkers for hepatocellular carcinoma related with hepatitis B virus. PLoS One. 2014;**9**(9):e107986

[5] Loosen SH, Schueller F, Trautwein C, Roy S, Roderburg C. Role of circulating microRNAs in liver diseases. World Journal of Hepatology. 2017;**9**(12):586-594

[6] Qi P, Cheng SQ, Wang H, Li N, Chen YF, Gao CF. Serum microRNAs as biomarkers for hepatocellular carcinoma in Chinese patients with chronic hepatitis B virus infection. PLoS One. 2011;**6**(12):e28486

[7] Sohn W, Kim J, Kang SH, Yang SR, Cho JY, Cho HC, Shim SG, Paik YH. Serum exosomal microRNAs as novel biomarkers for hepatocellular carcinoma. Experimental & Molecular Medicine. 2015;**47**:e184

[8] Ali HEA, Abdel Hameed R, Effat H, Ahmed EK, Atef AA, Sharawi SK, Ali M, Abd Elmageed ZY, Abdel Wahab AH. Circulating microRNAs panel as a diagnostic tool for discrimination of HCV-associated hepatovcellular carcinoma. Clinics and Research in Hepatology and Gastroenterology. 2017;**41**(4):e51-e62

[9] Zhang Y, Li T, Qiu Y, Zhang T, Guo P, Ma X, Wei Q, Han L. Serum microRNA panel for early diagnosis of the onset of hepatocellular carcinoma. Medicine (Baltimore). 2017;**96**(2):e5642

[10] Zekri AN, Youssef AS, El-Desouky ED, Ahmed OS, Lotfy MM, Nassar AA, Bahnassey AA. Serum microRNA panels as potential biomarkers for early detection of hepatocellular carcinoma on top of HVCV infection. Tumour Biology. 2016;**37**(9):12273-12286

[11] Khairy A, Hamza I, Shaker O, Yosry A. Serum miRNA panel in Egyptian patients with chronic hepatitis C related hepatocellular carcinoma. Asian Pacific Journal of Cancer Prevention. 2016;**17**(5):2699-2703

[12] Bimonte S, Leongito M, Barbieri A, Del Vecchio V, Falco M, Giudice A, Palaia R, Albino V, Di Giacomo R, Petrillo A, Granata V, Izzo F. The therapeutic targets of miRNA in hepatic cancer stem cells. Stem Cells International. 2016;**2016**:1065230

[13] Ohki S, Shibata M, Gonda K, Machida T, Shimura T, Nakamura I, Ohtake T, Koyama Y, Suzuki S, Ohto H, Takenoshita S. Circulating myeloid-deribved suppressor cells are increased and correlate to immune suppression, inflammation and hypoproteinemia in patients with cancer. Oncology Reports. 2012;**28**(2):453-458

[14] Rutkowski MR, Svoronos N, Perales-Puchalt A, Conejo-Garcia JR. The tumor macroenvironment: Cancer promoting networks beyond tumor beds. Advances in Cancer Research. 2015;**128**:235-262

[15] Olsson AK, Cederval J. NETosis in cancer – Platelet-neutrophil crosstalk promotes tumor-associated pathology. Frontiers in Immunology. 2016;**7**:373

[16] Cederval J, Dimberg A, Olsson AK. Tumor-induced local and systemic impact on blood vessel function. Mediators of Inflammation. 2015;**2015**:418290

[17] Mohri Y, Tanaka K, Toiyama Y, Ohi M, Yasuda H, Inoue Y, Kusunoki M. Impact of preoperative neutrophil to lymphocyte ratio and postoperative infectious complications on survival after curative gastrectomy for gastric cancer: A single institutional cohort study. Medicine (Baltimore). 2016;**95**(11):e3125. DOI: 10.1097/MD0000000000003125

[18] De Visser KE, Coussens LM. The interplay between innate and adaptive immunity regulates cancer development. Cancer Immunology, Immunotherapy. 2005;**54**(11):1143-1152

[19] Abdel-Razik A, Mousa N, Besheer TA, Eissa M, Elhelaly R, Arafa M, El-Wakeel N, Eldars W. Neutrophil to lymphocyte ratio as a reliable marker to predict insulin resistance and fibrosis stage in chronic hepatitis C virus infection. Acta Gastroenterologica Belgica. 2015;**78**(4):386-392

[20] Biyik M, Ucar R, Solak Y, Gungor G, Polat I, Gaipov A, Cakir OO, Ataseven H, Demir A, Turk S, Polat H. Blood neutrophil-to-lymphocyte ratio independently predicts survival

in patients with liver cirrhosis. European Journal of Gastroenterology & Hepatology. 2013;**25**(4):435-441

[21] Qi X, Li J, Deng H, Li H, Su C, Guo X. Neutrophil-to-lymphocyte ratio for the prognostic assessment of hepatocellular carcinoma: A systematic review and meta-analysis of observational studies. Oncotarget. 2016;**7**(29):45283-45301

[22] Sun XD, Shi XJ, Chen YG, Wang CL, Ma Q, Lv GY. Elevated preoperative neutrophil-lymphocyte ratio is associated with poor prognosis in hepatocellular carcinoma patients treated with liver transplantation: A meta-analysis. Gastroenterology Research and Practice. 2016;**2016**:4743808

[23] Xiao WK, Chen D, Li SQ, Fu SJ, Peng BG, Liang LJ. Prognostic significance of neutrophil-lymphocyte ratio in hepatocellular carcinoma: A meta-analysis. BMC Cancer. 2014;**14**:117

[24] Mano Y, Shirabe K, Yamashita Y, Harimoto N, Tsujita E, Takeishi K, Aishima S, Ikegami T, Yoshizumi T, Yamanaka T, Maehara Y. Preoperative neutrophil-to-lymphocyte ratio is a predictor of survival after hepatectomy for hepatocellular carcinoma: A retrospective analysis. Annals of Surgery. 2013;**258**(2):301-305

[25] Okamura Y, Ashida R, Ito T, Sugiura T, Mori K, Uesaka K. Preoperative neutrophil to lymphocyte ratio and prognostic nutritional index predict overall survival after hepatectomy for hepatocellular carcinoma. World Journal of Surgery. 2015;**39**(6):1501-1509

[26] Huang GQ, Zhu GQ, Liu YL, Wang LR, Braddock M, Zheng MH, Zhou MT. Stratified neutrophil-to-lymphocyte ratio accurately predict mortality risk in hepatocellular carcinoma patients following curative liver transplantation. Oncotarget. 2016;**7**(5):5429-5439

[27] Ji F, Fu S, Guo Z, Pang H, Chen D, Wang X, Ju W, Wang D, He X, Hua Y, Peng B. Prognostic significance of preoperative aspartate aminotransferase to neutrophil ratio index in patients with hepatocellular carcinoma after hepatic resection. Oncotarget. 2016;**7**(44):72276-72289

[28] Yamamura K, Sugimoto H, Kanda M, Yamada S, Nomoto S, Nakayama G, Fujii T, Koike M, Fujiwara M, Kodera Y. Comparison of inflammation-based prognostic scores as predictors of tumor recurrence in patients with hepatocellular carcinoma after curative resection. Journal of Hepato-Biliary-Pancreatic Sciences. 2014;**21**(9):682-688

[29] Hung HC, Lee JC, Cheng CH, Wu TH, Wang YC, Lee CF, Wu TJ, Chou HS, Chan KM, Lee WC. Impact of neutrophil to lymphocyte ratio on survival for hepatocellular carcinoma after curative resection. Journal of Hepato-Biliary-Pancreatic Sciences. 2017. DOI: 10.1002/jhbp.498 [Epub ahead of print]

[30] Strumfa I, Bogdanova T, Kalva A, Strumfs B, Rumba R, Vanags A, Drike I, Mezale D, Abolins A, Jakovlevs A, Balodis D, Gardovskis J. Systemic inflammatory reaction in gastric cancer: Biology and practical implications of neutrophil to lymphocyte ratio, Glasgow prognostic score and related parameters. In: Mozsik G, editor. Gastric Cancer. InTech; 2017. pp. 143-197. DOI: 10.5772/intechopen.69723

[31] Zheng J, Seier K, Gonen M, Balachandran VP, Kingham TP, D'Angelica MI, Allen PJ, Jarnagin WR, DeMatteo RP. Utility of serum inflammatory markers for predicting

microvascular invasion and survival for patients with hepatocellular carcinoma. Annals of Surgical Oncology. 2017. DOI: 10.1245/s10434-017-6060-7 [Epub ahead of print]

[32] Okamura Y, Sugiura T, Ito T, Yamamoto Y, Ashida R, Mori K, Uesaka K. Neutrophil to lymphocyte ratio as an indicator of the malignant behaviour of hepatocellular carcinoma. The British Journal of Surgery. 2016;**103**(7):891-898

[33] Liao R, Tang ZW, Li DW, Luo SQ, Huang P, Du CY. Preoperative neutrophil-to-lymphocyte ratio predicts recurrence of patients with single-nodule small hepatocellular carcinoma following curative resection: A retrospective report. World Journal of Surgical Oncology. 2015;**13**:265

[34] Lu SD, Wang YY, Peng NF, Peng YC, Zhong JH, Qin HG, Xiang BD, You XM, Ma L, Li LQ. Preoperative ratio of neutrophils to lymphocytes predicts postresection survival in selected patients with early or intermediate stage hepatocellular carcinoma. Medicine (Baltimore). 2016;**95**(5):e2722

[35] Goh BK, Kam JH, Lee SY, Chan CY, Allen JC, Jeyaraj P, Cheow PC, Chow PK, Ooi LL, Chung AY. Significance of neutrophil-to-lymphocyte ratio, platelet-to-lymphocyte ratio and prognostic nutrition index as preoperative predictors of early mortality after liver resection for huge (≥10 cm) hepatocellular carcinoma. Journal of Surgical Oncology. 2016;**113**(6):621-627

[36] Shimoda M, Tago K, Shiraki T, Mori S, Kato M, Aoki T, Kubota K. Risk factors for early recurrence of single lesion hepatocellular carcinoma after curative resection. World Journal of Surgery. 2016;**40**(10):2466-2471

[37] Chan AW, Chan SL, Wong GL, Wong vW, Chong CC, Lai PB, Chan HL, To KF. Prognostic nutritional index (PNI) predicts tumor recurrence of very early/early stage hepatocellular carcinoma after surgical resection. Annals of Surgical Oncology. 2015;**22**(13):4138-4148

[38] Li SH, Wang QX, Yang ZY, Jiang W, Li C, Sun P, Wei W, Shi M, Guo RP. Prognostic value of the neutrophil-to-lymphocyte ratio for hepatocellular carcinoma patients with portal/hepatic vein tumor thrombosis. World Journal of Gastroenterology. 2017;**23**(17):3122-3132

[39] Peng W, Li C, Wen TF, Yan LN, Li B, Wang WT, Yang JY, Xu MQ. Neutrophil to lymphocyte ratio changes predict small hepatocellular carcinoma survival. The Journal of Surgical Research. 2014;**192**(2):402-408

[40] Bertuzzo VR, Cescon M, Ravaioli M, Grazi GL, Ercolani G, Del Gaudio M, Cuccheti A, D'Errico-Grigioni A, Golfieri R, Pinna AD. Analysis of factors affecting recurrence of hepatocellular carcinoma after liver transplantation with a special focus on inflammation markers. Transplantation. 2011;**91**(11):1279-1285

[41] Fu SJ, Ji F, Han M, Chen MG, Wang XP, Ju WQ, Zhao Q, Wu LW, Ren QQ, Guo ZY, Wang DP, Zhu XF, Ma Y, He XS. Prognostic value of combined preoperative fibrinogen and neutrophil-lymphocyte ratio in patients with hepatocellular carcinoma after liver transplantation. Oncotarget. 2017;**8**(3):4301-4312

[42] Limaye AR, Clark V, Soldevila-Pico C, Morelli G, Suman A, Firpi R, Nelson DR, Cabrera R. Neutrophil-lymphocyte ratio predicts overall and recurrence-free survival after liver transplantation for hepatocellular carcinoma. Hepatology Research. 2013;**43**(7):757-764

[43] Wang W, Ye Y, Wang T, Zhang F, Geng L, Yu J, Zhou L, Yan S, Zheng S. Prognostic prediction of male recipients selected for liver transplantation: With special attention to neutrophil to lymphocyte ratio. Hepatology Research. 2016;**46**(9):899-907

[44] Harimoto N, Yoshizumi T, Shimagaki T, Nagatsu A, Motomura T, Harada N, Okabe H, Itoh S, Ikegami T, Uchiyama H, Soejima Y, Maehara Y. Inflammation-based prognostic score in patients with living donor liver transplantation for hepatocellular carcinoma. Anticancer Research. 2016;**36**(10):5537-5542

[45] Xiao GQ, Yang JY, Yan LN. Combined Hangzhou criteria with neutrophil-lymphocyte ratio is superior to other criteria in selecting liver transplantation candidates with HBV-related hepatocellular carcinoma. Hepatobiliary & Pancreatic Diseases International. 2015;**14**(6):588-595

[46] Halazun KJ, Najjar M, Abdelmessih RM, Samstein B, Griesemer AD, Guarrera JV, Kato T, Verna EC, Emond JC, Brown Jr RS. Recurrence after liver transplantation for hepatocellular carcinoma: A new MORAL to the story. Annals of Surgery. 2017;**265**(3):557-564

[47] Na GH, Kim DG, Han JH, Kim EY, Lee SH, Hong TH, You YK. Inflammatory markers as selection criteria of hepatocellular carcinoma in living-donor liver transplantation. World Journal of Gastroenterology. 2014;**20**(21):6594-6601

[48] Parisi I, Tsochatzis E, Wijewantha H, Rodriguez-Peralvarez M, De Luca L, Manousou P, Fatourou E, Pieri G, Papastergiou V, davies N, Yu D, Luong T, Dhillon AP, Thorburn D, Patch D, O'Beirne J, Meyer T, Burroughs AK. Inflammation-based scores do not predict post-transplant recurrence of hepatocellular carcinoma in patients within Milan criteria. Liver Transplantation. 2014;**20**(11):1327-1335

[49] Shindoh J, Sugawara Y, Nagata R, Kaneko J, Tamura S, Aoki T, Sakamoto Y, Hasegawa K, Tanaka T, Kokudo N. Evaluation methods for pretransplant oncologic markers and their prognostic impacts in patient undergoing living donor liver transplantation for hepatocellular carcinoma. Transplant International. 2014;**27**(4):391-398

[50] Sullivan KM, Groeschl RT, Turaga KK, Tsai S, Christians KK, White SB, Rilling WS, Pilgrim CH, Gamblin TC. Neutrophil-to-lymphocyte ratio as a predictor of outcomes for patients with hepatocellular carcinoma: A western perspective. Journal of Surgical Oncology. 2014;**109**(2):95-97

[51] Bruix J, Cheng AL, Meinhardt G, Nakajima K, De Sanctis Y, Llovet J. Prognostic factors and predictors of sorafenib benefit in patients with hepatocellular carcinoma: Analysis of two phase II studies. Journal of Hepatology. 2017. DOI: 10.1016/j.jhep.2017.06.026 [Epub ahead of print]

[52] Howell J, Pinato DJ, Ramaswami R, Arizumi T, Ferrari C, Gibbin A, Burlone ME, Guaschino G, Toniutto P, Black J, Sellers L, Kudo M, Pirisi M, Sharma R. Integration of

the cancer-related inflammatory response as a stratifying biomarker of survival in hepatocellular carcinoma treated with sorafenib. Oncotarget. 2017;**8**(22):36161-36170

[53] Wei K, Wang M, Zhang W, Mu H, Song TQ. Neutrophil-lymphocyte ratio as a predictor of outcomes for patients with hepatocellular carcinoma undergoing TAE combined with Sorafenib. Medical Oncology. 2014;**31**(6):969

[54] Zheng YB, Zhao W, Liu B, Lu LG, He X, Huang JW, Li Y, Hu BS. The blood neutrophil-to-lymphocyte ratio predicts survival in patients with advanced hepatocellular carcinoma receiving sorafenib. Asian Pacific Journal of Cancer Prevention. 2013;**14**(9):5527-5531

[55] Taussig MD, Irene Koran ME, Mouli SK, Ahmad A, Geevarghese S, Baker JC, Lipnik AJ, Banovac F, Brown DB. Neutrophil to lymphocyte ratio predicts disease progression following intra-arterial therapy of hepatocellular carcinoma. HPB: The Official Journal of the International Hepato Pancreato Biliary Association. 2017;**19**(5):458-464

[56] Xu X, Chen W, Zhang L, Miao R, Zhou Y, Wan Y, Dong Y, Liu C. Prognostic significance of neutrophil to lymphocyte ratio in patients with hepatocellular carcinoma after transcatheter arterial chemoembolization. Chinese Medical Journal. 2014;**127**(24):4204-4209

[57] Terashima T, Yamashita T, Iida N, Yamashita T, Nakagawa H, Arai K, Kitamura K, Kagaya T, Sakai Y, Mizukoshi E, Honda M, Kaneko S. Blood neutrophil to lymphocyte ratio as a predictor in patients with advanced hepatocellular carcinoma treated with hepatic arterial infusion chemotherapy. Hepatology Research. 2014. DOI: 10.1111/hepr.12436

[58] Tsunematsu S, Suda G, Yamasaki K, Kimura M, Takaaki I, Umemura M, Ito J, Sato F, Nakai M, Sho T, Morikawa K, Ogawa K, Kamiyama T, Taketomi A, Sakamoto N. Combination of neutrophil-to-lymphocyte ratio and early des-gamma-carboxyprothrombin change ratio as a useful predictor of treatment response for hepatic arterial infusion chemotherapy against advanced hepatocellular carcinoma. Hepatology Research. 2017;**47**(6):533-541

[59] Tajiri K, Kawai K, Minemura M, Yasumura S, Hosokawa A, Kawabe H, Tomizawa G, Sugiyama T. Neutrophil/lymphocyte ratio as a prognostic indicator of hepatic arterial infusion chemotherapy with arterial cisplatin plus continuous 5-fluorouracil. Hepatology Research. 2015;**45**(7):755-763

[60] Long J, Zheng JS, Sun B, Lu N. Microwave ablation of hepatocellular carcinoma with portal vein tumor thrombosis after transarterial chemoembolization: A prospective study. Hepatology International. 2016;**10**(1):175-184

[61] Li X, Han Z, Cheng Z, Yu J, Liu S, Yu X, Liang P. Preoperative neutrophil-to-lymphocyte ratio is a predictor of recurrence following thermal ablation for recurrent hepatocellular carcinoma: A retrospective analysis. PLoS One. 2014;**9**(10):e110546

[62] Chen TM, Lin CC, Huang PT, Wen CF. Neutrophil-to-lymphocyte ratio associated with mortality in early hepatocellular carcinoma patients after radiofrequency ablation. Journal of Gastroenterology and Hepatology. 2012;**27**(3):553-561

[63] Dan J, Zhang Y, Peng Z, Huang J, Gao H, Xu L, Chen M. Postoperative neutrophil-to-lymphocyte ratio change predicts survival of patients with small hepatocellular carcinoma undergoing radiofrequency ablation. PLoS One. 2013;**8**(3):e58184

[64] Tajiri K, Baba H, Kawai K, Minemura M, Yasumura S, Takahara T, Sugiyama T. Neutrophil-to-lymphocyte ratio predicts recurrence after radiofrequency ablation in hepatitis B virus infection. Journal of Gastroenterology and Hepatology. 2016;**31**(7):1291-1299

[65] Sukato DC, Tohme S, Chalhoub D, Han K, Zajko A, Amesur N, Orons P, Marsh JW, Geller DA, Tsung A. The prognostic role of neutrophil-to-lymphocyte ratio in patients with unresectable hepatocellular carcinoma treated with radioembolization. Journal of Vascular and Interventional Radiology. 2015;**26**(6):816-824

[66] He G, Zhang H, Zhou J, Wang B, Chen Y, Kong Y, Xie X, Wang X, Fei R, Wei L, Chen H, Zeng H. Peritumoural neutrophils negatively regulate adaptive immunity via the PD-L1/PD-1 signalling pathway in hepatocellular carcinoma. Journal of Experimental & Clinical Cancer Research. 2015;**34**:141

[67] Wang Q, Blank S, Fiel MI, Kadri H, Luan W, Warren L, Zhu A, Deaderick PA, Sarpel U, Labow DM, Hiotis SP. The severity of liver fibrosis influences the prognostic value of inflammation-based scores in hepatitis B-associated hepatocellular carcinoma. Annals of Surgical Oncology. 2015;**22**(Suppl 3):S1125-S1132

[68] Motomura T, Shirabe K, Mano Y, Muto J, Toshima T, Umemoto Y, Fukuhara T, Uchiyama H, Ikegami T, Yoshizumi T, Soejima Y, Maehara Y. Neutrophil-lymphocyte ratio reflects hepatocellular carcinoma recurrence after liver transplantation via inflammatory micro-environment. Journal of Hepatology. 2013;**58**(1):58-64

[69] Huang GQ, Zheng JN, Zou TT, Chen YR, Shi KQ, Poucke SV, Cheng Z, Ruan LY, Zheng MH. Stratified platelet-to lymphocyte ratio: A novel target for prognostic prediction of hepatocellular carcinoma after curative liver resection. Journal of Clinical and Translational Hepatology. 2017;**5**(1):35-42

[70] Yang HJ, Jiang JH, Liu QA, Zhou CM, Du YF, Wu T, Chen NZ, Xiang BD. Preoperative platelet-to-lymphocyte ratio is a valuable prognostic biomarker in patients with hepatocellular carcinoma undergoing curative liver resection. Tumour Biology. 2017;**39**(6). DOI: 1010428317707375

[71] Shen SL, Fu SJ, Chen B, Kuang M, Li SQ, Hua YP, Liang LJ, Guo P, Hao Y, Peng BG. Preoperative aspartate aminotransferase to platelet ratio is an independent prognostic factor for hepatitis B-induced hepatocellular carcinoma after hepatic resection. Annals of Surgical Oncology. 2014;**21**(12):3802-3809

[72] Lai Q, Castro Santa E, Rico Juri JM, Pinheiro RS, Lerut J. Neutrophil and platelet-to-lymphocyte ratio as new predictors of dropout and recurrence after liver transplantation for hepatocellular cancer. Transplant International. 2014;**27**(1):32-41

[73] Tian XC, Liu XL, Zeng FR, Chen Z, Wu DH. Platelet-to-lymphocyte ratio acts as an independent risk factor for patients with hepatitis B virus-related hepatocellular carcinoma who received transarterial chemoembolization. European Review for Medical and Pharmacological Sciences. 2016;**20**(11):2302-2309

[74] Li X, Han Z, Cheng Z, Yu J, Yu X, Liang P. Clinical significance of the preoperative platelet-to-lymphocyte ratio in recurrent hepatocellular carcinoma after thermal ablation: A retrospective analysis. International Journal of Hyperthermia. 2015;**31**(7):758-763

[75] Shiozawa K, Watanabe M, Ikehara T, Matsukiyo Y, Kogame M, Shinohara M, Kikuchi Y, Igarashi Y, Sumino Y. Plasma biomarkers as predictive factors for advanced hepatocellular carcinoma with sorafenib. [article in Japanese]. Gan to Kagaku Ryoho. 2016;**43**(7): 63-867

[76] Hu DH, Yu SM. Association between platelet to lymphocyte ratio (PLR) and overall survival (OS) of hepatocellular carcinoma (HCC): A meta-analysis. Cellular and Molecular Biology (Noisy-le-Grand, France). 2017;**63**(8):30-32

[77] Ma W, Zhang P, Qi J, Gu L, Zang M, Yao H, Shi X, Wang C, Jiang Y. Prognostic value of platelet to lymphocyte ratio in hepatocellular carcinoma: A meta-analysis. Scientific Reports. 2016;**6**:35378

[78] Song W, Wang K, Zhong FP, Fan YW, Peng L, Zou SB. Clinicopathological and prognostic significance of platelet-to-lymphocyte ratio in patients with hepatocellular carcinoma. Oncotarget. 2016;**7**(49):81830-81838

[79] Zhao Y, Si G, Zhu F, Hui J, Cai S, Huang C, Cheng S, Fathy AH, Xiang Y, Li J. Prognostic role of platelet to lymphocyte ratio in hepatocellular carcinoma: A systematic review and meta-analysis. Oncotarget. 2017;**8**(14):22854-22862

[80] Shiba H, Horiuchi T, Sakamoto T, Furukawa K, Shirai Y, Iida T, Fujiwara Y, Haruki K, Yanaga K. Glasgow prognostic score predicts therapeutic outcome after hepatic resection for hepatocellular carcinoma. Oncology Letters. 2017;**14**(1):293-298

[81] Abe T, Tashiro H, Kobayashi T, Hattori M, Kuroda S, Ohdan H. Glasgow prognostic score and prognosis after hepatectomy for hepatocellular carcinoma. World Journal of Surgery. 2017;**41**(7):1860-1870

[82] Li MX, Bi XY, Li ZY, Huang Z, Han Y, Zhou JG, Zhao JJ, Zhang YF, Zhao H, Cai JQ. Prognostic role of Glasgow prognostic score in patients with hepatocellular carcinoma: A systematic review and meta-analysis. Medicine (Baltimore). 2015;**94**(49):e2133

[83] Chen H, Hu N, Chang P, Kang T, Han S, Lu Y, Li M. Modified Glasgow prognostic score might be a prognostic factor for hepatocellular carcinoma: A meta-analysis. Panminerva Medica. 2017;**59**(4):302-307

[84] Pang S, Zhou Z, Yu X, Wei S, Chen Q, Nie S, Liang X, Liu L. The predictive value of integrated inflammation scores in the survival of patients with resected hepatocellular carcinoma: A retrospective cohort study. International Journal of Surgery. 2017;**42**:170-177

[85] Fujiwara Y, Shiba H, Furukawa K, Iida T, Haruki K, Gocho T, Wakiyama S, Hirohara S, Ishida Y, Misawa T, Ohashi T, Yanaga K. Glasgow prognostic score is related to blood transfusion requirements and post-operative complications in hepatic resection for hepatocellular carcinoma. Anticancer Research. 2010;**30**(12):5129-5136

[86] Abe T, Tashiro H, Hattori M, Kuroda S, Tahara H, Ohira M, Kobayashi T, Ide K, Ishiyama K, Ohdan H. Prediction of long-term survival by using the Glasgow prognostic score in patients with hepatocellular carcinoma after liver transplantation. Hepatology Research. 2016;**46**(7):622-633

[87] Aino H, Sumie S, Niizeki T, Kuromatsu R, Tajiri N, Nakano M, Satani M, Okamura S, Shimose S, Miyahara K, Torimura T. The systemic inflammatory response as a prognostic factor for advanced hepatocellular carcinoma with extrahepatic metastasis. Molecular and Clinical Oncology. 2016;**5**(1):83-88

[88] Morimoto M, Numata K, Moriya S, Kondo M, Nozaki A, Morioka Y, Maeda S, Tanaka K. Inflammation-based prognostic score for hepatocellular carcinoma patients on sorafenib treatment. Anticancer Research. 2012;**32**(2):619-623

[89] Zhou DS, Xu L, Luo YL, He FY, Huang JT, Zhang YJ, Chen MS. Inflammation scores predict survival for hepatitis B virus-related hepatocellular carcinoma patients after transarterial chemoembolization. World Journal of Gastroenterology. 2015;**21**(18):5582-5590

5

Genetic Single Nucleotide Polymorphisms (GSNPs) in the DNA Repair Genes and Hepatocellular Carcinoma Related to Aflatoxin B1 among Guangxiese Population

Xue-Ming Wu, Zhi-Feng Xi, Jun Lu, Xing-Zhizi Wang, Tian-Qi Zhang, Xiao-Ying Huang, Jin-Guang Yao, Chao Wang, Zhong-Heng Wei, Chun-Ying Luo, Bing-Chen Huang, Qun-Qing Xu, Wen-Pei Yang, Qiang Xia and Xi-Dai Long

Abstract

Aflatoxin B1 (AFB1) is an important environmental carcinogen for the development of hepatocellular carcinoma (HCC). HCC is a complex disease likely resulting from genetic single nucleotide polymorphisms (GSNPs) of multiple interacting genes and gene-environment interactions. Recent efforts have been made to analyze the associations between risk of this malignancy and GSNPs in genes involved in the repair of DNA damage induced by AFB1. Here, we reviewed the results of published case-control studies that have examined the effects of common alleles of all susceptible DNA repair genes, including XRCC1, XRCC3, XRCC4, XRCC7, XPC, and XPD, on risk of AFB1-related HCC among Guangxi population. Statistically significant differences in genotype frequencies found in case-control comparisons were rs25487, rs80309960, rs861539, rs7003908, rs28383151, rs3734091, rs13181, and rs2228001 polymorphism. The overall effects of these GNSPs were moderate in terms of relative risk, with ORs ranging from 2 to 10. Furthermore, some evidence of the interaction of GSNPs in DNA repair genes and AFB1 exposure modulate risk of this cancer was also found, although the results require confirmation with larger sample size studies.

Keywords: genetic single nucleotide polymorphism, hepatocellular carcinoma, DNA repair, DNA damage, aflatoxin B1, Guangxiese population

1. Introduction

In China, hepatocellular carcinoma (HCC) is the fourth most common malignant tumors and accounts for about 50% of the world's HCC cases [1, 2]. This malignancy occurs more often in some hot and humid areas such as Guangxi area, mainly because of high aflatoxin B1(AFB1) exposure [3, 4]. However, accumulating epidemiological evidence has shown that although many people are exposed to this risk factor, only a relatively small proportion of people with chronic AFB1 exposure develop HCC [3, 4]. This suggests that an individual susceptibility related to genetic factors including genetic single nucleotide polymorphisms (GSNPs) in DNA repair genes might be correlated with HCC tumorigenesis [3–5]. In past several decade years, evidence has been accumulated to support the hypothesis that GSNPs in DNA repair genes may be of importance in determining individual susceptibility to AFB1-related HCC [6–8]. Here, we review recent efforts in identifying genetic single nucleotide polymorphisms (SNPs) in DNA repair genes, which may have impact on AFB1-related HCC risk among Guangxiese population.

2. Epidemiology of AFB1-related HCC among Guangxi areas

In Guangxi, a known high AFB1 exposure area, HCC is the most common occurring cancer [5]. Epidemiologically, this type tumor is characterized as follows: (*a*) the incidence rate displaying a noticeable mountain shape, gradually increasing with age increasing before shape top and gradually decreasing with age increasing after shape top and (b) more than three times risk of HCC among males than among females, especially in the high AFB1-exposure areas (including Baise and Nanning) [5]. During 1990–1992, the incidence rates of this tumor in Guangxi area increased markedly compared between the late 1970s and the early 1980s (25.22 per 100,000 vs. 15.85 per 100,000), especially male Guangxiese population (**Figure 1A**) [9]. This might result from the increasing infective rate of hepatitis viruses and advance of diagnostic ability [10]. The following epidemiological investigations showed that the incidence rate of HCC among Guangxiese population significantly markedly decrease during 2004 and 2005 (mainly because of the control of hepatitis virus infection) (**Figure 1**) [9]. However, the incident rates of this tumor in high AFB1-exposure areas have little change. According to epidemiological investigation from AFB1-exposures areas, during May 2007–April 2008, incidence rates were 103.1/100,000 and 117.8/100,000 for Fusui in Nanning and Xiangzhou in Baise (two main high AFB1 exposure areas), respectively [11]. This is similar to the results before 10 years [11].

Because of the very poor prognosis, HCC is the first most common cause of death from cancer in Guangxi [9]. In the past 40 years, the total mortality rate of HCC gradually increased and followed by gradually decreased (**Figure 1B**), regardless of male or female population. Furthermore, this trend was not only associated with age but also more noticeable in male population than female population (**Figure 2**), possibly because male individuals featured more AFB1 exposure [4]. Supporting above-mentioned hypothesis, molecular epidemiological studies from high AFB1-exposure areas of Guangxi have exhibited that these individuals featuring more AFB1 exposure would face decreasing 5-year survival rate and increasing death risk [12–14].

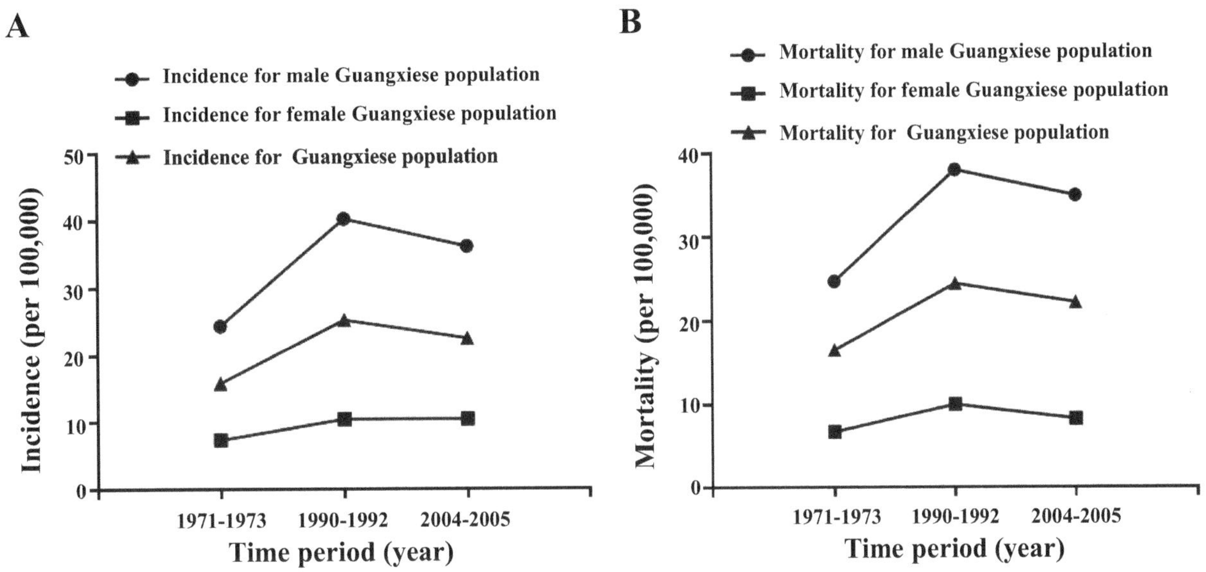

Figure 1. The incidence and mortality rates of hepatocellular carcinoma (HCC) in Guangxi during 1971 and 2005. Total incidence rate (A) and mortality rates (B), regardless of male or female population, were significantly increasing from during 1971 and 1973 to during 1990 and 1992. However, they would decrease during 2004 and 2005.

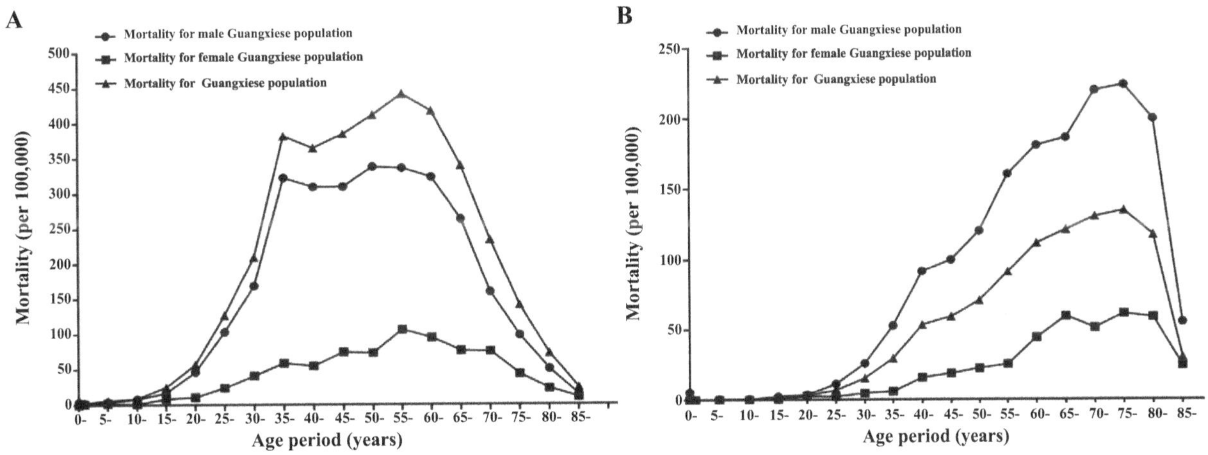

Figure 2. The gender and age distributions of hepatocellular carcinoma (HCC) mortality among Guangxiese population. (A) The gender and age distributions of HCC mortality between 1990 and 1992. (B) The gender and age distributions of HCC mortality between 2004 and 2005.

3. DNA damage induced byAFB1 and DNA repair

Several previous reviews have significantly summarized the toxicology of AFB1 [3–5, 15]. Generally, AFB1, an important mycotoxin and a category I known human carcinogen produced by *Aspergillus parasiticus* and *Aspergillus flavus* [4, 5], has been found as toxic contaminants of human food such as ground nuts and core in tropical areas as a result of fungal contamination during growth and after harvest which under hot and humid conditions [15]. Once this toxigenic agent is taken into body, it is metabolized by phase I detoxification enzymes to its reactive form, also called AFB1-8,9-epoxide (AFBO). This reactive product can also covalently bind to DNA and induce DNA damage, which might ultimately result to the development of HCC [16, 17].

AFB1-induced DNA damage types consist of DNA adducts, oxidative damage, and gene mutations. For AFB1-DNA adducts, AFB1-N^7-Gua adduct, the most common adduct type, is primarily identified and confirmed *in vivo* research studies [17–22], whereas the formamidopyridine AFB1 adduct (AFB1-FAPy) is a ring-opened DNA adduct [23, 24]. Because of the accumulations of AFB1-FAPy, it is characterized by a time-dependent and non-enzyme way and exhibits apparent persistence in DNA; it may be of biological basis of genes mutation. Furthermore, AFB1-N^7-Gua and AFB1-FAPy can induce error-prone DNA repair and result in the damage of DNA strands, including double-strand breaks (DSBs), single-strand breaks (SSBs), base pair substitution, frame shift mutations, and oxidation DNA damage such as 8-oxodeoxyguanosine (8-_{oxyG}) [25–28]. For genes mutations induced by AFB1 exposure, G:C > T:A mutation in codon 249 of TP53 gene has been frequently reported [29–36]. This mutation is tested in more than 40% of HCC from high-AFB1-exposure areas, but in either very rare or absent for those from low or null AFB1 exposure areas [36–39]. Therefore, G:C > T:A mutation in codon 249 of TP53 gene is regarded as the hotspot mutation caused by AFB1 and the molecular symbol of AFB1-related HCC [40–42].

DNA damage by AFB1 exposure, if not repaired, may cause genomic instability and ultimately result in cellular malignant transformation and tumor formation [20]. In human cells, several evolved surveillance mechanisms, including base excision repair (BER), nucleotide excision repair (NER), single-strand break repair (SSBR), and double-strand break repair (DSBR), can monitor the integrity of genome and repair and minimize the consequences of detrimental genome damage [3, 40]. DNA repair genes play an important role during aforementioned repair pathways of DNA damage; therefore, GSNPs in the DNA repair genes may be associated with risk of developing AFB1-related HCC [4].

4. Xeroderma pigmentosum C (XPC) GSNPs and AFB1-HCC among Guangxiese population

Xeroderma pigmentosum C (XPC) gene locates on chromosome 3p25 and spans 33kb. Its encoding protein consists of 940 amino acids and acts as a DNA damage recognition molecule during the global genome NER pathway [43, 44]. XPC can bind tightly with RAD23 homolog B (RAD23B, also called HR23B) to form a stable XPC/RAD23B complex. This complex can recognize DNA adducts formed by exogenous carcinogens such as AFB1 and binds to the DNA damage sites [44]. Thus, XPC may play a role in the pathogenesis of HCC-related AFB1. The pathological and cellular researches have shown that the abnormal expression of this gene is correlated with hepatocarcinogenesis [45]. Some studies have shown that GSNPs of XPC (rs2228001 (also called codon Lys939Gln polymorphism) can decrease DNA repair capacity related to AFB1-induced DNA damage [46–49]. In the past several decade years, a total of four studies from Guangxi area reported XPC rs2228001 polymorphism was involved in AFB1 detoxification (**Table 1**) [12, 49–51]. The first study

No.	Ref.	Year	AFB1 exposure[a]	Methods	Matching factor	Cases (*n*)	Controls (*n*)	Risk value[b] (OR)
1	Wu et al. [51]	2010	High	Case-control	Age, sex, HBV, HCV, race	98	157	1.46–2.08 ($P < 0.05$)
2	Long et al. [12]	2010	High	Case-control	Age, sex, HBV, HCV, race	1156	1402	1.25–1.81 ($P < 0.001$)
3	Li et al. [50]	2010	High	Case-control	No	500	507	1.20–1.81 ($P > 0.05$)
4	Yao et al. [49]	2014	High	Case-control	Age, sex, HBV, HCV, race	1486	1996	1.57–2.19 ($P < 0.001$)

[a]Defined by means of Henry et al. (Science, 1999).

[b]AFB1-related HCC risk will increase if OR > 1 and corresponding *P*-value < 0.05; will decrease if OR < 1 and corresponding *P*-value < 0.05; and will not change if OR is about 1 and/or corresponding *P*-value > 0.05.

Table 1. Characteristics of studies about GSNP at codon 939 of XPC and AFB1-related HCC risk.

conducted by Wu et al. [51] is from Baise area (a famous high AFB1 exposure area with high incidence rate of HCC). In this study, researchers investigated the association between XPC rs2228001 polymorphism and HCC risk via an hospital-based case-control study (including 98 HCC patients and 157 age-, sex-, race-, and hepatitis viruses-matching controls) method and found XPC rs2228001 polymorphism increased HCC risk of female individuals (odds ratios [ORs] were 5.44 with 95% CI 1.38–21.50), but not tumor risk of male population. Noticeably, they found a significant interaction of XPC variables and AFB1 exposure levels [51].

Results from the matching-design studies with large-size samples show that the mutant genotypes of XPC rs2228001 polymorphism increased about two times risk of HCC [12, 49]. The following quantitative analysis exhibited that AFB1 exposure interacted with risk genotypes of XPC rs2228001 polymorphism on HCC risk (22.33 > 1.88 × 8.69 for the interaction of AFB1-exposure years and XPC risk genotypes and 18.38 > 1.11 × 4.62 for the interaction of AFB1-exposure levels and XPC risk genotypes) [12, 49]. Furthermore, mutant alleles were correlated with the decrease of XPC expression levels in cancerous tissues and with the overall survival of HCC patients [12]. However, another study also from Nanning area (another high AFB1 exposure area in Guangxi) exhibited that this polymorphism does not change HCC risk [50], possibly because it bases on nonmatching design and some confounders might affect their results. Interestingly, a significant risk value for HCC among female population was observed in the stratified analyses (OR = 2.17, 95% CI = 1.01–4.64), similar with findings from Wu et al. [51]. Given these different effects, we accomplished meta-analysis and found XPC rs2228001 polymorphism increased AFB1-related risk (combined OR = 1.89, $P < 0.01$). Therefore, these results demonstrate that GSNP at codon 939 of XPC gene is not only a genetic determinant in the development of HCC caused by AFB1 in Guangxiese population but also an independent prognostic factor influencing the survival of HCC, like AFB1 exposure.

5. Xeroderma pigmentosum D (XPD) GSNPs and AFB1-HCC among Guangxiese population

Xeroderma pigmentosum gene, contains 22 introns and 23 exons, locates on 19q13.3 and spans about 20 kb [3, 52]. Its encoded product is one of the TFIIH complexes (a DNA-dependent ATPase/helicase complex), it has classically been linked to the damage verification and the opening of the DNA helix step of NER pathway [53]. To date, molecular epidemiological studies on two GSNPs in this gene, namely, rs369191500 polymorphism (codon 312, Asp to Asn) and rs13181 polymorphism (codon 751, Lys to Gln), have been conducted by different laboratories [54]. Genotype-phenotype analyses have shown that these two GSNPs are associated with low DNA repair ability, which might modify DNA-adduct levels, p53 gene mutation, and risk of cancer [55, 56]. For genetic polymorphisms among Guangxiese population, a total of four epidemiological studies have been conducted via case-control design (**Table 2**). In 2009, Zeng et al. [57] investigated the association between XPD GSNPs and HCC and observed about 2.60-time risk of HCC for these with mutant genotypes of XPD codon 751. After that, results from Long et al. [58] and Yao et al. [49] have exhibited that the variants of XPD rs13181 polymorphism (including rs13181-LG and -GG) was significantly different between controls and HCC cases (26.3 vs. 35.9% for rs13181-LG and 8.6 vs. 20.1% for rs13181-GG, respectively, $P < 0.001$). Mutant alleles increased the

No.	Ref.	Year	AFB1 exposure[a]	Methods	Matching factor	Cases	Controls	Risk value[b]
						(*n*)	(*n*)	(OR)
1	Zeng et al. [57]	2009	High	Case-control	No	300	312	About 2.60 ($P < 0.001$)
2	Long et al. [58]	2009	High	Case-control	Age, sex, HBV, HCV, race	618	712	1.75–2.47 ($P < 0.001$)
3	Yao et al. [49]	2014	High	Case-control	Age, sex, HBV, HCV, race	1486	1996	2.19–4.27 ($P < 0.001$)
4	Hu et al. [59]	2016	High	Case-control	No	178	178	2.33–3.38 ($P < 0.05$)

[a] Defined by means of Henry et al. (Science, 1999).

[b] AFB1-related HCC risk will increase if OR > 1 and corresponding P-value < 0.05; will decrease if OR < 1 and corresponding P-value < 0.05; and will not change if OR is about 1 and/or corresponding P-value > 0.05.

Table 2. Characteristics of studies about genetic polymorphism at codon 751 of XPD and AFB1-related HCC risk.

risk of developing the cancer with a risk value of 1.75 (1.30–2.37) for Lys/Gln and 2.47 (1.62–3.76) for Gln/Gln, respectively [58]. Furthermore, the interactive effects of mutant genotypes of rs13181 polymorphism in XPD gene and AFB1 exposure on HCC risk were also found ($P_{interaction} < 0.05$) [49]. Recently, Hu et al. [59] have reported higher frequency of XPD codon 751 Gln alleles among HCC families than among non-HCC families. This suggests that genetic susceptibility resulting from XPD GSNPs might have a potential effect on AFB1-related HCC risk among Guangxiese population. Meta-analysis further improved the above-mentioned hypothesis [56]. However, the studies from molecular epidemiological studies exhibit that another GSNP of XPD is not significantly correlate with the risk of HCC related to AFB1 [49, 58].

6. The human 8-oxoguanine DNA glycosylase (hOGG1) GSNPs and AFB1-HCC among Guangxiese population

As described previously [60], DNA glycosylases play a central role in the BER pathway because they can recognize and catalyze the removal of damaged bases. Among having been reported GSNPs in DNA glycosylase-encoded genes, only hOGG1 correlates with DNA repair capacity [5, 61]. This gene consists of 7 exons and 6 introns and spans 17 kb on chromosome 3p26.2. It encodes a 546-amino acid protein, a specific DNA glycosylase that catalyzes the release of 8-$_{oxy}$G and the cleavage of DNA at the AP site (**Figure 3**) [61, 62]. The presence of several polymorphisms within hOGG1 locus is identified and only rs1052133 polymorphism (at codon 326, Ser → Cys) is suggested to modify DNA repair capacity [63–65]. Therefore, low capacity of 8-$_{oxy}$G repair resulting from hOGG1 326Cys polymorphism might contribute to the persistence of 8-$_{oxy}$G in genomic DNA *in vivo*, which, in turn, could be associated with increased cancer risk [66]. Several reports imply this polymorphism may be associated with HCC related to AFB1 exposure [67–70]. Through a hospital-based case-control study (including 500 cases with HCC and 507 healthy controls) conducted in Nanning area from Guangxi, Ji et al. [67] investigated the relationship between hOGG1 rs1052133 polymorphism and HCC risk and found significantly different distribution of three genotypes (Ser/Ser, Ser/Cys, and Cys/Cys) between cases and controls (71.40, 8.00, and 20.60% for patients with HCC, 84.22, 10.06, and 5.72% for controls). Regression logistic analysis shows that mutant alleles of this polymorphism increase AFB1-related HCC risk (OR = 2.14, 95% CI = 1.57–2.91). Molecular epidemiological studies from other researchers have also proved higher frequencies of Cys alleles in HCC cases than controls and this change increased HCC risk among Guangxiese population featuring AFB1-exposure history [69, 70]. Given that hOGG1 expression is significantly related to HCC carcinogenesis [71, 72], Peng et al. [68] explored the effects of hOGG1 rs1052133 polymorphism on 8-$_{oxy}$G levels and hOGG1 expression in Guangxiese population with AFB1 exposure. They observed that Cys alleles downregulated hOGG1 expression and increased 8-$_{oxy}$G levels. These findings suggested the pathogenic role of hOGG1 Cys326Ser polymorphism in the carcinogenesis of AFB1-related HCC.

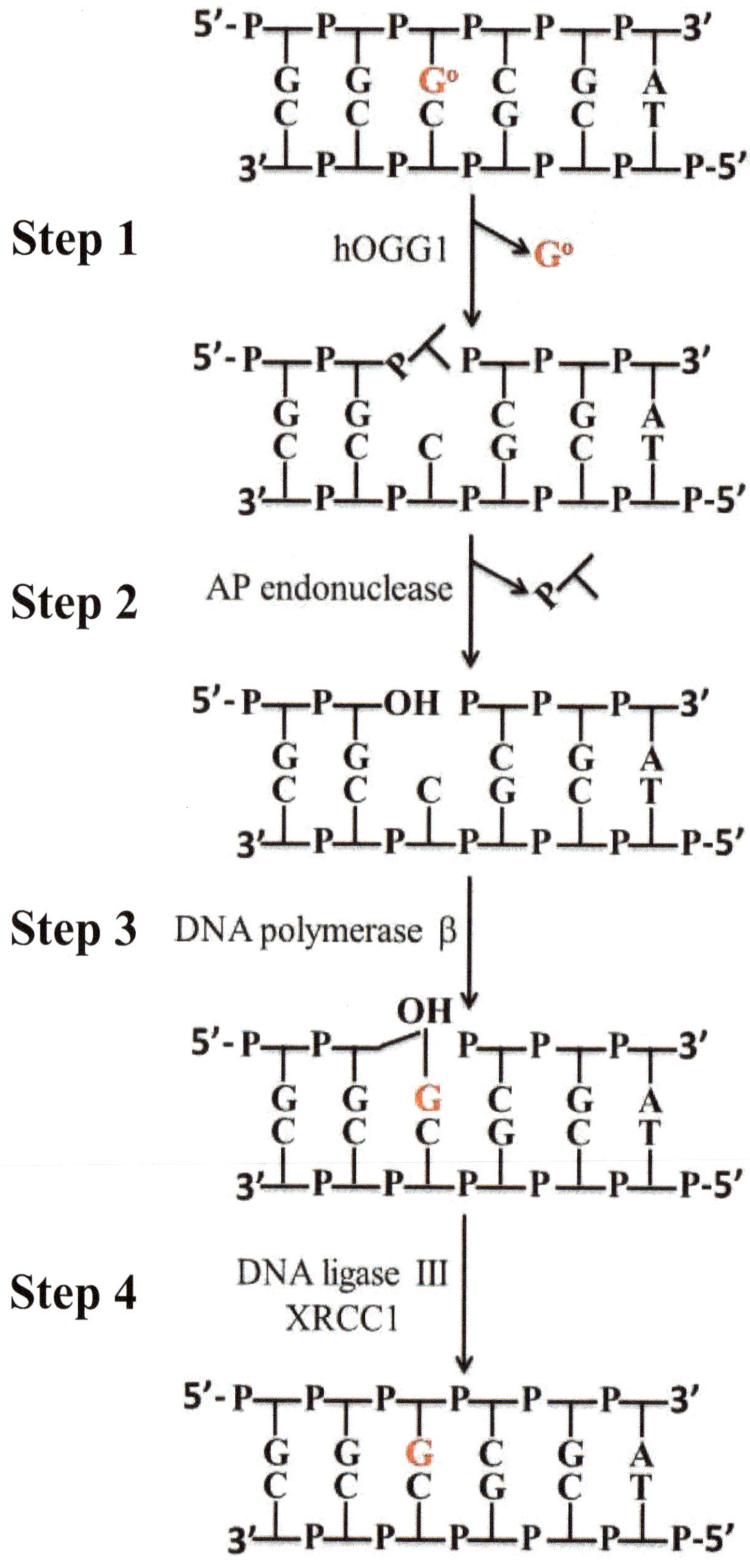

Figure 3. The base excision repair for oxidative DNA damage 8-oxyG in mammalian cells. In this repair pathway, human 8-oxoguanine DNA glycosylase (hOGG1) can catalyze the release of 8-oxyG (Red) and the cleavage of DNA at the AP site.

7. The XRCC1 GSNPs and AFB1-HCC among Guangxiese population

X-ray repair cross-complementing group 1 (XRCC1), also called RCC, spans about 32 kb on chromosome 19q13.2 and contains 17 exons and 16 introns. The encoding protein of XRCC1 acts as a scaffold protein in SSBR and BER pathways via the interaction with Pol β, DNA ligase III, and PARP [73]. According to data from SNP database, more than 50 GSNPs in the coding region of XRCC1 gene, which lead to amino acid substitution, have been identified. Of GSNPs, rs25487 polymorphism (at codon 399, Arg → Gln) is of special concern, because this GSNP resides in functionally significant regions and may decrease DNA repair activity and increase the risk of gene mutation cancers [3].

In Guangxi area, a total of five molecular epidemiological studies were found in PubMed Database, Web of Science Database, Wangfang Database, Google Database, and Weipu database (**Table 3**). In 2005, Long et al. [74] investigated the effects of XRCC1 rs25487 polymorphism on AFB1-related HCC risk. In their study, they included 140 patients with pathologically diagnosed HCC and 536 age-, sex-, race-, and hepatitis virus-matching controls and found significantly different distribution of three genotypes of XRCC1 rs25487 polymorphism (Arg/Arg, Arg/Gln, and Gln/Gln) between cases and controls (51.43, 45.00, and 3.57% for patients with HCC, 6.54, 29.66, and 2.88% for controls). Regression logistic analysis shows that mutant alleles of this polymorphism increase AFB1-related HCC risk (OR = 2.18, 95% CI = 1.27–3.74). They also observed more noticeable risk role for HCC under the conditions of individuals with both high AFB1 exposure and mutant genotypes of XRCC1 rs25487 polymorphism (risk value 1.84–10.87). The several following molecular epidemiological studies furthermore prove these results [49, 75, 77]. However, associations between

No.	Ref.	Year	AFB1 exposure[a]	Methods	Matching factor	Cases (n)	Controls (n)	Risk value[b] (OR)
1	Long et al. [74]	2005	High	Case-control	Age, sex, HBV, HCV, race	140	536	2.18 ($P = 0.0001$)
2	Long et al. [75]	2006	High	Case-control	Age, sex, HBV, HCV, race	257	649	2.47 ($P = 0.0001$)
3	Zeng et al. [76]	2010	High	Case-control	No	500	507	about 1 ($P > 0.05$)
4	He et al. [77]	2012	High	Case-control	Age, sex	119	119	2.50 ($P < 0.05$)
5	Yao et al. [49]	2014	High	Case-control	Age, sex, HBV, HCV, race	1486	1996	2.19–4.27 ($P < 0.001$)

Notes: [a] Defined by means of Henry et al. (Science, 1999, 286: 2453-2454).

[b] AFB1-related HCC risk will increase if OR > 1 and corresponding P-value < 0.05; will decrease if OR < 1 and corresponding P-value < 0.05; and will not change if OR is about 1 and/or corresponding P-value > 0.05.

Table 3. Characteristics of studies about genetic polymorphism at codon 399 of XRCC1 and AFB1-related HCC risk.

XRCC1 rs25487 polymorphism and individual susceptibility to HCC have been reported in a case-control study with the insignificant results [76]. This may be because of nonmatching design and the effects of confounders such as age, gender, race, and hepatitis viruses. Supporting aforementioned conclusions, meta-analysis from data in high AFB1 exposure areas also exhibited that these subjects with Gln alleles of XRCC1 rs25487 polymorphism had increasing HCC risk (OR > 1, $P < 0.01$) [78]. This suggests that XRCC1 rs25487 polymorphism should be a risk biomarker of Guangxiese HCC related to AFB1 exposure.

8. The XRCC3 GSNPs and AFB1-HCC among Guangxiese population

X-ray repair cross-complementing group 3 (XRCC3) is an important paralogs of the strand-exchange protein RAD51 and is primarily found and cloned by functional complementation in the Chinese hamster cell line irs1SF. This gene spans about 17.8 kb on chromosome 14q32.33 and contains 10 exons. Functionally, XRCC3 can bind directly with DNA breaks and facilitate the formation of the RAD51 nucleoprotein filament and protein-protein interaction of RAD51 family members in the SSBR pathway [79]. In XRCC3-defective irs1SF hamster cells, spontaneous chromosomal aberrations, high sensitivity to cross-linking agents, mild sensitivity to gamma rays, and significantly attenuated Rad51 focus formation after gamma ray exposure were observed, which suggests that XRCC3 is crucial for the SSBR pathway [80].

Recent molecular epidemiological studies have shown that the function of XRCC3 is modified by its GSNPs. Of the known GSNPs, only rs2228001 polymorphism (at codon 241, Thr → Met) is of special concern, because this GSNP results the change Thr to Met at codon 241 [81–83]. Up to now, three reports from high AFB1-exposure areas of Guangxi supported the above-mentioned conclusions [49, 84, 85]. In the first frequent case-control study in Guangxi population [85], higher mutant frequencies at codon 241 of XRCC3 are observed among cases with HCC than controls (33.01 vs. 61.48%, $P < 0.001$). The results from logistic regression analysis further prove that this mutate increases about 2- to 10-time risk of HCC. The following two relatively larger sample size molecular epidemiological studies (study 1 conducted by Long et al. [84] consisting of 491 patients with HCC and 862 healthy controls; study 2 from Yao et al. [49] including 1486 cases and 1996 controls) were accomplished in high AFB1 exposure. Similar to data from the first study, individuals having the mutant genotypes of XRCC3 rs2228001 polymorphism would feature higher risk of developing HCC. Interactive analysis of risk genotypes and AFB1 exposure further demonstrated that this allele multiplicatively interacted with AFB1 exposure in the process of hepatotumorigenesis [49]. Taken together, these results suggest that the GSNPs in XRCC3 gene, such as rs2228001 polymorphism, might a genetic determinant in the HCC carcinogenesis caused by AFB1 exposure among Guangxiese population.

9. The XRCC7 GSNPs and AFB1-HCC among Guangxiese population

X-ray repair cross-complementing 7 (XRCC7), also called protein kinase DNA-activated catalytic polypeptide (PRKDC), spans about 197 kb on 8q11.21 and contains 85 exons. Protein encoded by his gene is a member of the PI3/PI4-kinase family and acts as the catalytic subunit of the DNA-dependent protein kinase (DNA-PK). Functionally, it interacts with the Ku70/Ku80 heterodimer protein in the nonhomologous end joining (NHEJ) repair and recombination [86–88]. More than 200 of GSNPs have been reported in the XRCC7 gene, some of which are reported to affect tumorigenesis of malignant tumors [89–93]. In Guangxi area, several reports imply XRCC7 rs7003908 polymorphism (T to G) may be associated with HCC related to AFB1 exposure [49, 94]. Through a hospital-based case-control study (including 348 cases with HCC and 597 age-, gender-, race-, and hepatitis viruses-matched healthy controls) conducted in high AFB1 exposure area from Guangxi, Long et al. [94] investigated the association between XRCC7 rs7003908 polymorphism and HCC risk and found significantly different distribution of three genotypes (rs7003908-TT, -TG, and -GG) between cases and controls (25.9, 44.5, and 29.6% for patients with HCC, 58.1, 30.0, and 11.9% for controls). Regression logistic analysis shows that mutant alleles of this polymorphism increase AFB1-related HCC risk, with risk value of 3.45 (2.40–4.94) for rs7003908-TG and 5.04 (3.28–7.76) for rs7003908-GG, respectively. Furthermore, this GSNP was also related to higher the amounts of DNA adducts induced by AFB1 ($r = 0.142$) [94]. Interestingly, it also multiplicatively interacts with AFB1-exposure variable (interactive value: OR = 1.74; 95% CI = 1.66–1.82; $P = 2.21 \times 10^{-133}$) [49]. Taken together, these data exhibited that the XRCC7 rs7003908 polymorphism might modify AFB1-related HCC risk via decreasing NHEJ capacity. However, more studies are inquired to support this conclusion.

10. The XRCC4 GSNPs and AFB1-HCC among Guangxiese population

X-ray repair cross-complementing 4 (XRCC4, also known as SSMED) is an important NHEJ pathway gene locating on 5q14.2 and spanning about 293 kb. This gene is a generally expressed protein of 334 amino acids residues and functions together with DNA ligase IV and DNA-PK in the repair of DNA double-strand breaks. XRCC4 plays an important role in both nonhomologous end joining and the completion of V(D)J recombination [95, 96]. Increasing evidence has shown that mutations in XRCC4 can cause short stature, microcephaly, and endocrine dysfunction (SSMED) resulting from more-deficient NHEJ capacity [97, 98]. This suggests that the low repair capacity of this gene from genetic changes might be associated with cancer risk [99, 100]. Up to now, only two GSPs in the XRCC4 gene, namely, rs28383151 (at codon 56, Ala to Thr) and rs3734091 (at codon 247, Ala to Ser), have reported to be correlated with risk of AFB1-related HCC among Guangxiese population [13, 14, 49]. In these studies, Long et al. [13, 14] have examined the association between genetic polymorphisms (Ala56Thr and Ala247Ser) in XRCC4 and risk of HCC in a large case-control study in at-risk Guangxiese population. Genotypes were determined in 1499 patients with HCC and 2045 individually matched controls. We observed that individuals with Thr/Thr genotype at Arg194Trp site and Ser/Ser genotype at Ala247Ser site of XRCC4 had about twofold and threefold increased risk for the cancer compared with wild types, respectively. Furthermore, when risk genotypes of XRCC4 and AFB1-exposure were combined, this risk role was more noticeable, with the adjusted OR being11.26 (95% CI, 8.36–15.18) for rs28383151 polymorphism and 14.43 (95% CI, 7.98–26.09) for rs3734091 polymorphism, respectively. Interactive analysis further exhibited this multiplicative interaction (interactive OR = 1.64, 95% CI = 1.55–1.73, 6.41×10^{-73}) [49].

Functional exploration showed that these two polymorphisms increased AFB1-DNA adducts levels and TP53M risk, and AFB1-related HCC prognosis, suggesting they should be important modified factors of AFB1 toxicological effects [5, 13, 14]. Together, these results imply that XRCC4 rs28383151 and rs3734091 polymorphisms might play a role in the carcinogenesis of the liver under the conditions of AFB1 exposure.

11. Future directions

In the past decades, great progress has been made in understanding the molecular mechanisms of the GSNPs affecting risk of AFB1-related HCC. However, we are still far from a comprehensive view of this effect. The molecular mechanism about GSNPs in the DNA repair genes modifying the risk of HCC caused by AFB1 remains largely unknown. Although several reports have displayed that GSNPs may progress tumorigenesis of AFB1-related HCC via downregulating expression of DNA repair genes, breaking the structure of DNA repair proteins, or decreasing the function of DNA repair genes, more direct evidence is still missing. Disclosing the roles of different phenotypes of DNA repair genes will greatly benefit our understanding of pathological mechanisms of GSNPs affecting AFB1-related HCC risk, and will shed important light on the prevention values for individuals with risk types.

12. Conclusion

Like most other human cancers, HCC is a complex disease attributed to environment variation and genetic susceptive factors. In high incidence areas of HCC in Guangxi, AFB1 is an important environment variation. In the process of AFB1 hepatocarcinogenesis, DNA damage induced by AFB1 exposure plays a central role because of their genotoxicity and interactions with genetic susceptive factors. Numerous studies reviewed in this chapter have demonstrated that the hereditary variations in DNA repair genes (including XRCC1, XRCC3, XRCC4, XRCC7, hOGG1, XPC, and XPD) are related to the susceptibility to AFB1-related HCC among Chinese population. These molecular epidemiological studies have significantly contributed to our knowledge of the importance of genetic polymorphisms in DNA repair genes in the etiology of HCC related to AFB1 exposure. It would be expected that genetic susceptibility factors involved in DNA repair genes for HCC could serve as useful biomarkers for identifying at-risk individuals and, therefore, targeting prevention of this malignant tumor.

However, there are several issues to be noted. Because of conflicting data existing in the same ethnic population in view of between some genotypes of DNA repair genes and the risk of HCC related to AFB1, the conclusions should first be drawn carefully. For example, whether the XRCC1 Arg399Gln polymorphism is a risk factor or not remains controversial and further studies are needed. Second, because of the difference in population frequencies corresponding to genetic polymorphisms that depend on ethnicity, caution should be taken, particularly in extrapolating these data to other ethnic populations, especially from other high AFB1-exposure areas. Third, when risk of a specific polymorphism is considered, AFB1 exposure should be stressed because AFB1 exposure may differ from areas to areas and from individuals to individuals. Last, in view of that fact the development of AFB1-related HCC is "polygenic," a panel of susceptive biomarkers are warranted to define individuals at high risk for this cancer.

Acknowledgements

This study was supported in part by the National Natural Science Foundation of China (Nos. 81572353, 81372639, 81472243, 81660495, and 81460423), the Innovation Program of Guangxi Municipal Education Department (Nos. 201204LX674 and 201204LX324), the Natural Science Foundation of Guangxi (Nos. 2016GXNSFDA380003, 2015GXNSFAA139223, 2013GXNSFAA019251, 2014GXNSFDA118021, and 2014GXNSFAA118144), Innovation Program of Guangxi Health Department (No. Z2013781), Research Program of Guangxi Clinic Research Center of Hepatobiliary Diseases (No. 2016-11), and Open Research Program from Molecular Immunity Study Room Involving in Acute & Severe Diseases in Guangxi Colleges and Universities (Nos. kfkt20160062 and kfkt20160063).

Abbreviations

8-_{oxyG}	8-oxodeoxyguanosine
AFB1	aflatoxin B1
AFBO	AFB1-8,9-epoxide
AFB1-FAPy	8,9-dihydro-8-(2,6-diamino-4-oxo-3,4-dihydropyrimid-5-yl formamide)-9-hydroxy-AFB1
AFB1-N^7-Gua	(8,9-dihydro-8-N^7-guanyl-9-hydroxy-AFB1)
BER	base excision repair
DSBR	double-strand break repair
DSBs	double-strand breaks
GSNP	genetic single nucleotide polymorphism
HCC	hepatocellular carcinoma
HR	hazard ratio
hOGG1	human 8-oxoguanine DNA glycosylase
NER	nucleotide excision repair
NHEJ	nonhomologous end joining
OR	odds ratio
SSBs	single-strand breaks
SSBR	single-strand break repair
SSMED	short stature, microcephaly, and endocrine dysfunction

TP53M	the hotspot mutation at codon 249 of TP53 gene;
XPC	xeroderma pigmentosum C
XPD	xeroderma pigmentosum D
XRCC1	X-ray repair cross-complementing group 1
XRCC3	X-ray repair cross-complementing group 3
XRCC4	X-ray repair cross-complementing group 4
XRCC7	X-ray repair cross-complementing group 7

Author details

Xue-Ming Wu[1†], Zhi-Feng Xi[2†], Jun Lu[2†], Xing-Zhizi Wang[1†], Tian-Qi Zhang[1†], Xiao-Ying Huang[1†], Jin-Guang Yao[1†], Chao Wang[3†], Zhong-Heng Wei[4†], Chun-Ying Luo[1†], Bing-Chen Huang[1†], Qun-Qing Xu[5†], Wen-Pei Yang[6†], Qiang Xia[2*] and Xi-Dai Long[1,2*]

*Address all correspondence to: sjtulongxd@263.net or xiaqiang@sjtu.edu.cn

1 Department of Pathology, the Affiliated Hospital of Youjiang Medical College for Nationalities (AHYMCN), Baise, China

2 Department of Liver Surgery, Ren Ji Hospital, School of Medicine, Shanghai Jiao Tong University, Shanghai, China

3 Department of Medicine, AHYMCN, Baise, China

4 Department of Tumor, AHYMCN, Baise, China

5 Department of Central Test, Youjiang Medical College for Nationalities, Baise, China

6 Department of Basic Medicine, Youjiang Medical College for Nationalities, Baise, China

† These authors contributed equally to this work.

References

[1] Torre LA, Bray F, Siegel RL, Ferlay J, Lortet-Tieulent J, Jemal A. Global cancer statistics, 2012. CA A Cancer Journal for Clinicians. 2015;**65**:87-108. DOI: 10.3322/caac.21262

[2] Chen W, Zheng R, Baade PD, Zhang S, Zeng H, Bray F, Jemal A, Yu XQ, He J. Cancer statistics in China, 2015. CA A Cancer Journal for Clinicians. 2016;**66**:115-132. DOI: 10.3322/caac.21338

[3] Xia Q, Huang XY, Xue F, Zhang JJ, Zhai B, Kong DC, Wang C, Huang ZQ, Long XD. Genetic polymorphisms of DNA repair genes and DNA repair capacity related to aflatoxin b1 (AFB1)-induced DNA damages. In: Chen C, editor. New Research Directions in DNA Repair. 1st ed. Rijeka: InTech; 2013. pp. 377-412. DOI: 10.5772/53967

[4] Long XD, Yao JG, Zeng Z, Huang CH, Huang ZS, Huang YZ, Ban FZ, Huang XY, Yao LM, Fan LD, Fu GH. DNA repair capacity-related to genetic polymorphisms of DNA repair genes and aflatoxin B1-related hepatocellular carcinoma among Chinese population. In: Kruman I, editor. DNA Repair. Rijeka: InTech; 2011. pp. 505-524. DOI: 10.5772/20792

[5] Long XD, Yao JD, Yang Q, Huang CH, Liao P, Nong LG, Tang YJ, Huang XY, Wang C, Wu XM, Huang BC, Ban FZ, Zeng LX, Ma Y, Zhai B, Zhang JQ, Xue F, Lu CX, Xia Q. Polymorphisms of DNA repair genes and toxicological effects of aflatoxin B1 exposure In: Faulkner AG, editor. Aflatoxins: Food Sources, Occurrence and Toxicological Effects. 1st ed. New York: Nova Science Publishers; 2014. pp. 107-124. DOI: 978-1-63117-298-4

[6] Clifford RJ, Zhang J, Meerzaman DM, Lyu MS, Hu Y, Cultraro CM, Finney RP, Kelley JM, Efroni S, Greenblum SI, Nguyen CV, Rowe WL, Sharma S, Wu G, Yan C, Zhang H, Chung YH, Kim JA, Park NH, Song IH, Buetow KH. Genetic variations at loci involved in the immune response are risk factors for hepatocellular carcinoma. Hepatology. 2010;**52**:2034-2043. DOI: 10.1002/hep.23943

[7] Dominguez-Malagon H, Gaytan-Graham S. Hepatocellular carcinoma: An update. Ultrastructural Pathology. 2001;**25**:497-516. DOI: 10.1080/25.497516

[8] Long XD, Tang YH, Qu DY, Ma Y. The toxicity and role of aflatoxin B1 and DNA repair (corresponding DNA repair enzymes). Youjiang Medical College for Nationalities Xue Bao. 2006;**28**:278-280. DOI: 10.3969/j.issn.1001-5817.2006.02.092

[9] Zhang CY, Huang TR, Yu JH, Zhang ZQ, Li JL, Deng W, Ye SY, Zhou DN, He ZF. Epidemiological analysis of primary liver cancer in the early 21st century in Guangxi province of China. Chinese Journal of Cancer. 2010;**29**:545-550. DOI: 10.3969/j.issn.0253-4304.2000.04.003

[10] Huang ZB, Wu ZB, Xu GC. A study on serum epidemiology of several hepatitis viruses in Guangxi areas with high incident areas of liver cancer. Guangxi Medical Unveristy Xue Bao. 2000;**17**:79. DOI: 10.3969/j.issn.1005-930X.2000.01.037

[11] Ma AM, Luo YX, Wan JL, Long XD, Huang YZ. An investigative analysis of incidence, prevention, and treatment of hepatocellular carcinoma in Xiangzhou, Baise, Guangxi Autonomous Region, China. Youjiang Minzu Yixueyuan Bao. 2010;**32**:165-166. DOI: 10.3969/j.issn.1001-5817.2010.02.024

[12] Long XD, Ma Y, Zhou YF, Ma AM, Fu GH. Polymorphism in xeroderma pigmentosum complementation group C codon 939 and aflatoxin B1-related hepatocellular carcinoma in the Guangxi population. Hepatology. 2010;**52**:1301-1309. DOI: 10.1002/hep.23807

[13] Long XD, Zhao D, Wang C, Huang XY, Yao JG, Ma Y, Wei ZH, Liu M, Zeng LX, Mo XQ, Zhang JJ, Xue F, Zhai B, Xia Q. Genetic polymorphisms in DNA repair genes XRCC4 and XRCC5 and aflatoxin B1-related hepatocellular carcinoma. Epidemiology. 2013;**24**:671-681. DOI: 10.1097/EDE.0b013e31829d2744

[14] Long XD, Yao JG, Zeng Z, Ma Y, Huang XY, Wei ZH, Liu M, Zhang JJ, Xue F, Zhai B, Xia Q. Polymorphisms in the coding region of X-ray repair complementing group 4 and aflatoxin B1-related hepatocellular carcinoma. Hepatology. 2013;**58**:171-181. DOI: 10.1002/hep.26311

[15] Kensler TW, Roebuck BD, Wogan GN, Groopman JD. Aflatoxin: A 50-year odyssey of mechanistic and translational toxicology. Toxicological Sciences: An Official Journal of the Society of Toxicology. 2011;**120**(Suppl 1):S28–S48. DOI: 10.1093/toxsci/kfq283

[16] Guengerich FP, Johnson WW, Shimada T, Ueng YF, Yamazaki H, Langouet S. Activation and detoxication of aflatoxin B1. Mutation Research. 1998;**402**:121-128. DOI: S0027-5107(97)00289-3

[17] Ben Rejeb I, Arduini F, Arvinte A, Amine A, Gargouri M, Micheli L, Bala C, Moscone D, Palleschi G. Development of a bio-electrochemical assay for AFB1 detection in olive oil. Biosensors and Bioelectronics. 2009;**24**:1962-1968. DOI: 10.1016/j.bios.2008.10.002

[18] Giri I, Stone MP. Wobble DC. dA pairing 5' to the cationic guanine N7 8,9-dihydro-8-(N7-guanyl)-9-hydroxyaflatoxin B1 adduct: Implications for nontargeted AFB1 mutagenesis. Biochemistry. 2003;**42**:7023-7034. DOI: 10.1021/bi020688n

[19] Habib SL, Said B, Awad AT, Mostafa MH, Shank RC. Novel adenine adducts, N7-guanine-AFB1 adducts, and p53 mutations in patients with schistosomiasis and aflatoxin exposure. Cancer Detection and Prevention. 2006;**30**:491-498. DOI: 10.1016/j.cdp.2006.10.006

[20] Wang JS, Groopman JD. DNA damage by mycotoxins. Mutation Research. 1999;**424**:167-181. DOI: 01.2013/0027-5107.10064859

[21] Essigmann JM, Croy RG, Nadzan AM, Busby WF, Jr, Reinhold VN, Buchi G, Wogan GN. Structural identification of the major DNA adduct formed by aflatoxin B1 in vitro. Proceedings of the National Academy of Sciences of the United States of America. 1977;**74**:1870-1874. DOI: 10.2013/0027-8424.266709

[22] Croy RG, Essigmann JM, Reinhold VN, Wogan GN. Identification of the principal aflatoxin B1-DNA adduct formed in vivo in rat liver. Proceedings of the National Academy of Sciences of the United States of America. 1978;**75**:1745-1749. DOI: 10.2013/0027-8427.273905

[23] Croy RG, Wogan GN. Temporal patterns of covalent DNA adducts in rat liver after single and multiple doses of aflatoxin B1. Cancer Research. 1981;**41**:197-203. DOI: 10.2013/0008-5472.7448760

[24] Groopman JD, Croy RG, Wogan GN. In vitro reactions of aflatoxin B1-adducted DNA. Proceedings of the National Academy of Sciences of the United States of America. 1981;**78**:5445-5449. DOI: 10.2013/0027-8424.6795633

[25] Chen JD, Liu CJ, Lee PH, Chen PJ, Lai MY, Kao JH, Chen DS. Hepatitis B genotypes correlate with tumor recurrence after curative resection of hepatocellular carcinoma. Clinical Gastroenterology and Hepatology. 2004;**2**:64-71. DOI: S1542356503002933

[26] Gradelet S, Le Bon AM, Berges R, Suschetet M, Astorg P. Dietary carotenoids inhibit aflatoxin B1-induced liver preneoplastic foci and DNA damage in the rat: Role of the modulation of aflatoxin B1 metabolism. Carcinogenesis. 1998;**19**:403-411. DOI: 10.2013/0143-3334. 9525273

[27] Farombi EO, Adepoju BF, Ola-Davies OE, Emerole GO. Chemoprevention of aflatoxin B1-induced genotoxicity and hepatic oxidative damage in rats by kolaviron, a natural bioflavonoid of Garcinia kola seeds. European Journal of Cancer Prevention: The Official Journal of the European Cancer Prevention Organisation. 2005;**14**:207-214. DOI: 10.2013/0959-8278. 15901988

[28] Liu J, Yang CF, Lee BL, Shen HM, Ang SG, Ong CN. Effect of *Salvia miltiorrhiza* on aflatoxin B1-induced oxidative stress in cultured rat hepatocytes. Free Radical Research. 1999;**31**:559-568. DOI: 10.2013/1071-5762.10630680

[29] Wild CP, Montesano R. A model of interaction: Aflatoxins and hepatitis viruses in liver cancer aetiology and prevention. Cancer Letters. 2009;**286**:22-28. DOI: 10.1016/j.canlet.2009.02.053

[30] Shen HM, Ong CN. Mutations of the p53 tumor suppressor gene and ras oncogenes in aflatoxin hepatocarcinogenesis. Mutation Research. 1996;**366**:23-44. DOI: 10.2013/0027-5107.8921985

[31] Golli-Bennour EE, Kouidhi B, Bouslimi A, Abid-Essefi S, Hassen W, Bacha H. Cytotoxicity and genotoxicity induced by aflatoxin B1, ochratoxin A, and their combination in cultured Vero cells. Journal of Biochemical and Molecular Toxicology. 2010;**24**:42-50. DOI: 10.1002/jbt.20310

[32] Paget V, Sichel F, Garon D, Lechevrel M. Aflatoxin B1-induced TP53 mutational pattern in normal human cells using the FASAY (functional analysis of separated alleles in yeast). Mutation Research. 2008;**656**:55-61. DOI: 10.1016/j.mrgentox.2008.07.009

[33] Van Vleet TR, Watterson TL, Klein PJ, Coulombe Jr. RA. Aflatoxin B1 alters the expression of p53 in cytochrome P450-expressing human lung cells. Toxicological Sciences. 2006;**89**:399-407. DOI: 10.1093/toxsci/kfj039

[34] Vahakangas K. TP53 mutations in workers exposed to occupational carcinogens. Human Mutation. 2003;**21**:240-251. DOI: 10.1002/humu.10182

[35] Staib F, Hussain SP, Hofseth LJ, Wang XW, Harris CC. TP53 and liver carcinogenesis. Human Mutation. 2003;**21**:201-216. DOI: 10.1002/humu.10176

[36] Chan KT, Hsieh DP, Lung ML. In vitro aflatoxin B1-induced p53 mutations. Cancer Letters. 2003;**199**:1-7. DOI: S0304383503003379

[37] Long XD, Ma Y, Huang HD, Yao JG, Qu de Y, Lu YL. Polymorphism of XRCC1 and the frequency of mutation in codon 249 of the p53 gene in hepatocellular carcinoma among Guangxi population, China. Molecular Carcinogenesis. 2008;**47**:295-300. DOI: 10.1002/mc.20384

[38] Li D, Cao Y, He L, Wang NJ, Gu JR. Aberrations of p53 gene in human hepatocellular carcinoma from China. Carcinogenesis. 1993;**14**:169-173. DOI: 10.2013/0143-3334. 8382111

[39] Kirk GD, Camus-Randon AM, Mendy M, Goedert JJ, Merle P, Trepo C, Brechot C, Hainaut P, Montesano R. Ser-249 p53 mutations in plasma DNA of patients with

hepatocellular carcinoma from the Gambia. Journal of the National Cancer Institute. 2000;**92**:148-153. DOI: 10.2013/0027-8874.10639517

[40] Aguilar F, Hussain SP, Cerutti P. Aflatoxin B1 induces the transversion of G-->T in codon 249 of the p53 tumor suppressor gene in human hepatocytes. Proceedings of the National Academy of Sciences of the United States of America. 1993;**90**:8586-8590. DOI: 10.2013/0027-8424.8397412

[41] Denissenko MF, Koudriakova TB, Smith L, O'Connor TR, Riggs AD, Pfeifer GP. The p53 codon 249 mutational hotspot in hepatocellular carcinoma is not related to selective formation or persistence of aflatoxin B1 adducts. Oncogene. 1998;**17**:3007-3014. DOI: 10.1038/sj.onc.1202214

[42] Duflot A, Hollstein M, Mehrotra R, Trepo C, Montesano R, Cova L. Absence of p53 mutation at codon 249 in duck hepatocellular carcinomas from the high incidence area of Qidong (China). Carcinogenesis. 1994;**15**:1353-1357. DOI: 10.2017/0143-3334.8033311

[43] Sugasawa K. XPC: Its product and biological roles. Advances in Experimental Medicine and Biology. 2008;**637**:47-56. DOI: 10.2016/0065-2598.19181110

[44] Nemzow L, Lubin A, Zhang L, Gong F. XPC: Going where no DNA damage sensor has gone before. DNA Repair (Amst). 2015;**36**:19-27. DOI: 10.1016/j.dnarep.2015.09.004

[45] Fautrel A, Andrieux L, Musso O, Boudjema K, Guillouzo A, Langouet S. Overexpression of the two nucleotide excision repair genes ERCC1 and XPC in human hepatocellular carcinoma. Journal of Hepatology. 2005;**43**:288-293. DOI: 10.1016/j.jhep.2005.02.020

[46] Strom SS, Estey E, Outschoorn UM, Garcia-Manero G. Acute myeloid leukemia outcome: Role of nucleotide excision repair polymorphisms in intermediate risk patients. Leuk Lymphoma. 2010;**51**:598-605. DOI: 10.3109/10428190903582804

[47] Khan SG, Yamanegi K, Zheng ZM, Boyle J, Imoto K, Oh KS, Baker CC, Gozukara E, Metin A, Kraemer KH. XPC branch-point sequence mutations disrupt U2 snRNP binding, resulting in abnormal pre-mRNA splicing in xeroderma pigmentosum patients. Human Mutation. 2010;**31**:167-175. DOI: 10.1002/humu.21166

[48] Gangwar R, Mandhani A, Mittal RD. XPC gene variants: A risk factor for recurrence of urothelial bladder carcinoma in patients on BCG immunotherapy. Journal of Cancer Research and Clinical Oncology. 2010;**136**:779-786. DOI: 10.1007/s00432-009-0717-y

[49] Yao JG, Huang XY, Long XD. Interaction of DNA repair gene polymorphisms and aflatoxin B1 in the risk of hepatocellular carcinoma. International Journal of Clinical and Experimental Pathology. 2014;**7**:6231-6244. DOI: 10.2016/1936-2625.25337275

[50] Li LM, Zeng XY, Ji L, Fan XJ, Li YQ, Hu XH, Qiu XQ, Yu HP. Association of XPC and XPG polymorphisms with the risk of hepatocellular carcinoma. Zhonghua gan zang bing za zhi = Zhonghua ganzangbing zazhi = Chinese Journal of Hepatology. 2010;**18**:271-275. DOI: 10.3760/cma.j.issn.1007-3418.2010.04.009

[51] Wu XM, Ma Y, Deng ZL, Long XD. The polymorphism at codon 939 of xeroderma pigmentosum C gene and hepatocellular carcinoma among Guangxi population. Zhonghua Xiaohua Zazhi. 2010;**30**:846-848. DOI: 10.3760/cma.j.issn.0254-1432.2010.11.018

[52] Van Houten B, Kuper J, Kisker C. Role of XPD in cellular functions: To TFIIH and beyond. DNA Repair (Amst). 2016;**44**:136-142. DOI: 10.1016/j.dnarep.2016.05.019

[53] Manuguerra M, Saletta F, Karagas MR, Berwick M, Veglia F, Vineis P, Matullo G. XRCC3 and XPD/ERCC2 single nucleotide polymorphisms and the risk of cancer: A HuGE review. American Journal of Epidemiology. 2006;**164**:297-302. DOI: 10.1093/aje/kwj189

[54] Sandoval-Carrillo A, Mendez-Hernandez EM, Vazquez-Alaniz F, Aguilar-Duran M, Tellez-Valencia A, Barraza-Salas M, Castellanos-Juarez FX, Llave-Leon OL, Salas-Pacheco JM. Polymorphisms in DNA repair genes (APEX1, XPD, XRCC1 and XRCC3) and risk of preeclampsia in a Mexican mestizo population. International Journal of Molecular Sciences. 2014;**15**:4273-4283. DOI: 10.3390/ijms15034273

[55] Guo XF, Wang J, Lei XF, Zeng YP, Dong WG. XPD Lys751Gln polymorphisms and the risk of esophageal cancer: An updated meta-analysis. Internal Medicine Journal. 2015;**54**:251-259. DOI: 10.2169/internalmedicine.54.3256

[56] Peng Q, Li S, Lao X, Chen Z, Li R, Qin X. Association between XPD Lys751Gln and Asp312Asn polymorphisms and hepatocellular carcinoma risk: A systematic review and meta-analysis. Medicine (Baltimore). 2014;**93**:e330. DOI: 10.1097/MD.0000000000000330

[57] Zeng XY, Qiu XQ, Ji L, Yu HP. Study on the relationship between hepatoceilular carcinoma and the interaction between polymorphisms in DNA repair gene XPD and environmental factors. Zhong Hua Liu Xing Bing Xue Za Zhi. 2009;**30**:702-705. DOI: 10.3760/cma.j.issn.0254-6450.2009.07.014

[58] Long XD, Ma Y, Zhou YF, Yao JG, Ban FZ, Huang YZ, Huang BC. XPD Codon 312 and 751 polymorphisms, and AFB1 exposure, and hepatocellular carcinoma risk. BMC Cancer. 2009;**9**:400. DOI: 10.1186/1471-2407-9-400

[59] Hu HB, Tang CL, Li YB, Qin WB, Lu WX. Genic polymorphisms of XPD and risk of liver cancer among Guangxi Zhuang population. Shan Dong Yi Yao. 2016;**56**:33-35. DOI: 10.3969/j.issn.1002-266X.2016.13.012

[60] Wallace SS. Base excision repair: A critical player in many games. DNA Repair (Amst). 2014;**19**:14-26. DOI: 10.1016/j.dnarep.2014.03.030

[61] Kuznetsov NA, Koval VV, Fedorova OS. Mechanism of recognition and repair of damaged DNA by human 8-oxoguanine DNA glycosylase hOGG1. Biochemistry (Mosc). 2011;**76**:118-130. DOI: 10.2016/1608-3040.21568844

[62] Boiteux S, Radicella JP. The human OGG1 gene: Structure, functions, and its implication in the process of carcinogenesis. Archives of Biochemistry and Biophysics. 2000;**377**:1-8. DOI: 10.1006/abbi.2000.1773

[63] Weiss JM, Goode EL, Ladiges WC, Ulrich CM. Polymorphic variation in hOGG1 and risk of cancer: A review of the functional and epidemiologic literature. Molecular Carcinogenesis. 2005;**42**:127-141. DOI: 10.1002/mc.20067

[64] Kohno T, Shinmura K, Tosaka M, Tani M, Kim SR, Sugimura H, Nohmi T, Kasai H, Yokota J. Genetic polymorphisms and alternative splicing of the hOGG1 gene, that is involved in the repair of 8-hydroxyguanine in damaged DNA. Oncogene. 1998;**16**:3219-3225. DOI: 10.1038/sj.onc.1201872

[65] Kamali M, Kargar S, Heiranizadeh N, Zare M, Kargar S, Zare Shehneh M, Neamatzadeh H. Lack of any Association between the Hogg1 Ser326Cys polymorphism and breast cancer risk: A systematic review and meta-analysis of 18 studies. Asian Pacific Journal of Cancer Prevention. 2017;**18**:245-251. DOI: 10.22034/APJCP.2017.18.1.245

[66] Wang W, Dang S, Li Y, Sun M, Jia X, Wang R, Liu J. hOGG1 Ser326Cys polymorphism and risk of hepatocellular carcinoma among East Asians: A meta-analysis. PLoS One. 2013;**8**:e60178. DOI: 10.1371/journal.pone.0060178

[67] Ji L, Zeng XY, Li LM, Qiu XQ, Chen SX, Yu HP. Interaction between the single-nucleotide polymorphism of DNA repair gene hOGG1 and HBV infection and its susceptibility to hepatocellular carcinoma. Journal of Hygiene Research. 2011;**40**:705-708. DOI: 10.2017/1000-8020.2011.06.017

[68] Peng T, Shen HM, Liu ZM, Yan LN, Peng MH, Li LQ, Liang RX, Wei ZL, Halliwell B, Ong CN. Oxidative DNA damage in peripheral leukocytes and its association with expression and polymorphisms of hOGG1: A study of adolescents in a high risk region for hepatocellular carcinoma in China. World Journal of Gastroenterology. 2003;**9**:2186-2193. DOI: 10.2016/1007-9327.14562375

[69] Yuan T, Wei J, Luo J, Liu M, Deng S, Chen P. Polymorphisms of base-excision repair genes hOGG1 326cys and XRCC1 280His increase hepatocellular carcinoma risk. Digestive Diseases and Sciences. 2012;**57**:2451-2457. DOI: 10.1007/s10620-012-2192-6

[70] Zhang H, He BC, He FC. Impact of DNA repair gene hOGG1 Ser326Cys polymorphism on the risk of hepatocellular carcinoma. Shijie Huaren xiaohua zazhi. 2006;**14**:2311-2314. DOI: 10.3969/j.issn.1009-3079.2006.23.010

[71] Cheng B, Jungst C, Lin J, Caselmann WH. Potential role of human DNA-repair enzymes hMTH1, hOGG1 and hMYHalpha in the hepatocarcinogenesis. Journal of Huazhong University of Science and Technology. Medical sciences. 2002;**22**:206-211, 215. DOI: 10.2016/1672-0733.12658805

[72] Su ZX, Li LQ, Peng T, Ye XP, Xiao KY, Shang LM. The implications of hOGG1 expression in hepatocellular carcinoma and cirrhosis tissues. China Medical Abstracts: Oncology. 2009;**1**:3-6. DOI: 10.3969/j.issn.1674-5671.2009.01.003

[73] London RE. The structural basis of XRCC1-mediated DNA repair. DNA Repair (Amst). 2015;**30**:90-103. DOI: 10.1016/j.dnarep.2015.02.005

[74] Long XD, Ma Y, Wei YP, Deng ZL. X-ray repair cross-complementing group 1 (XRCC1) Arg 399 Gln polymorphism and aflatoxin B1 (AFB1)-related hepatocellular carcinoma (HCC) in Guangxi population. Chinese Journal of Cancer Research. 2005;**17**:17-21. DOI: 10.1007/s11670-005-0004-7

[75] Long XD, Ma Y, Wei YP, Deng ZL. The polymorphisms of GSTM1, GSTT1, HYL1*2, and XRCC1, and aflatoxin B1-related hepatocellular carcinoma in Guangxi population, China. Hepatology Research. 2006;**36**:48-55. DOI: 10.1016/j.hepres.2006.06.004

[76] Zeng XY, Yu HP, Qiu XQ, Ji L, Li LM. A case-control study of polymorphism of XRCC1 gene and the risk of hepatocellular carcinoma. Zhonghua Ji Bing Kong Zhi Za Zhi. 2010;**14**:760-763. DOI: 10.3760/cma.j.issn.0254-6448.2010.11.018

[77] He GZ, Huang TR, Deng JH, Zhang CY, Li JL. Research on association between XRCC1Arg399Gln polymorphism and liver cancer. Guangxi Zhongyi Xueyuan Xuebao. 2012;**15**:1-3. DOI: 10.3969/j.issn.1008-7486.2012.03.001

[78] Chen BP, Long XD, Fu GH. Meta-analysis of XRCC1 Codon 399 polymorphism and susceptibility of hepatocellular carcinoma. Journal of Shanghai Jiao Tong University (Medical Science). 2011;**31**:1588-1602. DOI: 10.3969/j.issn.1674-8115.2011.11.018

[79] Bishop DK, Ear U, Bhattacharyya A, Calderone C, Beckett M, Weichselbaum RR, Shinohara A. Xrcc3 is required for assembly of Rad51 complexes in vivo. Journal of Biological Chemistry. 1998;**273**:21482-21488. DOI: 10.2016/0021-9258. 9705276

[80] Kawabata M, Kawabata T, Nishibori M. Role of recA/RAD51 family proteins in mammals. Acta Medica Okayama. 2005;**59**:1-9. DOI: 10.2016/0386-300X.PMID.15902993

[81] Cheng S, Wang L, Wang L, Wang Z. Association of XRCC3 gene rs861539 polymorphism with gastric cancer risk: Evidence from a case-control study and a meta-analysis. International Journal of Clinical and Experimental Pathology. 2015;**8**:1911-1919. DOI: 10.2016/1936-2625.10086

[82] Bei L, Xiao-Dong T, Yu-Fang G, Jian-Ping S, Zhao-Yu Y. DNA repair gene XRCC3 Thr241Met polymorphisms and lung cancer risk: A meta-analysis. Bull Cancer. 2015;**102**:332-339. DOI: 10.1016/j.bulcan.2015.02.003

[83] Zhang X, Zhang L, Tian C, Yang L, Wang Z. Genetic variants and risk of cervical cancer: Epidemiological evidence, meta-analysis and research review. British Journal of Obstetrics and Gynaecology. 2014;**121**:664-674. DOI: 10.1111/1471-0528.12638

[84] Long XD, Ma Y, Qu de Y, Liu YG, Huang ZQ, Huang YZ, Lin ZH, Wei NB, Zhou SC. The polymorphism of XRCC3 codon 241 and AFB1-related hepatocellular carcinoma in Guangxi population, China. Annals of Epidemiology. 2008;**18**:572-578. DOI: 10.1016/j.annepidem.2008.03.003

[85] Long XD, Ma Y, Deng ZL, Huang YZ, Wei NB. Association of the Thr241Met polymorphism of DNA repair gene XRCC3 with genetic susceptibility to AFB1-related

hepatocellular carcinoma in Guangxi population. Zhonghua Yi Xue Yi Chuan Xue Za Zhi. 2008;**25**:268-271. DOI: 940625058

[86] Chen BP, Li M, Asaithamby A. New insights into the roles of ATM and DNA-PKcs in the cellular response to oxidative stress. Cancer Letters. 2012;**327**:103-110. DOI: 10.1016/j.canlet.2011.12.004

[87] Shrivastav M, De Haro LP, Nickoloff JA. Regulation of DNA double-strand break repair pathway choice. Cell Research. 2008;**18**:134-147. DOI: 10.1038/cr.2007.111

[88] Jolly CJ, Cook AJ, Manis JP. Fixing DNA breaks during class switch recombination. The Journal of Experimental Medicine. 2008;**205**:509-513. DOI: 10.1084/jem.20080356

[89] Zhou C, Tang H, Yu J, Zhuang D, Zhang H. Blood-based DNA methylation of DNA repair genes in the non-homologous end-joining (NEHJ) pathway in patient with glioma. International journal of Clinical and Experimental Pathology. 2015;**8**:9463-9467. DOI: 10.2016/1936-2625.PMID.26464705

[90] Xiao M, Shen Y, Chen L, Liao Z, Wen F. The rs7003908 (T>G) polymorphism in the XRCC7 gene and the risk of cancers. Molecular Biology Reports. 2014;**41**:3577-3582. DOI: 10.1007/s11033-014-3220-8

[91] Jahantigh D, Salimi S, Mousavi M, Moossavi M, Mohammadoo-Khorasani M, Narooei-nejad M, Sandoughi M. Association between functional polymorphisms of DNA Double-Strand breaks in repair genes XRCC5, XRCC6 and XRCC7 with the risk of systemic lupus erythematosus in South East Iran. DNA Cell Biology. 2015;**34**:360-366. DOI: 10.1089/dna.2014.2465

[92] Hsieh YH, Chang WS, Tsai CW, Tsai JP, Hsu CM, Jeng LB, Bau DT. DNA double-strand break repair gene XRCC7 genotypes were associated with hepatocellular carcinoma risk in Taiwanese males and alcohol drinkers. Tumour Biology. 2015;**36**:4101-4106. DOI: 10.1007/s13277-014-2934-5

[93] Hsia TC, Chang WS, Chen WC, Liang SJ, Tu CY, Chen HJ, Liang JA, Tsai CW, Hsu CM, Tsai CH, Bau DT. Genotype of DNA double-strand break repair gene XRCC7 is associated with lung cancer risk in Taiwan males and smokers. Anticancer Research. 2014;**34**:7001-7005. DOI: 10.2016/0250-7005.PMID.25503126

[94] Long XD, Yao JG, Huang YZ, Huang XY, Ban FZ, Yao LM, Fan LD. DNA repair gene XRCC7 polymorphisms (rs#7003908 and rs#10109984) and hepatocellular carcinoma related to AFB1 exposure among Guangxi population, China. Hepatology Research. 2011;**41**:1085-1093. DOI: 10.1111/j.1872-034X.2011.00866.x

[95] Koike M, Yutoku Y, Koike A. Cloning, localization and focus formation at DNA damage sites of canine XRCC4. The Journal of Veterinary Medical Science. 2017;**78**:1865-1871. DOI: 10.1292/jvms.16-0381

[96] Hammel M, Yu Y, Radhakrishnan SK, Chokshi C, Tsai MS, Matsumoto Y, Kuzdovich M, Remesh SG, Fang S, Tomkinson AE, Lees-Miller SP, Tainer JA. An intrinsically disordered APLF links Ku, DNA-PKcs, and XRCC4-DNA Ligase IV in an extended flexible Non-homologous end joining complex. Journal of Biological Chemistry. 2016;**291**:26987-27006. DOI: 10.1074/jbc.M116.751867

[97] Mizuta R, Cheng HL, Gao Y, Alt FW. Molecular genetic characterization of XRCC4 function. International Immunology. 1997;**9**:1607-1613. DOI: 10.2016/0953-8178.PMID. 9352367

[98] Li Z, Otevrel T, Gao Y, Cheng HL, Seed B, Stamato TD, Taccioli GE, Alt FW. The XRCC4 gene encodes a novel protein involved in DNA double-strand break repair and V(D)J recombination. Cell. 1995;**83**:1079-1089. DOI: 0092-8674(95)90135-3

[99] Yang CH, Lin YD, Yen CY, Chuang LY, Chang HW. A systematic Gene-Gene and Gene-Environment interaction analysis of DNA repair genes XRCC1, XRCC2, XRCC3, XRCC4, and oral cancer risk. OMICS. 2015;**19**:238-247. DOI: 10.1089/omi.2014.0121

[100] Jung SW, Park NH, Shin JW, Park BR, Kim CJ, Lee JE, Shin ES, Kim JA, Chung YH. Polymorphisms of DNA repair genes in Korean hepatocellular carcinoma patients with chronic hepatitis B: Possible implications on survival. Journal of Hepatology. 2012;**57**:621-627. DOI: 10.1016/j.jhep.2012.04.039

6

Minimally Invasive Therapies for Hepatocellular Carcinoma: Mechanisms of Local Control and Systemic Immunologic Response

Andrew W. Ritchey, Joshua D. Kuban and Rahul A. Sheth

Abstract

Minimally invasive treatments for hepatocellular carcinoma (HCC) are a cornerstone in the management of this challenging disease. For many years, percutaneously guided ablative techniques, such as radiofrequency ablation (RFA), cryoablation, and microwave ablation (MWA), have successfully treated many different solid malignancies including HCC. Since the initial implementation of these ablative techniques, there have been many advances in the design, technique, and patient selection as well as investigation into the body's response to treatment. The mechanisms of thermal-based ablative techniques, advantages and disadvantages of each technique, subsequent immunologic response following ablation, and advances in care that utilize combination therapy to potentiate the immunologic response creating a robust and long-term immunity to HCC are outlined in this chapter.

Keywords: hepatocellular carcinoma (HCC), immunotherapy, immunologic, response, immune, cancer, carcinoma, oncology, radiofrequency, microwave, ablation, cryoablation

1. Introduction

Hepatocellular carcinoma (HCC) is the most rapidly increasing type of cancer in the United States due to viral hepatitis and various forms of liver cirrhosis. HCC is resistant to traditional chemotherapy and often is not amenable to surgical resection due to factors involving the primary tumor or patient comorbidities [1, 2]. Thus, minimally invasive therapies for the treatment of malignant liver tumors have become a cornerstone of treatment. These minimally invasive techniques, including radiofrequency ablation (RFA), microwave ablation (MWA), and cryoablation (cryo), have been shown to have distinct advantages over traditional treatment methods. These methods are not only able to locally control the malignancy through cellular necrosis and apoptosis but also potentially trigger systemic immune responses [3–6]. Additionally, these minimally invasive techniques offer other advantages such as lower morbidity, preservation of healthy tissues, lower cost, and decreased hospitalization time relative to surgical resection [5]. In this chapter, the mechanisms, advantages, disadvantages, synergism, and immunologic responses to the techniques outlined above are discussed.

2. Radiofrequency ablation

2.1. Overview

Radiofrequency ablation (RFA) is a minimally invasive technique used to thermally ablate targeted lesions in a variety of tissues. RFA is performed by percutaneously inserting one or more probes using various forms of image guidance, such as computed tomography (CT) or ultrasound (US). RFA may also be performed through other approaches such as laparoscopy and open surgery. The number of probes used is based on multiple factors such as the size of the lesion, the impedance of the targeted region, and surrounding structures such as blood vessels and lymphatic channels. In addition to the placement of RFA probes, one or more grounding pads are also placed on the patient. These grounding pads are located at a distant site from the probes. For example, a common practice is to place multiple grounding pads on both thighs when using RFA to ablate lesions located in the liver. Once the placement of the RFA probes has been confirmed with image guidance, an alternating current is generated by a power source between the probes and the grounding pads. This alternating current creates the thermal ablative region by causing ions to oscillate, generating frictional heat. RFA can reliably generate temperatures of 60–100°C in the targeted region leading to focal hyperthermic injury to the nearby cells. When temperatures reach 60°C or higher, instant cell death occurs, and at temperatures above 100°C, charring of surrounding tissues occurs. These two temperature points are crucial to the procedure because the operator can be certain that cell death has occurred in the regions >60°C, but it is also important to monitor the temperatures so that they do not increase too quickly or reach >100°C. If the temperature becomes too high, charring of the tissues occurs, which increases the impedance significantly and causes the technique to lose efficacy by diminishing the ablative zone substantially [7]. Additionally, at temperatures above 110°C, vaporization of the tissues occurs. Vaporization also increases the impedance of the tissues limiting the ablative zone [8].

The ablated area with RFA can be divided into three zones: central, transitional, and the unaffected surrounding parenchyma [8]. The central zone is the area directly surrounding the RFA probe. In this zone, the temperatures are the highest, typically >50–60°C, leading to coagulative necrosis of the cells in this region. The cells in this zone immediately undergo irreversible injury through protein denaturation of both the cytosolic, nucleic, and mitochondrial enzymes leading to coagulative necrosis. In addition to protein denaturation, the cell membrane integrity is also compromised. The higher temperatures in the central zone lead to changes in fluid permeability through destruction of the membrane actin filaments. These membrane changes result in an intracellular fluid shift and subsequent cytolysis [5, 8].

Cells in the transitional zone are heated through conductive heat transfer from tissues in the central zone. This conductive heat transfer produces a sharp temperature gradient with average lower temperatures ranging from 40 to 45°C [5]. Cells within the transitional zone experience thermal injury, but since temperatures of 50°C are not reached, these cells do not undergo immediate cellular death [9]. Rather, the cells' metabolic processes and DNA repair mechanisms are impaired, which trigger specific changes that eventually lead to apoptosis or eventual cellular recovery. Other proposed mechanisms of cellular death include ischemia from vascular damage, reperfusion injury, and cytokine release and subsequent immunologic response to the damaged cells. Due to these changes, a complete response to ablation in this region will take several days to fully develop. This region also undergoes reactive hyperemia in response to the damage. The combination of hyperemia and increased cellular susceptibility creates a favorable environment to use liposomal chemotherapeutics. Liposomal chemotherapeutics will accumulate in the region due to the hyperemia and have increased activity on the already susceptible tumor cells. Since very few of the cells in this region are completely denatured, the transitional zone plays a critical role in the immunologic response, which will be discussed in more detail [5, 6, 8].

Surrounding parenchyma is not left totally unaffected by RFA. While the cells within this zone will not undergo cellular changes, necrosis, or apoptosis, there are several processes that will occur. There is an upregulation of various factors, presentation of antigens to antigen-presenting cells (APCs), and stimulation of the immune system, which will be discussed more in depth in later sections. Additionally, hyperemia occurs which can result in reperfusion injury [5, 6].

All of the above processes are dependent on a multitude of different factors such as the tumor composition, the surrounding parenchyma, the rate at which the energy is applied, and surrounding anatomic structures. The majority of the data on the effects of hyperthermia have been generated from literature on low-temperature hyperthermia that was applied uniformly over longer periods.

2.2. Patient selection

Traditionally, hepatic resection (HR) has been regarded as the first-line treatment for HCC, and RFA was typically reserved for patients with non-resectable disease. However, RFA has become a first-line treatment for early-stage HCC in patients with non-resectable disease, metastatic disease, recurrent HCC after HR, and for patients who are unable or are unwilling to undergo surgery [10]. RFA is best used in patients who have a solitary nodule <5 cm measured in the greatest dimension or less than three nodules all measuring <3 cm in the greatest dimension. RFA is most effective when treating HCC lesions that are ≤2 cm measured from the largest dimension. The reason it is more effective in these smaller lesions is that ablation margins of >4–5 mm can be easily obtained [1, 10]. Histologic and prospective studies have shown that the sensitivity of CT for detecting remnant neoplasm is anywhere between 36 and

44% [11, 12]. Thus, the clinician cannot readily rely on imaging to confirm that the lesion has been fully treated during or after the procedure making pre-procedure planning and patient selection crucial. Meta-analysis and systematic reviews have also shown that the efficacy of RFA and HR when used to treat lesions <5 cm is similar. There is no difference in 1-year overall survival; however, there is a difference in the 3- and 5-year survival. HR offers greater 3- and 5-year survival when compared to RFA as well as 1-, 3-, and 5-year disease-free rates. It has been postulated that these findings are due to how each treatment method works. With RFA, the primary lesion is directly targeted with minimal damage to the surrounding tissues, which may leave satellite lesions that would have been removed with HR. Additionally other factors come into play with RFA such as the shape and distribution of the ablation zone. However, RFA has been shown to have fewer complications during and after the procedure, shorter hospital stays, and is considered safer and less invasive than HR. While HR has a significant role in the treatment of HCC, there are limited studies comparing RFA to HR [10, 13, 14]. At the current time, it cannot be confirmed which treatment is superior to the other in treating early-stage HCC. It is up to the treating clinician to determine which treatment is best. RFA should be considered as a first-line treatment in specific patients with small solitary lesions <5 cm; patients with less than three lesions that are <3 cm; patients with non-resectable, metastatic, or recurrent disease; patients who elect for non-operative or a minimally invasive approach; and patients who are non-operative due to medical comorbidities [10].

2.3. Advantages and disadvantages of RFA

Of all the thermal ablative techniques for treating HCC, RFA has been the most researched. There are many technical advantages using RFA for the treatment of HCC. The most obvious advantage of RFA as well as other thermal ablative techniques is the ability to treat a wide variety of patients while sparing normal liver parenchyma.

However, an important consideration with RFA and other thermal ablative techniques is the "heat sink effect" of surrounding anatomic structures. The heat sink effect is caused when the desired ablative region contains or is abutted by larger vessels that result in heat dissipation. This dissipation can ultimately lead to temperatures not reaching cytotoxic levels in the lesion [15–17]. Animal studies have shown that the heat sink effect is not significant until the vessel diameter is ≥3 mm [15]. Additional studies have shown a clinically significant increase in tumor recurrence when abutted by a vessel at least 3 mm in diameter [16]. Another concern is damage and thrombosis of surrounding vessels. It has been shown that there is minimal damage and thrombosis to surrounding vessels if the size of those vessels is greater than 3 mm [15]. The implication of these studies is that if a lesion contains a vessel greater than 3 mm, the RFA probe should be placed close to, but not in, the vessel to achieve the best outcome [15, 16]. This placement will move the tumor cells surrounding the vessel into the central ablation zone increasing the likelihood of cell death without significantly increasing damage to the vascular structure.

Other methods to mitigate the heat sink effect have also been studied. One method to overcome the heat sink effect is to occlude the blood supply to the region being ablated with a balloon catheter or gel foam [18]. Since the majority of the blood supply to HCC lesions is derived from the hepatic artery, temporary occlusion of this artery with a balloon catheter will reduce the heat sink effect and increase the size of the ablative region. Another method of occlusion is embolization of feeding vessels with gel foam. These methods enable the generation of a larger ablative zone. Risks of hepatic artery occlusion and gel foam embolization do exist and should be considered [16].

Injection of NaCl-containing solutions has also been explored to overcome the heat sink effect [16, 19–21]. Pre-treatment with hypertonic saline, 5–36%, results in significantly higher temperatures and a significantly larger ablation zone when compared to no pre-treatment [19, 20]. The NaCl solutions can be injected at any point during the procedure to expand the size of the ablation zone [21].

Transarterial chemoembolization (TACE) combined with RFA is another widely studied technique for overcoming the heat sink phenomenon. Combining these two techniques has multiple benefits that have been shown in both animal and human models [22–24]. First, TACE reduces the amount of conductive cooling by reducing blood flow to the targeted region. The reduction in blood flow increases the size of the central ablation zone, thus increasing the amount of coagulative necrosis. In addition, the amount of tissue that receives sublethal hyperthermia is increased and simultaneously exposed to a chemotherapeutic agent. The synergy is created by increased membrane permeability, intratumoral accumulation of the pharmacologic agent, and increased drug sensitivity of the cells within the transitional zone [5, 6, 8, 24]. Liposomal doxorubicin has been well studied in the setting of liver malignancies and is a good choice of chemotherapeutic agent [22, 24]. The wider ablation margin with increased volume of both the central and transitional zone and high local concentration of chemotherapeutic agent results in destruction of microscopic satellite lesions surrounding the lesion consequently improving local control of the tumor [18, 24].

2.4. Immunologic response to RFA

To adequately discuss the immunologic response to RFA, the basic immunologic response must first be discussed. The immune system is composed of two basic parts, the innate and the adaptive immune systems. Both of these systems work in concert to mount a defense to pathogens, such as viruses and bacteria, and prevent unregulated cell growth. The immune system is able to recognize and eliminate both dangerous self and non-self cells through a system of complex interactions and "danger signals." However, in HCC and other malignancies, the cells evade the immune system through numerous mechanisms [4, 25].

Typically, the first response by the immune system that occurs is by the non-specific or innate immune system. The non-specific immune system is composed of natural killer cells (NK), mast cells, eosinophils, basophils, macrophages, neutrophils, and dendritic cells (DC). These cells are the first to mobilize and produce signals initiating the specific immune response. The specific or adaptive immune system is composed of B and T lymphocytes. With co-stimulation from the innate system, the adaptive system generates a robust and lasting immune response through the formation of antibodies and memory B and T cells. The basic process that must occur to achieve a full immune response is antigen recognition and presentation by antigen-presenting cells (APCs), subsequent recognition of the antigen by T-cells through interaction with APCs, cellular interaction generating costimulatory signals, and the presence of danger signals [4, 6]. It is important to mention the roles of CD4 or T helper cells (Th) and CD8 T cells or cytotoxic T cells (CTLs). In regards to antitumor immunity, the most important role of CD4 cells is to assist in the activation and proliferation of CD8 T cells. It is currently theorized that a high ratio of CD4:CD8 is important to forming lasting immunity to malignancies because of the role of CD4 cells in stimulating CD8 cells [30]. CD8 T cells have been the focus of antitumor immunity due to their ability to recognize MHC I molecules. MHC I molecules are used to display intracellular antigens on the surface of cells infected by viruses and malignant cells. CD8 cells bind to cells expressing specific MHC I molecule complexes and then destroy the targeted cells through the apoptotic cascade [26].

In contrast to HR where the objective is to completely remove the HCC lesion and occasionally remove local lymphoid tissues, minimally invasive techniques such as RFA leave necrosed tumor cells and their spilled intracellular materials behind. The retained intracellular materials, which were previously invisible to the immune system, can now act as antigens that trigger local and systemic immune responses to HCC. In addition to the release of antigenic material from the remaining necrotic tissues, danger signals, such as DNA, RNA, pro-inflammatory cytokines, uric acid, and heat-shock proteins (HSPs), are released. These damage-associated molecular pattern molecules (DAMPs) are then picked up by DCs and presented to T-cells starting the immune cascade. All of these DAMPs are inflammatory mediators and have the potential to trigger a robust tumor suppressing immune response but are only released by cells undergoing necrosis. Cells, which undergo apoptosis, may actually lead to tolerance if the ratio of apoptosis to necrosis within the lesion becomes too high [4, 25].

One class of DAMP of particular importance to RFA and other thermal ablative techniques is the heat shock protein (HSP) family. HSPs have special roles and are involved in protein folding, cellular signaling, cellular transport, and survival. HSPs are produced within cells in response to thermal injury and play a role as chaperones enabling the refolding of denatured proteins. Additionally, HSPs participate in the initiation of the adaptive immune response by presenting antigens to DCs, modulating DAMP-induced immune stimulation, and function as danger signals [25, 27]. HSPs' ability to chaperone peptides and provide maturation signals to dendritic cells causes the ultimate cross-presentation of antigen to CD8+ T cells. Independent of the adaptive response, HSPs induce local necrosis through stimulation of the innate immune system. HSPs' ability to efficiently stimulate both the innate and adaptive immune system holds great potential; therefore, upregulation of HSPs represents a potential approach to eliminate HCC and other malignancies [28].

In patients treated with RFA, there is a decreased response by CD25+ T-regulatory (Treg) cells [29]. Treg cells or T suppressor cells, a specific subset of T-cells, are responsible for downregulating the immune response. The Treg cell's role is to prevent autoimmune disease and create tolerance to self-antigens. Tregs achieve immunosuppression by downregulating CD4 and CD8 T cells, thus decreasing the tumoricidal immunologic response. In fact, high levels of CD25 T cells are associated with poorer outcomes in patients with malignancy [26]. Thus, patients with HCC can benefit from treatments that decrease the number of Treg cells and subsequent decreased immune tolerance of malignant cells. Indeed, RFA results in decreased counts of suppressive T cells, but additionally RFA shows increased survival benefit due to improved CD8 T-cell counts. The post ablation increase in CD8 T-cells is strongly associated with decreased recurrence and increased survival in patients with HCC [30]. Patients who will undergo HR or liver transplantation can also benefit from RFA-induced stimulation of CD8 cells. One major issue these patients face long term is disease recurrence. Unitt et al. showed improved survival in patients who demonstrate strong CD4 and CD8 T cell responses after undergoing resection surgery [31]. The response by CD4 and CD8 T cells as well as the increase of specific antibodies has been seen weeks to months following RFA [32].

Most of our knowledge about the immune response to RFA is based on animal models and small human trials. One of the first studies to show a significant immune response to RFA was conducted in 2003. In this animal study, tumors were implanted into rabbits that were then either untouched or treated with RFA. The RFA-treated animals showed at least a threefold increase in specific T-cell infiltration compared to the untreated animals. The treated animals also showed an increase in survival rate. This study suggested that an anticancer immunologic effect could be created through RFA [33]. This study was then further augmented by blocking CTLA-4 with monoclonal antibody at the time of RFA. This strongly enhanced antitumor immunity and provided protection against tumor rechallenge. This demonstrated that a lasting systemic memory response is achievable with combination therapy. Furthermore, a 20-fold increase in specific cytotoxic T-cells (CTLs) was achieved when RFA + blocking antibody was used compared to RFA + control antibody demonstrating that the increased immune response to RFA can be potentiated [34]. Zerbini et al. were the first to demonstrate an increased immunologic response in human subjects. The effect of RFA on 20 patients with HCC was studied and found to have a significant increase in tumor-specific T-cell response. Circulating T and natural killer (NK) cells showed increased activation and expression of specific cytotoxic surface markers. Although an upregulated immune response was demonstrated in these subjects, the effect was not associated with increased protection to HCC relapse [35]. Later, Zerbini and colleagues showed that the immunologic effects post RFA are dependent on maturation of DCs driven by the release of intracellular debris [36]. In a murine urothelial carcinoma model, subtotal RFA was used to induce an immunologic response. In response to subtotal RFA, there was an increase in CD4 and CD8 responses and significant tumor regression with rechallenge [37].

It is clear that numerous benefits of RFA exist and that there is great potential for targeted stimulation of the immune system using RFA in conjunction with immune modulators. Nevertheless, the possibility of causing rapid growth of metastases exists [38–40]. Recent accounts of RFA and other forms of ablation causing growth of distant metastases have been reported. These reports in conjunction with the fact that RFA will induce mediators such as cytokines, including interleukin-6 (IL-6) and factors such as hepatocyte growth factor (HGF), vascular endothelial growth factor (VEGF), hypoxia-induced factor-1α (HIF-1α), and HSPs, all have potential to cause tumor growth locally and distantly [38–42]. It is theorized that damage to the surrounding healthy liver parenchyma and following regeneration is the source of the pro-growth factors. Ahmed et al. [40] showed using a rat model that damaging normal hepatic tissue with RFA will induce distant tumor growth, which is mediated by VEGF and the HGF/c-Met pathway. Interestingly, multiple studies have shown that incomplete ablation of HCC will also promote not only distant growth but also local invasion [41, 43–45].

While increased local and distant growth of tumor cells is a real possibility, there are multiple studies investigating how to mitigate the pro-growth effects created by RFA. Studies have investigated c-Met and VEGF inhibitors to attenuate the tumorigenic effects [38, 40]. Additionally, studies have looked at non-specific anti-inflammatory drugs to mitigate the effects of RFA-induced inflammation on tumorigenesis. Both aspirin and celecoxib have been investigated to prevent tumorigenesis [41, 42]. In animal models, each of these drugs when used in conjunction with RFA reduced local inflammation and subsequent effects on distant tumor cells. Furthermore, it is crucial to note that while there is information about distant tumorigenesis following RFA, clinically RFA has not been shown to worsen survival compared to untreated patients and remains an effective first-line treatment in appropriate patients [46].

3. Cryoablation

3.1. Overview

Cryoablation is a thermal ablative technique that has been used since the nineteenth century. While other thermal ablative techniques add heat to the surrounding tissue, cryoablation removes heat. In its earliest form, a salt and ice solution was applied to breast and skin cancers. This treatment resulted in decreased pain and lesion size. In its current form, cryoablation is performed similarly to other ablative techniques. It can be used in either a percutaneous fashion, with image guidance, or through an open or laparoscopic surgical approach. Cryoablation is used to treat numerous types of cancers, but is most commonly used to treat liver, kidney, lung, prostate, and breast malignancies [47].

Modern cryoablation requires the use of a specialized cryoprobe that is inserted into the targeted lesion (**Figure 1**). Once in the desired location, the probe is rapidly cooled beginning the freeze cycle for a specified length of time. After the freeze cycle is completed, the probe is warmed up to start the thaw cycle. These freeze/thaw cycles are repeated one or more times depending on the lesion and preference of the clinician [47]. The mechanism of cooling relies on the Joule-Thompson effect that describes how a gas that does not work expands (adiabatic expansion) and results in a decrease in temperature [48]. All gases except hydrogen, helium, and neon will decrease in temperature when expanded through the Joule-Thompson process. Commonly used gases for the freeze cycle are nitrogen and argon. One of these gases is pumped into the cryoprobe, and when the gas reaches the distal tip of the probe, the gas is throttled and then allowed to rapidly expand to atmospheric pressure. The result is a rapid decrease in temperature and cooling of the surrounding tissues via conduction. During the freeze cycles, temperatures can reach as low as −160°C, well below the −20 to −40°C required to cause cell death [49]. As mentioned above, helium does not undergo this effect, rather than cooling when rapidly expanded helium will increase the temperature. For this reason, helium is used in the thaw cycle to heat the surrounding tissues [47].

Cryoablation results in direct and indirect cellular injury and death. When the freeze cycle begins, the tissues are cooled and ice starts to form in the extracellular space. Since the formation of ice occurs in the extracellular space before the intracellular space, an osmotic gradient

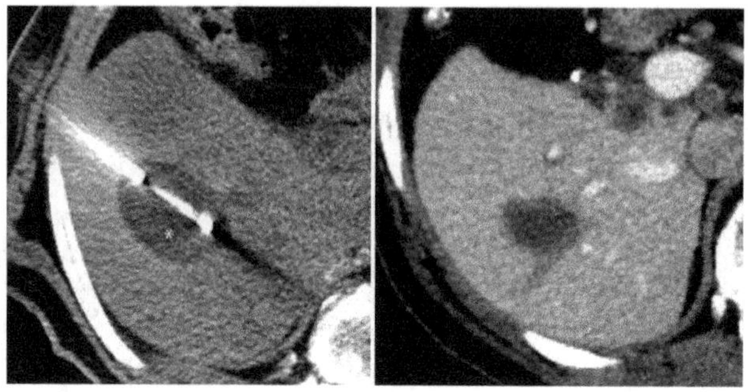

Figure 1. Hepatic cryoablation. A cryoablation needle was advanced into a focal hepatic lesion (left), with a resultant ice ball visible on CT (asterisk). Follow-up imaging demonstrated a focal defect at the site of the previous lesion (right), consistent with a complete ablation.

forms. This gradient pulls free water into the extracellular space increasing the solute concentration and dehydrating the cells. The high concentration of solutes intracellularly results in damage to enzymes and destabilizes membranes of both intracellular organelles and the cell [47]. Intracellular proteins are denatured as well, but return to their original conformation once thawing is completed [50]. Cells at the periphery of the ablation will remain intact and are not immediately killed by cryoablation. These cells will eventually undergo apoptosis that is triggered by damage to organelles [47].

When cells are frozen rapidly, there is no enough time for fluid shifts to occur, and cell death occurs via physical damage to organelles and the cellular membrane from intracellular ice formation. In both cases, pore formation in the membrane occurs, which allows for fluid shifts during the thaw cycle resulting in swelling and rupture [51]. The intracellular fluid shift during the thaw cycle occurs since extracellular ice melts before intracellular ice creating an osmotic gradient into the cell. It is important to note that intracellular ice will continue to grow during the thaw cycle reaching a maximum at −20 to −25°C. This formation of ice during the thaw cycle occurs due to the influx of free water. Additionally, the rate of thawing determines the amount of cellular death. Rapid thawing will decrease the biocidal effect by reducing the amount of intracellular ice formation. A greater degree of cellular death is seen in passive thawing when compared to active thawing. The highest degree of necrosis is seen with repeated freeze thaw cycles [52].

Indirect injury to cells occurs via vascular damage. During the freeze cycle, the endothelium of vessels is damaged, and when thawed, this injury triggers platelet aggregation. This aggregation leads to thrombosis and subsequent ischemia of the tissues [53]. The ischemia is twofold, not only does it lead to cellular death, but it also triggers inflammation. This leads to an influx of neutrophils and macrophages to the ablated zone [54]. The entire process can take months to complete, resulting in a zone of necrosis surrounded by a peripheral band of neutrophils [47].

3.2. Advantages and disadvantages of cryoablation

The one of the best advantages of cryoablation is the ability to monitor the ablation zone in real time. As the ablation proceeds, formation of an ice-ball occurs that is visible on ultrasound (US), magnetic resonance (MR), and CT. This occurs because the water molecules undergo a phase change and subsequent change in density. For example, during a cryoablation, the ablative zone will become hypoattenuating on CT. The leading edge of the ablation marks 0°C, since this region is where the phase change from liquid to solid is occurring [47].

In contrast to other modalities, such as RFA, each cryoprobe acts independently from the others and can be used simultaneously to tailor the shape of the ablation to the tumor. This is in sharp contrast to ablating with multiple RF probes where only one probe can be active at a time and they must be operated sequentially. Cryoablation additionally offers better pain control when compared to RFA [47]. The cooling of the tissues can create a level of analgesia not offered by hyperthermic ablative techniques. Cryoablation significantly reduces the amount of opioids used in the 24 hours following the procedure leading to shorter hospital stays [55]. In regards to HCC, it has been shown that RFA can induce ischemia-reperfusion injury of the liver resulting in cancer growth. With cryoablation, there is a lower potential for this type of injury decreasing the risk of cancer growth [56]. Cryoablation can also be used in patients who are candidates for RFA. Patients who are candidates are those with tumors <5 cm, single lesions, or multiple lesions <3 cm with a Child-Pugh class A or B liver function [57].

Cryoablation results in a robust inflammatory response following the procedure. This in combination with the fact that the released proteins return to their native conformation produces a large potential to create beneficial antitumor immunologic responses. The large amount of unaltered tumor antigen coupled with a large inflammatory response creates a scenario in which significant numbers of DCs are able to present a large amount of antigen to T cells [47, 50, 54]. The potential immunologic response will be discussed in detail later. This robust inflammatory response also presents a significant disadvantage, cryoshock [47, 57–59].

Cryoshock is a systemic immune response that leads to hypotension, respiratory distress, multiorgan failure, and disseminated intravascular coagulation. Similar reactions are not seen in patients treated with hyperthermic ablations. Cryoshock occurs in up to 1% of patients who undergo hepatic cryotherapy. Of this 1%, up to 18% of patients can die because of cryoshock [57, 58]. Cryoshock is thought to be mediated by the production of cytokine, such as IL-1β, IL-6, and tumor necrosis factor (TNF), from the robust immune response created by cryoablation [47, 57–60]. These are similar to the mediators found in patients with septic shock [59, 65]. Cryoshock typically occurs when large volume liver ablations are attempted [47]. An additional disadvantage of cryoablation is bleeding complications. Typically, these occur when performing large ablations within the liver. Frozen tissues are extremely brittle and may fracture leading to significant bleeding. For this reason, the user must be careful to not torque or reposition the probes once the ablation has started [61]. Although cryoablation has various disadvantages, it has a similar complication rate compared to RFA and remains a relatively safe and effective procedure for the treatment of HCC [57–60, 62].

3.3. Immunologic response to cryoablation

For several decades, the immune response to cryoablation has been known. In the 1970s, antitumor antibodies were first seen in humans following cryoablation [63]. Since then, it has been shown that cryoablation will induce specific anti-tumor cytotoxic effects post ablation. Lymphocytes produced post-ablation show specific affinity for tumor cells when rechallenged, whereas lymphocytes in patients post HR do not. Reintroduced tumor cells are also rendered less effective by the immunologic response [64].

Cryoablation is proven to create a more robust immunological response than hyperthermic ablative techniques such as RFA and MWA. Higher DC antigen loading due to hypothermic cytotoxicity generates the more robust immunologic response. Increased antigen presentation and subsequent heightened immune response are due to two main factors: increased antigen in the native conformation and less coagulation in the ablation zone [47]. The hypothermic mechanism of cryoablation leads to less regional coagulative effect when compared to hyperthermic ablations. This allows the antigens produced by cryoablation to more readily enter circulation and regional lymph nodes for presentation to DCs. The ability of cryoablation to preserve circulation is beneficial for stimulating the immune system but can be detrimental. The spilling of tumor antigens into circulation and subsequent cytokine release is also believed to be responsible for cryoshock.

Heightened levels of cytokines such as IL-1β, IL-6, TNF-α, and NF-κB are seen after cryoablation [65, 66]. Cryoablation used on hepatic malignancy will increase the levels of these specific cytokines up to 15–25 times more when compared to RFA. Interestingly, Erinjeri et al. found that the changes in WBC count increased linearly with ablation size but the levels of IL-6 did not [65], suggesting that larger ablative zones could trigger higher tumor-specific immune responses without added increased risk for cryoshock. Additionally, this group found that the predominant cytokines that are released post cryoablation, IL-6 and IL-10, stimulate a Th2 response.

According to the Th1/Th2 model, each subset triggers a different type of immunity. Th1 triggers cytotoxic lymphocytes and cellular immunity, whereas Th2 stimulates B-cells and antibody production. Signals that stimulate the Th1 response include IL-2, IL-12, IFN-γ, and TNF, and the cytokines that trigger the Th2 response include IL-4, IL-5, IL-6, IL-9, IL-10, and IL-13 [65, 67]. In addition, IL-6, which activates NF-κB and STAT3, has been implicated in hepatic regeneration and increased tumor regeneration post ablation. Regeneration is mediated by NF-κb and STAT3, both of which are activated by IL-6 [65]. Since, both IL-6 and IL-10 are increased after not only cryoablation but also hyperthermic ablation, they are potential targets for adjuvant immunologic therapy. Decreasing IL-6 could potentially increase the Th1 response (cellular-mediated tumor immunity) and decrease the growth of primary and metastatic hepatic malignancy post ablation [68].

Immune checkpoint inhibitor therapy, a new oncologic therapy that uses monoclonal antibody to target and block the T cell surface receptor CTLA-4, has potential use in combination therapy with cryoablation. The function of CTLA-4 is to inhibit self-reactive T-cells in order to prevent autoimmune diseases. However, in the case of cancer, it is beneficial for T cells to be able to recognize specific "self" cells. It has been shown that blockade of CTLA-4 will increase the CD8 T cell response as well as CD4 T cell memory when used as a monotherapy or combination immune therapy [69, 70]. Phase 3 trials using ipilimumab, a CTLA-4 blocking monoclonal antibody, have showed improved recurrence-free survival when used as an adjuvant treatment in patients with high-risk melanoma [71]. Combination cryotherapy with CTLA-4 blockade has been studied in prostate cancer. While cryoablation alone has not been shown to mediate the rejection of metastatic lesions, when combined with CTLA-4 blockade, it can mediate rejection of metastatic lesions and prevent disease recurrence [72].

While cryoablation has been strongly shown to activate the immune system, the opposite has also been seen. Multiple animal models have shown susceptibility to rechallenge and increased metastasis post ablation [73–75]. A possible explanation for these results is variation in the technical factors of cryoablation. Differing animal models, methods of freezing, length, number of freeze-thaw cycles, differences in minimum temperature achieved as well as differing ablation zone size and position all contribute to different clinical outcome and immunologic stimulation or anergy [73]. Sabel et al. established that variation in the technical parameters of cryoablation indeed affect the ratio of apoptosis to necrosis and subsequent immune response. Sabel et al. investigated the rate of freezing in an animal model using either a low or high rate of freezing. They found that a high rate of freezing induced a higher amount of necrosis when compared to a low rate of freezing. The high rate induced more danger signals stimulating a strong anti-tumor response [73]. A high ratio of apoptosis to necrosis has been shown to downregulate the immunologic response and even induce anergy [76]. When apoptotic cells are presented to DCs, a lower amount of TNF-α, IL-1β, IL-8, IL-10, IL-12, and granulocyte macrophage colony-stimulating factor (GM-CSF) produce inhibitory effects on these cells [77, 78]. The ablation zone size and percentage of tumor encompassed may play a role in the immunologic response. An experiment conducted in a murine metastatic liver tumor model demonstrated that smaller volume ablations show a significant decrease in metastasis [79].

4. Microwave ablation

4.1. Overview

Microwave ablation (MWA) is a hyperthermic ablative technique that is similar in many ways to RFA. MWA was introduced in the 1980s and 1990s and showed potential, but suffered from problems controlling the emitted field. There was a relatively high complication rate with MWA, thus RFA became the dominant ablative technique [80, 81]. While the early MWA systems had higher complication rates, since then newer designs have significantly decreased the complication rates. Recent retrospective and prospective studies have proven the efficacy and safety of MWA for not only HCC lesions but also other hepatic lesions [82–85].

From a procedural point of view, MWA and RFA are performed similarly under image guidance. The operator guides a MWA antenna toward the targeted lesion using their favored imaging modality (**Figure 2**). Unlike RFA, MWA does not require the use of grounding pads to establish an electrical circuit. MWA uses dielectric hysteresis to produce heat. An oscillating field, typically 900–2500 MHZ, is applied forcing polar molecules (such as water) to continuously move and realign in the field creating kinetic energy and ultimately raising the temperature of the tissue. Microwaves are able to propagate through a variety of tissues, even those with low electrical conductivity, high impedance, or low thermal conductivity. This makes MWA more versatile [86].

4.2. Advantages and disadvantages of MWA

MWA has the distinct advantage of being able to penetrate through high impedance tissues, meaning that even if charred or desiccated tissues build up near the probe, the field is able to penetrate and continue enlarging the ablation zone. Since MWA does not rely on conduction of tissue, heat is able to penetrate tissues with a high impedance such as lung or bone [86].

Multiple MWA antennas are able to be used synergistically to enlarge the ablation zone, achieve higher temperatures, or concomitantly ablate multiple lesions [87]. While RFA using multiple probes requires the probes to be used in series, MWA with multiple antennas can be used simultaneously with one power source. Due to the properties of MWA, there is future potential use ablating larger lesions than is currently possible.

The peak temperatures achieved in the central zone can readily exceed 100°C. The ability to achieve higher temperatures and use multiple probes simultaneously means shorter treatment times and larger area of coagulative necrosis and lethal hyperthermia. Higher temperatures and larger central zone lessen the effect of nearby heat sinks. It has been shown that large vessels <10 mm in size will not affect the ablation, making it possible to ablate lesions in regions that are not possible with RFA [88].

While MWA has many advantages, its ability to deliver a high amount of energy comes with several trade-offs. Coaxial cables have excellent properties for this application and are thus used to connect the antenna to the microwave generator. However, the coaxial cables used have a large diameter in order to avoid dangerous cable overheating. Larger diameter decreases the risk of overheating but becomes cumbersome and inflexible leading to difficulties while manipulating the antennas and performing the procedure [89]. The microwave antennas are likewise made using coaxial cable and also suffer from the same problem. In order for the antenna to handle higher power levels, the diameter must be increased or an active cooling system needs to be employed [86, 89].

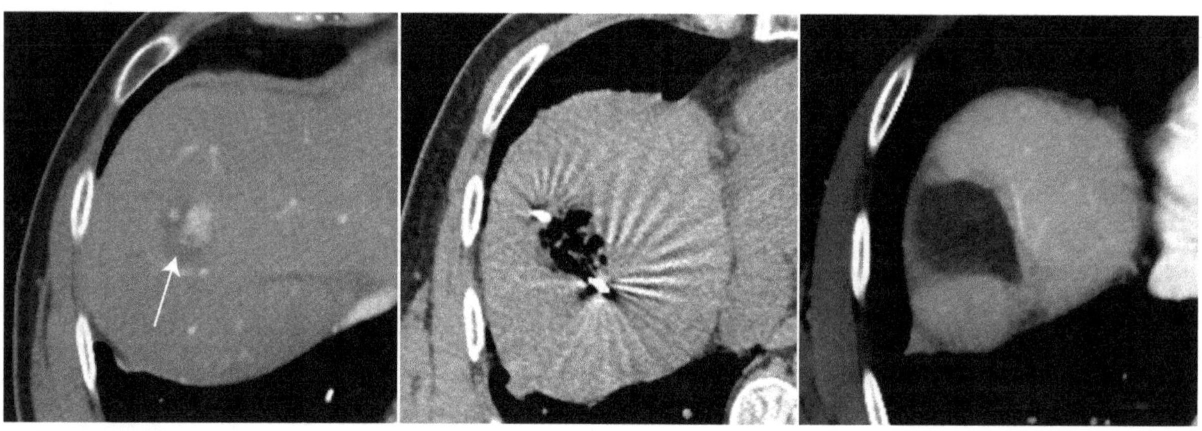

Figure 2. Hepatic microwave ablation. Pre-procedure imaging demonstrates a focal HCC lesion at the hepatic dome (left, arrow). Two microwave needles were advanced into the lesion, with gas bubbles developing during the ablation (middle). Follow-up imaging demonstrates a focal defect without enhancing viable tissue consistent with a complete ablation (right).

Active cooling systems have helped eliminate several problems. They allow a smaller diameter antenna to handle higher power and eliminate the risk of ablating healthy tissues along the proximal antenna tract, increase the size of the ablation, increase the amount of power delivered, and can prevent the probe from backing out. Various cooling methods have been employed from chilled saline to cooling with compressed gas utilizing the Joule-Thomson phenomenon [86]. Some newer probes that use the Joule-Thompson phenomenon are able to be locked into place by freezing the antenna tract to prevent it from moving or backing out.

Since the primary advantage of MWA is the ability to deliver, a significant amount of power safety concerns arises. With MWA, it is harder to predict the size of the ablation zone, which can lead to damage of surrounding structures. The shape of the ablation zone produced can be relatively thin and long increasing this risk. While problems with MWA exist, currently these issues should not limit its use ablating HCC and other lesions in the liver. MWA has been proven effective and comparatively safe to RFA when measuring complication rates [82–85].

4.3. Immunologic response to MWA

The immunologic response to MWA is less well characterized compared to other methods of ablation, such as RFA and cryoablation. The vast majority of the research regarding the immune response and immunologic stimulation has been studied with either RFA or cryoablation. Recently specific immunologic mechanisms and the effects following MWA have been studied in more detail. It has been assumed that the immunologic response to MWA is similar to the mechanism and response to RFA [90, 91]. Currently, our knowledge about the immune response to MWA comes from both animal and clinical trials of various tumor types from breast to hepatic carcinomas [92–94].

In regards to patient management and future treatment, the goal of therapy is to generate a lasting immune response that results in regression of distant lesions and generate protection from disease recurrence. As detailed in previous sections, the aim of treatment is to generate specific cytokines triggering the Th1 response and activating the cellular immune system. Similar to other ablative techniques, MWA alone is not powerful enough to trigger the desired immune response, but holds potential with combination therapy [90, 91].

The specific immune response to MWA in patients with HCC has been analyzed by Zhang et al. In their study, 45 patients with HCC treated with MWA had peripheral blood analysis following treatment. The results showed significant increases in IL-12 and decreases in IL-4 and IL-10 [91]. These results are promising since IL-12 is involved in the differentiation of Th1 cells and generation of cellular immunity. Furthermore, patients showed decreased levels of IL-4 and IL-10, which are involved in activation of humoral immunity. While MWA alone is not enough to create a significantly different clinical response, the cytokine profile produced is advantageous.

Various combination therapies have been studied ranging from OK-432, immunotherapy, GM-CSF, and CTLA-4 blockade [92–94]. OK-432, also known as picibanil, is a low virulence mixture of *Streptococcus pyogenes* that has been used as an antitumor agent since 1975 [95].

OK-432 is able to induce pro-inflammatory cytokines and activate the T-cell–mediated immunity. Li et al. demonstrated that MWA and OK-432 used in combination resulted in prolonged survival and a strong immunologic response to rechallenge in a murine model of breast cancer. The results showed that a dominant Th1 response is generated. The cytokines IL-12, IL-2, and IFN-γ were significantly increased with no effect on Th2-type cytokines. Additionally, immunohistochemical analysis showed that a predominance of CD8+ T cells infiltrating the treated tumors.

Immunotherapy combined with MWA for the treatment of HCC has been investigated in both phase I and phase II trials [93, 96]. This combination was shown to increase the absolute number of circulating lymphocytes. When analyzed for specific subgroups, patients showed increased levels of cytotoxic subsets of T cells and decreased suppressive subsets. Additionally, patients treated with immunotherapy had significantly improved liver function. However, the disease-free survival and overall survival rate were not significantly improved.

CTLA-4 blockade holds great promise when combined with cryoablation, but could also be used in with MWA. CTLA-4 blocking antibodies and GM-CSF combined with MWA were shown to induce tumor-specific cellular immune response in a murine model [94]. The combination of the three resulted in a 90% rejection upon tumor rechallenge and 50% of the animals treated showed distant tumor regression. Since both of these drugs are currently available for human use, this combination represents one that could be clinically used today.

5. Conclusion

Minimally invasive thermal-based therapy has become a reliable method for the treatment of HCC. Many advances in ablative therapy have occurred since their initial implementation ranging from design to technical implementation. The most promising of these advances is combination therapies that create a tumor-specific immunologic response. Combination therapy has shown great promise in the treatment and prevention of not only HCC, but also other malignancies. There is much more to learn about the immunologic reaction to ablative therapy creating an exciting time of investigation and discovery.

Author details

Andrew W. Ritchey[1], Joshua D. Kuban[2] and Rahul A. Sheth[2]*

*Address all correspondence to: rasheth@mdanderson.org

1 University of Texas Health Science Center Houston – McGovern Medical School, Houston, Texas, USA

2 MD Anderson Cancer Center, Houston, Texas, USA

References

[1] Li G, Staveley-O'Carroll K, Kimchi E. Potential of radiofrequency ablation in combination with immunotherapy in the treatment of hepatocellular carcinoma. Journal of Clinical Trials. Apr 2016;**6**(2):1-9. DOI: 10.4172/2167-0870.1000257

[2] Cui J, Wang N, Zhao H, Haofan J, Wang G, Niu C, Terunuma H, He H, Li W. Combination of radiofrequency ablation and sequential cellular immunotherapy improves progression-free survival for patients with hepatocellular carcinoma. International Journal of Cancer. 2014;**134**:342-351. DOI: 10.1002/ijc.28372

[3] Takaki H et al. Thermal ablation and immunomodulation: From preclinical experiments to clinical trials. Diagnostic and Interventional Imaging. 2017;**98**:651-659

[4] Bastianpillai C, Petrides N, Shah T, Guillaumier S, Ahmed H, Arya M. Harnessing the immunomodulatory effect of thermal and non-thermal ablative therapies for cancer treatment. Tumour Biology. Dec 2015;**36**(12):9137-9146. DOI: 10.1007/s13277-015-4126-3

[5] Chu K, Dupuy D. Thermal ablation of tumours: Biological mechanisms and advances in therapy. Nature Reviews Cancer. Mar 2014;**14**(3):199-208. DOI: 10.1038/nrc3672

[6] Mehta A, Oklu R, Sheth R. Thermal ablative therapies and immune checkpoint modulation: Can locoregional approaches effect a systemic response? Gastroenterology Research and Practice. 2016;**2016**:9251375. DOI: 10.1155/2016/9251375

[7] Goldberg SN, Ahmed M, Gazelle GS, Kruskal JB, Huertas JC, Halpern EF, Oliver BS, Lenkinski RE. Radio-frequency thermal ablation with NaCl solution injection: Effect of electrical conductivity on tissue heating and coagulation-phantom and porcine liver study. Radiology. 2001;**219**(1):157-165. DOI: 10.1148/radiology.219.1.r01ap27157

[8] Ahmed M, Brace C, Lee F, Goldberg S. Principles of and advances in percutaneous ablation. Radiology. 2011;**258**(2):351-369. DOI: 10.1148/radiol.10081634

[9] Thompson SM, Callstrom MR, Butters KA, Knudsen B, Grande JP, Roberts LR, Woodrum DA. Heat stress induced cell death mechanisms in hepatocytes and hepatocellular carcinoma: In vitro and in vivo study. Lasers in Surgery and Medicine. 2014; **46**(4):290-301. DOI: 10.1002/lsm.2223

[10] Duan C, Liu M, Zhang Z, Ma K, Bie P. Radiofrequency ablation versus hepatic resection for the treatment of early-stage hepatocellular carcinoma meeting Milan criteria: A systematic review and meta-analysis. World Journal of Surgical Oncology. 2013;**11**(1):190. DOI: 10.1186/1477-7819-11-190

[11] DS L, NC Y, Raman SS, Limanond P, Lassman C, et al. Radiofrequency ablation of hepatocellular carcinoma: Treatment success as defined by histologic examination of the explanted liver. Radiology. 2005;**234**(3):954-960. DOI: 10.1148/radiol.2343040153

[12] Dromain C, de Baere T, Elias D, et al. Hepatic tumors treated with percutaneous radiofrequency ablation: CT and MR imaging follow-up. Radiology. 2002;**223**(1):255-262. DOI: 10.1148/radiol.2231010780

[13] Molinari M, Helton S. Hepatic resection versus radiofrequency ablation for hepatocellular carcinoma in cirrhotic individuals not candidates for liver transplantation: A Markov model decision analysis. American Journal of Surgery. 2009;**198**(3):396-406. DOI: 10.1016/j.amjsurg.2009.01.016

[14] Cho YK, Kim JK, Kim WT, Chung JW. Hepatic resection versus radiofrequency ablation for very early stage hepatocellular carcinoma: A Markov model analysis. Hepatology. 2010;**51**(4):1284-1290. DOI: 10.1002/hep.23466

[15] DS L, Raman SS, Vodopich DJ, Wang M, Sayre J, Lassman C. Effect of vessel size on creation of hepatic radiofrequency lesions in pigs: Assessment of the "heat sink" effect. American Journal of Roentgenology. 2002;**178**(1):47-51. DOI: 10.2214/ajr.178.1.1780047

[16] DS L, Raman SS, Limanond P, Aziz D, Economou J, Busuttil R, Sayre J. Influence of large peritumoral vessels on outcome of radiofrequency ablation of liver tumors. Journal of Vascular and Interventional Radiology. 2003;**14**(10):1267-1274

[17] Rossi S, Garbagnati F, De Francesco I, Accocella F, Leonardi L, Quaretti P, Zangrandi A, Paties C, Lencioni R. Relationship between the shape and size of radiofrequency induced thermal lesions and hepatic vascularization. Tumori. 1999;**85**(2):128-132

[18] Rossi S, Garbagnati F, Lencioni R, Allgaier HP, Marchianò A, Fornari F, Quaretti P, Tolla GD, Ambrosi C, Mazzaferro V, Blum HE, Bartolozzi C. Percutaneous radio-frequency thermal ablation of nonresectable hepatocellular carcinoma after occlusion of tumor blood supply. Radiology. 2000;**217**(1):119-126. DOI: 10.1148/radiology.217.1.r00se02119

[19] Ahmed M, Lobo SM, Weinstein J, Kruskal JB, Gazelle GS, Halpern EF, Afzal SK, Lenkinski RE, Goldberg SN. Improved coagulation with saline solution pretreatment during radiofrequency tumor ablation in a canine model. Journal of Vascular and Interventional Radiology. 2002;**13**(7):717-724

[20] Lee JM, Han JK, Kim SH, Shin KS, Lee JY, Park HS, Hur H, Choi BI. Comparison of wet radiofrequency ablation with dry radiofrequency ablation and radiofrequency ablation using hypertonic saline preinjection: Ex vivo bovine liver. Korean Journal of Radiology. 2004;**5**(4):258-265. DOI: 10.3348/kjr.2004.5.4.258

[21] A1 S, Ishizaka H, Awata S, Shiraishi A, Hirasawa S, Tatezawa T, Kano M, Shimodaira K, Taketomi-Takahashi A, Tsushima Y, Endo K. Expansion of radiofrequency ablation volume by saturated NaCl saline injection in the area of vaporization. Acta Radiologica. 2009;**50**(1):61-64. DOI: 10.1080/02841850802562071

[22] Ahmed M, Goldberg SN. Combination radiofrequency thermal ablation and adjuvant IV liposomal doxorubicin increases tissue coagulation and intratumoural drug accumulation. International Journal of Hyperthermia. 2004;**20**(7):781-802

[23] Goldberg SN, Kamel IR, Kruskal JB, Reynolds K, Monsky WL, Stuart KE, Ahmed M, Raptopoulos V. Radiofrequency ablation of hepatic tumors: Increased tumor destruction with adjuvant liposomal doxorubicin therapy. AJR – American Journal of Roentgenology. 2002;**179**(1):93-101. DOI: 10.2214/ajr.179.1.1790093

[24] Higgins M, Soulen M. Combining locoregional therapies in the treatment of hepatocellular carcinoma. Seminars in Interventional Radiology. 2013;**30**(1):74-81. DOI: 10.1055/s-0033-1333656

[25] Pradeu T, Cooper EL. The danger theory: 20 years later. Frontiers in Immunology. 2015; **3**(287):56-61

[26] Adeegbe DO, Nishikawa H. Natural and induced T regulatory cells in cancer. Frontiers in Immunology. 2013;**4**:190. DOI: https://doi.org/10.3389/fimmu.2013.00190

[27] Calderwood SK, Ciocca DR. Heat shock proteins: Stress proteins with Janus-like properties in cancer. International Journal of Hyperthermia. 2008;**24**(1):31-39

[28] Milani V, Noessner E, Ghose S, Kuppner M, Ahrens B, Scharner A, Gastpar R, Issels RD. Heat shock protein 70: Role in antigen presentation and immune stimulation. International Journal of Hyperthermia. 2002;**18**(6):563-575. DOI: 10.1080/02656730210166140

[29] Fietta AM, Morosini M, Passadore I, Cascina A, Draghi P, Dore R, Rossi S, Pozzi E, Meloni F. Systemic inflammatory response and downmodulation of peripheral CD25+Foxp3+ T-regulatory cells in patients undergoing radiofrequency thermal ablation for lung cancer. Human Immunology. 2009;**70**(7):477-486. DOI: 10.1016/j.humimm.2009.03.012 Epub 2009 Mar 27

[30] Hiroishi K, Eguchi J, Baba T, Shimazaki T, Ishii S, Hiraide A, Sakaki M, Doi H, Uozumi S, Omori R, Matsumura T, Yanagawa T, Ito T, Imawari M. Strong CD8(+) T-cell responses against tumor-associated antigens prolong the recurrence-free interval after tumor treatment in patients with hepatocellular carcinoma. Journal of Gastroenterology. 2010; **45**(4):451-458. DOI: 10.1007/s00535-009-0155-2

[31] Unitt E, Marshall A, Gelson W, Rushbrook SM, Davies S, Vowler SL, Morris LS, Coleman N, Alexander GJ. Tumour lymphocytic infiltrate and recurrence of hepatocellular carcinoma following liver transplantation. Journal of Hepatology. 2006;**45**(2):246-253. DOI: 10.1016/j.jhep.2005.12.027

[32] Widenmeyer M, Shebzukhov Y, Haen SP, Schmidt D, Clasen S, Boss A, Kuprash DV, Nedospasov SA, Stenzl A, Aebert H, Wernet D, Stevanović S, Pereira PL, Rammensee HG, Gouttefangeas C. Analysis of tumor antigen-specific T cells and antibodies in cancer patients treated with radiofrequency ablation. International Journal of Cancer. 2011; **128**(11):2653-2662. DOI: 10.1002/ijc.25601

[33] Wissniowski TT, Hänsler J, Neureiter D, Frieser M, Schaber S, Esslinger B, Voll R, Strobel D, Hahn EG, Schuppan D. Activation of tumor-specific T lymphocytes by radio-frequency ablation of the VX2 hepatoma in rabbits. Cancer Research. 2003;**63**(19):6496-6500

[34] Den Brok MH, Sutmuller RP, van der Voort R, Bennink EJ, Figdor CG, Ruers TJ, et al. In situ tumor ablation creates an antigen source for the generation of antitumor immunity. Cancer Research. 2004;**64**(11):4024-4029

[35] Zerbini A, Pilli M, Penna A, Pelosi G, Schianchi C, Molinari A, et al. Radiofrequency thermal ablation of hepatocellular carcinoma liver nodules can activate and enhance tumor-specific T-cell responses. Cancer Research. 2006;**66**(2):1139-1146

[36] Zerbini A, Pilli M, Fagnoni F, Pelosi G, Pizzi MG, Schivazappa S, et al. Increased immunostimulatory activity conferred to antigen-presenting cells by exposure to antigen extract from hepatocellular carcinoma after radiofrequency thermal ablation. Journal of Immunotherapy. 2008;**31**(3):271-282. DOI: 10.1097/CJI.0b013e318160ff1c

[37] Dromi SA, Walsh MP, Herby S, Traughber B, Xie J, Sharma KV, et al. Radiofrequency ablation induces antigen-presenting cell infiltration and amplification of weak tumor-induced immunity. Radiology. 2009;**251**(1):58-66

[38] Rozenblum N, Zeira E, Scaiewicz V, Bulvik B, Gourevitch S, Yotvat H, Galun E, Goldberg SN. Oncogenesis: An "off-target" effect of radiofrequency ablation. Radiology. 2015;**276**(2):426-432. DOI: 10.1148/radiol.2015141695

[39] Nijkamp M, Borren A, Govaert K, et al. Radiofrequency ablation of colorectal liver metastases induces an inflammatory response in distant hepatic metastases but not in local accelerated outgrowth. Journal of Surgical Oncology. 2010;**101**(7):551-556

[40] Ahmed M, Kumar G, Moussa M, et al. Hepatic radiofrequency ablation-induced stimulation of distant tumor growth is suppressed by c-Met inhibition. Radiology. 2016;**279**(1):103-117. DOI: 10.1148/radiol.2015150080

[41] Jiang T, Zhang X, Ding J, Duan B, Inflammation LS. Cancer: Inhibiting the progression of residual hepatic VX2 carcinoma by anti-inflammatory drug after incomplete radiofrequency ablation. International Journal of Clinical and Experimental Pathology. 2015;**8**(11):13945-13956

[42] Kumar G, Goldberg SN, Wang Y, Velez E, Gourevitch S, Galun E, Ahmed M. Hepatic radiofrequency ablation: Markedly reduced systemic effects by modulating periablational inflammation via cyclooxygenase-2 inhibition. European Radiology. 2017;**27**(3):1238-1247. DOI: 10.1007/s00330-016-4405-4

[43] Zhang N, Wang L, Chai ZT, Zhu ZM, Zhu XD, Ma DN, Zhang QB, Zhao YM, Wang M, Ao JY, Ren ZG, Gao DM, Sun HC, Tang ZY. Incomplete radiofrequency ablation enhances invasiveness and metastasis of residual cancer of hepatocellular carcinoma cell HCCLM3 via activating β-catenin signaling. PLoS One. 2014;**9**(11):e115949. DOI: 10.1371/journal.pone.0115949

[44] Kong J, Kong L, Ke S, Gao J, Ding X, Zheng L, Sun H, Sun W. After insufficient radiofrequency ablation, tumor-associated endothelial cells exhibit enhanced angiogenesis and promote invasiveness of residual hepatocellular carcinoma. Journal of Translational Medicine. 2012;**10**:230. DOI: 10.1186/1479-5876-10-230

[45] Kong J, Pan B, Ke S, Dong S, Li X, Zhou A, Zheng L, Sun WB. Insufficient radiofrequency ablation promotes angiogenesis of residual hepatocellular carcinoma via HIF-1alpha/VEGFA. PLoS One. 2012;**7**:e37266. DOI: 10.1371/journal.pone.0037266

[46] Lencioni R, Cioni D, Crocetti L, et al. Early-stage hepatocellular carcinoma in patient with cirrhosis: Long-term results of percutaneous image-guided radiofrequency ablation. Radiology. 2005;**234**(3):961-967. DOI: 10.1148/radiol.2343040350

[47] Erinjeri JP, Clark TW. Cryoablation: Mechanism of action and devices. Journal of Vascular and Interventional Radiology. 2010;**21**(8):187-191. DOI: 10.1016/j.jvir.2009.12.403

[48] O'Rourke AP, Haemmerich D, Prakash P, Converse MC, Mahvi DM, Webster JG. Current status of liver tumor ablation devices. Expert Review of Medical Devices . 2014;**4**(4):523-537. DOI: http://dx.doi.org/10.1586/17434440.4.4.523

[49] Baust J, Gage A, Ma H, Zhang CM. Minimally invasive cryosurgery—Technological advances. Cryobiology. 1997;**34**(4):373-384. DOI: https://doi.org/10.1006/cryo.1997.2017

[50] Privalov P. Cold denaturation of protein. Critical Reviews in Biochemistry and Molecular Biology. 1990;**25**(4):281-306. DOI: http://dx.doi.org/10.3109/10409239009090612

[51] Baust J, Gage A. The molecular basis of cryosurgery. BJU International. 2005;**95**(9):1187-1191. DOI: 10.1111/j.1464-410X.2005.05502.x

[52] Woolley M, Schulsinger D, Durand D, Zeltser I, Waltzer W. Effect of freezing parameters (freeze cycle and thaw process) on tissue destruction following renal Cryoablation. Journal of Endourology. 2004;**16**(7):519-522. DOI: https://doi.org/10.1089/089277902760367494

[53] Finelli A, Rewcastle J, Jewett M. Cryotherapy and radiofrequency ablation: Pathophysiologic basis and laboratory studies. Current Opinion in Urology. 2003;**13**(3):187-191

[54] Weber S, Lee F, Chinn D, Warner T, Chosy S, Mahvi D. Perivascular and intralesional tissue necrosis after hepatic cryoablation: Results in a porcine model. Surgery. 1997;**122**(4):742-747. DOI: https://doi.org/10.1016/S0039-6060(97)90082-9

[55] Thacker PG, Callstrom MR, Curry TB, Mandrekar JN, Atwell TD, Goetz MP, Rubin J. Palliation of painful metastatic disease involving bone with imaging-guided treatment: Comparison of patients' immediate response to radiofrequency ablation and cryoablation. AJR – American Journal of Roentgenology. 2011;**197**(2):510-515. DOI: 10.2214/AJR.10.6029

[56] Song K. Percutaneous cryoablation for hepatocellular carcinoma. Clinical and Molecular Hepatology. 2016;**22**(4):509-515. DOI: 10.3350/cmh.2016.0079

[57] Yang Y, Wang C, Lu Y, Bai W, An L, Qu J, Gao X, Chen Y, Zhou L, Wu Y, Feng Y, Zhang M, Chang X, Ly J. Outcomes of ultrasound-guided percutaneous argon-helium cryoablation of hepatocellular carcinoma. Journal of Hepato-Biliary-Pancreatic Sciences. 2012;**19**(6):674-684. DOI: 10.1007/s00534-011-0490-6

[58] Seifert JK, Morris DL. World survey on the complications of hepatic and prostate cryotherapy. World Journal of Surgery. 1999;**23**(2):109-113

[59] Seifert JK, Stewart GJ, Hewitt PM, Bolton EL, Junginger T, Morris DL. Interleukin-6 and tumor necrosis factor-α levels following hepatic Cryotherapy: Association with volume and duration of freezing. World Journal of Surgery. 1999;**23**(10):1019-1026

[60] Sheen AJ, Poston GJ, Sherlock DJ. Cryotherapeutic ablation of liver tumours. The British Journal of Surgery. 2002;**89**(11):1396-1401. DOI: 10.1046/j.1365-2168.2002.02292.x

[61] Hruby G, Edelstein A, Karpf J, et al. Risk factors associated with renal parenchymal fracture during laparoscopic cryoablation. BJU International. 2008;**102**(6):723-726. DOI: 10.1111/j.1464-410X.2008.07735.x

[62] Adam R, Hagopian EJ, Linhares M, Krissat J, Savier E, Azoulay D, Kunstlinger F, Castaing D, Bismuth H. A comparison of percutaneous cryosurgery and percutaneous radiofrequency for unresectable hepatic malignancies. Archives of Surgery. 2002;**137**(12):1332-1339

[63] Soanes WA, Ablin RJ, Gonder MJ. Remission of metastatic lesions following cryosurgery in prostatic cancer: Immunologic considerations. The Journal of Urology. 1970;**104**(1): 154-159

[64] Neel HB, Ketcham AS, Hammond WG. Experimental evaluation of in situ oncocide for primary tumor therapy: Comparison of tumor-specific immunity after complete excision, cryonecrosis and ligation. The Laryngoscope. 1973;**83**(3):376-387. DOI: 10.1288/00005537-197303000-00009

[65] Erinjeri JP, Thomas CT, Samoilia A, Fleisher M, Gonen M, Sofocleous CT, Thornton RH, Siegelbaum RH, Covey AM, Brody LA, Alago W Jr, Maybody M, Brown KT, Getrajdman GI, Solomon SB. Image-guided thermal ablation of tumors increases the plasma level of interleukin-6 and interleukin-10. 2013. Journal of Vascular and Interventional Radiology. 2013;**24**(8):1105-1112. DOI: 10.1016/j.jvir.2013.02.015

[66] Ahmad F, Gravante G, Bhardwaj N, et al. Changes in interleukin-1β and 6 after hepatic microwave tissue ablation compared with radiofrequency, cryotherapy and surgical resections. American Journal of Surgery. 2010;**200**(4):500-506

[67] Schwacha MG, Schneider CP, Chaudry IH. Differential expression and tissue compartmentalization of the inflammatory response following thermal injury. Cytokine. 2002; **17**(5):266-274. DOI: https://doi.org/10.1006/cyto.2001.1003

[68] Trikha M. Targeted anti-interleukin-6 monoclonal antibody therapy for cancer: A review of the rationale and clinical evidence. Clinical Cancer Research. 2003;**9**(13):4653-4665

[69] Hokey DA, Yan J, Hirao LA, Dai A, Boyer JD, Jure-Kunkel MN, Weiner DB. CLTA-4 blockade in vivo promotes the generation of short-lived effector CD8 T cells and a more persistent central memory CD4 T cell response. Journal of Medical Primatology. 2008;**37**(8):62-68. DOI: 10.1111/j.1600-0684.2008.00324.x

[70] Spranger S, Koblish HK, Horton B, Scherle PA, Newton R, Gajewski TF. Mechanism of tumor rejection with doublets of CTLA-4, PD-1/PD-L1, or IDO blockade involves restored IL-2 production and proliferation of CD8(+) T cells directly within the tumor microenvironment. Journal for ImmunoTherapy of Cancer. 2014;**2**(1):3. DOI: 10.1186/2051-1426-2-3

[71] Eggermont AM, Chiarion-Sileni V, Grob JJ, Dummer R, Wolchok JD, Schmidt H, O7 H, Robert C, Ascierto PA, Richards JM, Lebbé C, Ferraresi V, Smylie M, Weber JS, Maio M, Konto C, Hoos A, de Pril V, Gurunath RK, de Schaetzen G, Suciu S, Testori A. Adjuvant ipilimumab versus placebo after complete resection of high-risk stage III melanoma (EORTC 18071): A randomised, double-blind, phase 3 trial. The Lancet Oncology. 2015;**16**(5):522-530. DOI: 10.1016/S1470-2045(15)70122-1

[72] Waitz R, Solomon SB, Petre EN, Trumble AE, Fasso M, Norton L, Allison JP. Potent induction of tumor immunity by combining tumor Cryoablation with anti–CTLA-4 therapy. Cancer Research. 2012;**72**(2):430-439. DOI: 10.1158/0008-5472.CAN-11-1782

[73] Sabel MS, Su G, Griffith KA, Chang AE. Rate of freeze alters the immunologic response after cryoablation of breast cancer. Annals of Surgical Oncology. 2010;**17**(4):1187-1193. DOI: 10.1245/s10434-009-0846-1

[74] Yamashita T, Hayakawa K, Hosokawa M, Kodama T, Inoue N, Tomita K, et al. Enhanced tumor metastases in rats following cryosurgery of primary tumor. Gann. 1982;**73**:222-228

[75] Shibata T, Yamashita T, Suzuki K, Takeichi N, Micallef M, Hosokawa M, et al. Enhancement of experimental pulmonary metastasis and inhibition of subcutaneously transplanted tumor growth following cryosurgery. Anticancer Research. 1998;**18**(4):4443-4448

[76] Savill J, Dransfield I, Gregory C, Haslett C. A blast from the past: Clearance of apoptotic cells regulates immune responses. Nature Reviews. Immunology. 2002;**2**(12):965-975

[77] Stuart LM, Lucas M, Simpson C, Lamb J, Savill J, Lacy-Hulbert A. Inhibitory effects of apoptotic cell ingestion upon endotoxin-driven myeloid dendritic cell maturation. Journal of Immunology. 2002;**168**(4):1627-1635

[78] Fadok VA, Bratton DL, Konowal A, Freed PW, Westcott JY, Henson PM. Macrophages that have ingested apoptotic cells in vitro inhibit proinflammatory cytokine production through autocrine/paracrine mechanisms involving TGF-beta, PGE2, and PAF. The Journal of Clinical Investigation. 1998;**101**(4):890-898. DOI: 10.1172/JCI1112

[79] Urano M, Tanaka C, Sugiyama Y, Miya K, Saji S. Antitumor effects of residual tumor after cryoablation: The combined effect of residual tumor and a protein-bound polysaccharide on multiple liver metastases in a murine model. Cryobiology. 2003;**46**(3): 238-245

[80] Poggi G, Tosoratti N, Montagna B, Picchi C. Microwave ablation of hepatocellular carcinoma. World Journal of Hepatology. 2015;**7**(25):2578-2589. DOI: 10.4254/wjh.v7.i25.2578

[81] Ohmoto K, Yoshioka N, Tomiyama Y, Shibata N, Kawase T, Yoshida K, Kuboki M, Yamamoto S. Comparison of therapeutic effects between radiofrequency ablation and percutaneous microwave coagulation therapy for small hepatocellular carcinomas. Journal of Gastroenterology and Hepatology. 2009;**24**(2):223-227. DOI: 10.1111/j.1440-1746.2008.05596.x

[82] Poggi G, Montagna B, DI Cesare P, Riva G, Bernardo G, Mazzucco M, Riccardi A. Microwave ablation of hepatocellular carcinoma using a new percutaneous device: Preliminary results. Anticancer Research. 2013;**33**(3):1221-1227

[83] Ziemlewicz T, Hinshaw JL, Lubner MG, Brace CL, Alexander ML, Agarwal P, Lee FT. Percutaneous microwave ablation of hepatocellular carcinoma with a gas-cooled system: initial clinical results with 107 tumors. Journal of Vascular and Interventional Radiology. 2015;**26**(1):62-68. DOI: 10.1016/j.jvir.2014.09.012

[84] Ierardi AM, Mangano A, Floridi C, Dionigi G, Biondi A, Duka E, Lucchina N, Lianos GD, Carrafiello G. A new system of microwave ablation at 2450 MHz: Preliminary experience. Updates in Surgery. 2015;**67**(1):39-45. DOI: 10.1007/s13304-015-0288-1

[85] Martin RC, Scoggins CR, McMasters KM. Safety and efficacy of microwave ablation of hepatic tumors: A prospective review of a 5-year experience. Annals of Surgical Oncology. 2010;**17**(1):171-178. DOI: 10.1245/s10434-009-0686-z

[86] Lubner MG, Brace CL, Hinshaw JL, Lee FT Jr. Microwave tumor ablation: Mechanism of action, clinical results, and devices. Journal of Vascular and Interventional Radiology. 2010;**21**(8):192-203. DOI: 10.1016/j.jvir.2010.04.007

[87] Trembly BS, Douple EB, Ryan TP, Hoopes PJ. Effect of phase modulation on the temperature distribution of a microwave hyperthermia antenna array in vivo. International Journal of Hyperthermia. 1994;**10**(5):691-705. DOI: http://dx.doi.org/10.3109/02656739409022448

[88] Yu NC, Raman SS, Kim YJ, Lassman C, Chang X, Lu DS. Microwave liver ablation: Influence of hepatic vein size on heat-sink effect in a porcine model. Journal of Vascular and Interventional Radiology. 2008;**19**(7):1087-1092. DOI: https://doi.org/10.1016/j.jvir.2008.03.023

[89] Brace CL. Microwave ablation technology: What every user should know. Current Problems in Diagnostic Radiology. 2009;**38**(2):61-67. DOI: https://doi.org/10.1067/j.cpradiol.2007.08.011

[90] Li X, Liang P. Immunotherapy for hepatocellular carcinoma following thermal ablation. Journal of BUON. 2014;**19**(4):867-871

[91] Zhang H, Hou X, Cai H, Zhuang X. Effects of microwave ablation on T-cell subsets and cytokines of patients with hepatocellular carcinoma. Minimally Invasive Therapy & Allied Technologies. 2017;**26**(4):207-211. DOI: 10.1080/13645706.2017.1286356

[92] Li L, Wang W, Pan H, Ma G, Shi X, Xie H, Liu X, Ding Q, Zhou W, Wang S. Microwave ablation combined with OK-432 induces Th1-type response and specific antitumor immunity in a murine model of breast cancer. Journal of Translational Medicine. 2017;**15**(1):23. DOI: 10.1186/s12967-017-1124-9

[93] MA Y, Liang P, XL Y, Han ZY, Dong XJ, Wang YU, Chenq C, Li X. Multiple courses of immunotherapy with different immune cell types for patients with hepatocellular carcinoma after microwave ablation. Experimental and Therapeutic Medicine. 2015; **10**(4):1460-1466. DOI: 10.3892/etm.2015.2681

[94] Chen Z, Shen S, Peng B, Tao J. Intratumoural GM-CSF microspheres and CTLA-4 blockade enhance the antitumour immunity induced by thermal ablation in a subcutaneous murine hepatoma model. International Journal of Hyperthermia. 2009;**25**(5):374-382. DOI: 10.1080/02656730902976807

[95] Ryoma Y, Moriya Y, Okamoto M, Kanaya I, Saito M, Sato M. Biological effect of OK-432 (picibanil) and possible application to dendritic cell therapy. Anticancer Research. 2004; **25**(5):3295-3301

[96] Zhou P, Liang P, Dong B, Yu X, Han Z, Xu Y. Phase I clinical study of combination therapy with microwave ablation and cellular immunotherapy in hepatocellular carcinoma. Cancer Biology & Therapy. 2011;**11**(5):450-456

7

Cellular Senescence and their Role in Liver Metabolism in Health and Disease: Overview and Future Directions

Matthew Schade, Jacqueline A Sanabria, Milad Modarresi, Bryan Gillon, Zach Hunter, Jacqueline Fannin, Amrita Mallick, Henri Brunengraber and Juan Sanabria

Abstract

Chronic liver disease has globally risen mainly due to a prevalent hepatitis C virus (HCV) infection rate and an epidemic of obesity. It is estimated by the year 2030, 2.2 billion people around the world will be overweight and 1.1 billion people will be obese. Diabetes and obesity are the main risk factors for the development of the metabolic syndrome and in the liver of non-alcoholic fatty liver disease (NAFLD) which could progress to non-alcoholic fatty steatohepatitis (NASH) related cirrhosis and liver malignancy. At present there is not effective therapy for NASH besides loss of weight and exercise. Furthermore, optimal management of HCC with curative intent includes resection or liver transplantation. Nevertheless, these therapies are limited because the degree of liver dysfunction or the medical conditions at the time of diagnosis and the scarcity of available liver grafts. The role of cellular lipid management and metabolism in human health and disease is taking a center stage. The present overview articulates the current pathophysiology of fatty liver disease under the aging processes, potential biological markers of liver disease diagnosis and progression and future therapies.

Keywords: review, senescence, cell aging, mitochondrial function, cancer, obesity, NASH, ROS, lipids, metabolism

1. Introduction

1.1. Global burden of chronic liver disease

Chronic liver disease has globally risen due to mainly a prevalent hepatitis C virus (HCV) infection rate and an epidemic of obesity [1–7]. During the last 2 decades, global viral hepatitis has increased by 163% (from 0.89 million to 1.45 million) and in 2013, viral hepatitis infections became the 7th leading cause of death [7]. While HBV infection is decreasing in most endemic areas due to successful vaccination policies, HCV infection lacks the benefits of a vaccine [7]. Even though HVC antiviral therapies recently introduced in clinical practice are highly successful, its implementation is limited due to access and/or financial constraints. Morphological studies in HCV showed hepatocyte lipid accumulation similar to the one that occurs in obesity.

Our group has estimated that 2.2 billion people will be overweight and 1.1 billion people will be obese globally by 2030 [8, 9]. In addition, 36.1% of adult men and 32.4% of adult women were diagnosed with the metabolic syndrome in 2010 [10]. Obesity represents the core component of the metabolic syndrome, a cluster of metabolic disarrangements including dyslipidemias, insulin resistance status, hypertension, diabetes and organ metabolic disturbances such as non-alcoholic fatty liver disease (NAFLD) and its inflammatory component non-alcoholic fatty steatohepatitis (NASH), nephropathy, cardiomyopathy and muscle dysfunction [10]. Hepatocellular carcinoma (HCC) has been reported more often in non-cirrhotic livers in the background of NASH and its risks factors include male gender, older age, cigarette smoking, obesity and insulin-resistant states [3, 4, 11]. Overweight and obesity are associated with an overall increase in liver primary cancers of 17% and 89%, respectively [2, 11, 12] and males with a BMI > 35 had a 3.5–4 increase risk of liver malignancy [12] (**Figure 1**). Optimal management of HCC with curative intent includes resection or liver transplantation. Nevertheless, these therapies are limited because the

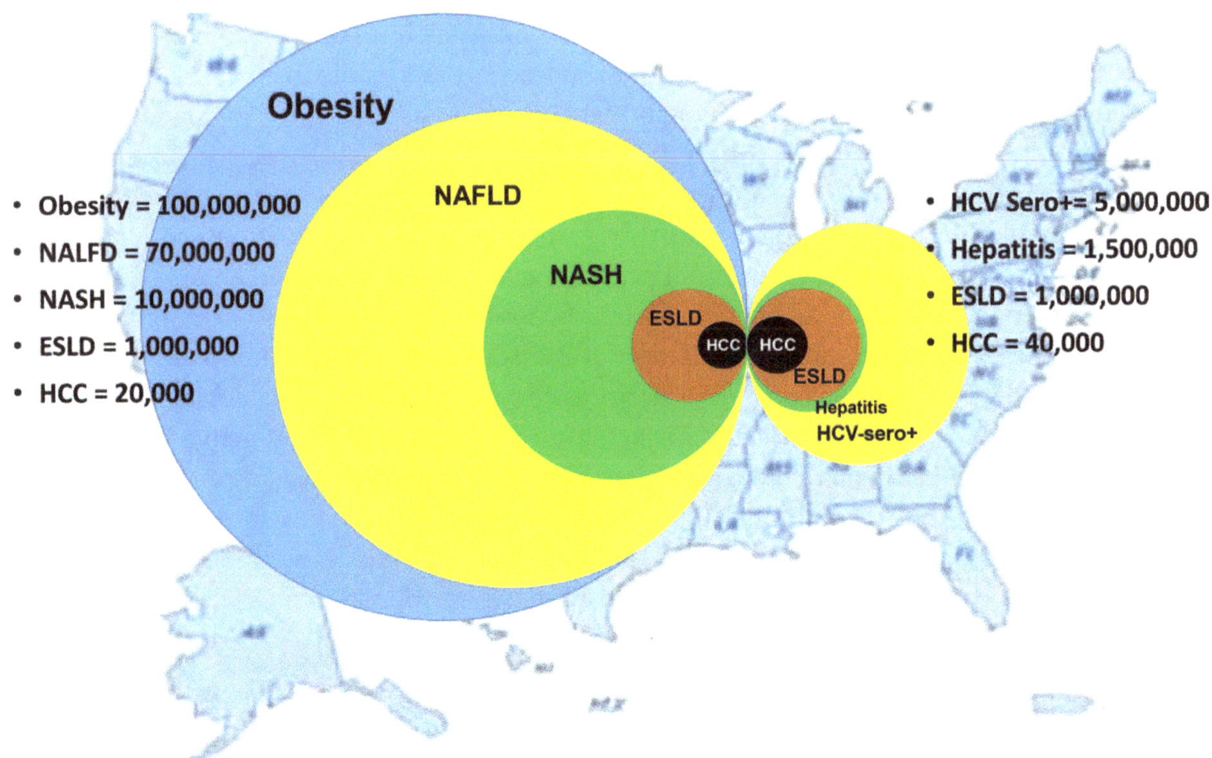

Figure 1. *Main causes of end stage liver disease (ESLD) and hepatocellular carcinoma (HCC).* Hepatitis C virus infection (HCV) and obesity are the main cause of the global and Western increase in ESLD and HCC. In USA 1 out of 3 adults is overweight and approximately 5 M people is HCV seropositive. While prevention relays in stopping virus transmission and implementing programs of healthy caloric intake and exercise programs, treatments of established ESLD and its malignant consequence are similar. Nevertheless, the most effective surgical treatment, liver transplantation is limited due to scarcity of donors and loco-regional therapies have limited survival effect due to malignant recurrence or progression of liver dysfunction.

degree of liver dysfunction or additional medical conditions at the time of diagnosis and the scarcity of available liver grafts. The role of cellular lipid management and metabolism in human health and disease is taking a center stage [13]. Higher fat intake, lower physical activity and a progressively aging population are among the behavioral and social factors of this phenomenon that add to the genetic load [1]. An overview of the role of cell aging and senescence in liver metabolic responses to high caloric intake will be performed in the pages to follow.

1.2. Regeneration, necrosis, apoptosis and senescent: a constant changing balance

The liver is a unique organ with an innate ability to regenerate through mass compensation to satisfy portal flow and metabolic demands [14]. After injury and cell necrosis, immune recall of resting cells occurs and activation of oval-precursor cells in conjunction with platelets migration switch to a cell division renewal cycle [15, 16]. Mitosis is more prominent at the peri-portal stem cell niche site (zone 1) assuring clonal expansion until reaching zone 3 (peri-central vein) [15, 16]. In health, liver mass homeostasis is closely regulated through a delicate balance among regeneration, apoptosis (programmed cell termination), and senescence. During states of acute liver injury, the pendulum moves towards a regenerative and repair phase, however, during chronic states of liver injury collagen synthesis and deposition persists leading to organ fibrosis. In addition, natural processes of organ aging play a main role in organ response to both acute and chronic injuries. Primary cell life span is determined by a limited number of cell duplications, the so called Hayflick limit [17]. After such limited divisions, cells enter a state of cell replicative senescence which is believed to be triggered by shortening of telomere ends. Replicative cellular senescence is a stable form of cell arrest characterized by a lack of cell proliferation activity and apoptosis resistance mediated through a lack of mitogen response even though the cells remain metabolically active. On the other hand, cells can be induced to a senescence status by a variety of cellular stressors such as DNA damage, UV light, radiation, oncogene activation, increased H_2O_2 production and heat stress [17, 18]. Senescent cells undergo morphological changes as they acquire an enlarged and flattened morphology, in addition to an increase expression of the senescence associated markers ß-galactosidase (SA-ß-GAL), an accumulation of the senescence associated heterochromatic foci (SAHF) and DNA damage foci, and the expression of the senescence associated secretary phenotype (SASP) [18]. Senescent status is achieved and maintained by active signaling of p53, a tumor suppressor gene that exercises its effects through activation of p21, a potent cell cycle inhibitor, and the p16-retinoblastoma protein [18]. Cells induced into an irreversible cell cycle arrest at the G1 phase will undergo metabolic disturbances with an increase reactive oxygen species (ROS) production, decrease adenosine triphosphate (ATP) synthesis and accumulation of lipofuscin [17].

Changes in the content of daily oral intake can influence life span and thus cell aging. The cell death-inducing DNA fragmentation factor α-subunit-like effector A (Cidea), is a transcriptional coactivator implicated in lipid accumulation, cell stress and cell aging. Authors showed in rodents, that a high lipid diet up-regulated Cidea with hepatic lipid accumulation, cell stress, mitochondrial dysfunction and genetic upregulation of aging [19]. Other studies, in support of this findings have shown a life span reduction up to 30% in genetically obese mice (ob/ob) and this reduction was reversed by a caloric restricted diet [19]. Lipid enriched diets are associated in humans with DM type 2, HTN and cardiovascular events all

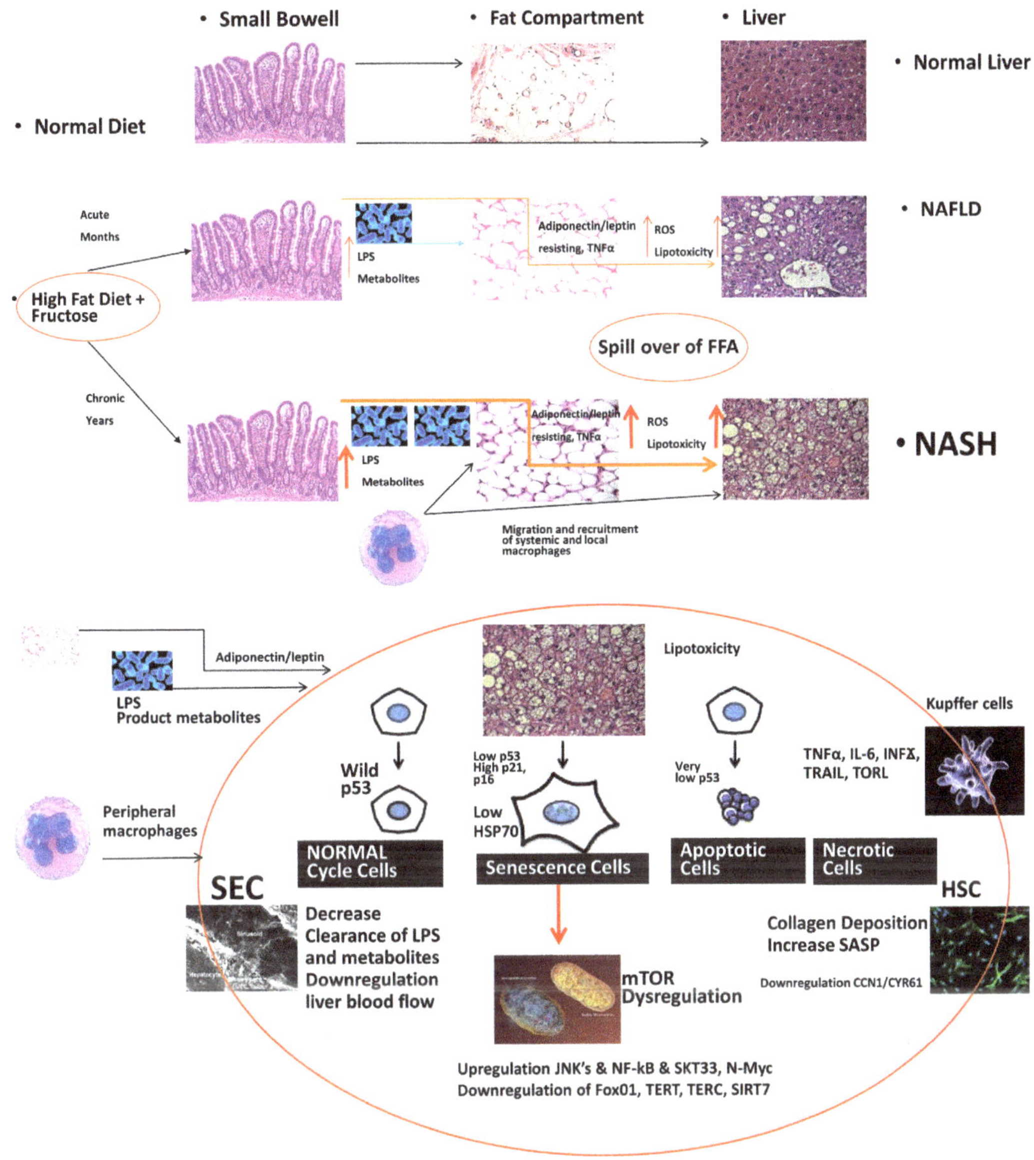

Figure 2. (A) *Morphological changes observed in the mice model of high fat diet (HFD) plus fructose (Western Diet) in the microbiota, fat content tissue and liver.* Liver cells accumulate FA in form of TG from the spill-over of lipid excess in the fat compartment and after saturated the normal processes of liver lipid metabolism. (B) *Local liver inflammatory response from lipid excess.* Lipotoxicity an addition to increase LPS activates SEC, HSC and Kupffer cells inducing more parenchymal cells into senescence and apoptosis which changes the local mielue into an inflammatory microenvironment. Continuous HFD decreased further mitochondrial function with lower ATP production and increase collagen deposition leading to progressive liver fibrosis, liver dysfunction. The state of progressive liver fibrosis due to a local and systemic inflammatory state results in an increasing insulin resistance status with the full metabolic syndrome phenotype. Its progression results in decompensated ESLD and the development of malignancy.

of which limit life span. Caloric restriction without malnutrition can extend life span while caloric excess has the opposite effect [20]. Thus, the choice of oral intake has a profound impact on life span.

The free radical intermediates hypothesis of cell aging still remains the most reasonable in the induction and maintenance of the senescent status [17, 21]. ROS, reactive nitrogen sp., and lipid peroxide are important regulators of cell signaling that provides reliable maintenance of cellular components, support redox-state and regulate the function of highly metabolic active cells as in hepatocyte and immune cells [20, 21]. ROS in excess from over-oxidation of lipids, proteins, nucleic acids and other macromolecules is associated with a misalignment of their functional activity, reactions that if they last through the cell cycle can lead to permanent cell dysfunction and/or accelerated aging cell process. Thus, an excess of food intake in form of continuous lipid charge will test the oxi-redox systems that keeps the fragile mitochondrial equilibrium in balance. Continuous metabolic stress changes the equilibrium towards lower levels of antioxidants (glutathione sp.) with further increase of ROS that in turn accelerates processes of apoptosis and senescence. Former processes further lead to arrest of regeneration and activation of hepatic stellate cells (HSC) and therefore fibrogenesis (**Figure 2A**).

The hormonal mielau modulates cellular response to caloric intake. Insulin and somatotropin signaling are critical not only in the control of cell aging and longevity under conditions of abundant food supply but also in mediating the effects of caloric restriction on life span. In a rodent model of thyroxine induced aging, thermogenesis was directly correlated with increased mitochondrial function, increased ROS production, decreased concentration of glutathione reduced, downregulation in the activity of antioxidants enzymes and increased senescent marker expression in the liver as well as in other organs [21]. Estrogen influences lipid metabolism through nuclear receptors which enhances apoptosis of mutated cells, improves mitochondrial function, and decreases the metabolic syndrome phenotype [10, 22]. Actions that may explain, at least in part the constant disparity of overall life expectancy by gender.

Lifestyle changes such as exercise and caffeine supplementation have shown to increase the ratio of reduced/oxidized glutathione in liver and muscle tissue in the rodent model [23]. Although liver enzymes were identical in experimental and controls groups, plasma levels of cytokines associated with inflammation (IL-1ß, IL-6, TNF-α and INF-α) and cell aging were found to be significantly decreased in the experimental group when compared to controls [23]. It was noted that although exercise increased the production of ROS, exercise also evoked a beneficial increase in levels of cell antioxidants, and lowered levels of oxidative damage when cells were exposed to a second injury, i.e. lipid charge. Thus, the concept of exercise inducing gene expression of antioxidant enzymes that may protect the cell from other insults was called 'hormesis' [23]. Although caffeine, a member of the methyl-xanthine family increased the ratio of reduced-oxidized glutathione, no other markers of cell stress were modified. Perhaps, caffeine potentiates further the beneficial effects of exercise.

2. Liver metabolism in health and disease

The reduced tri-peptide glutathione (GSH) is the major antioxidant in the body responsible for maintaining the intracellular redox balance. 90% of the GSH in plasma derives from the liver [24] and aging is associated with a progressive decline in the levels of GSH in humans and rodents [25]. Senescent liver cells in culture showed elevated ROS leading to a state of chronic oxidative stress. In addition, age associated decline in GSH has been linked to an activation of neural sphingolipid hydrolase enzyme (NSMase) and the accumulation of bioactive ceramide, a precursor of inflammation [25]. The availability of L-cysteine is the rate-limiting factor of GSH synthesis and oral supplementation of cysteine alleviates GSH deficiencies in humans and rodents [25]. GSH deficiency can be alleviated by the oral intake of cysteine and its restoration rates appears to be age and sex dependent. Older animal models are associated with increased cellular stress and an enhanced subcellular injury after heat stress associated with an increased iron intracellular deposition [26]. These cause damages to mitochondria and lysosomes. Although a more precise mechanism of organelle damage was not enunciated, iron deposition mediated a decrease in Transferrin-receptor-1 which upregulates the iron storage protein ferritin after heat stress. Nevertheless, the synthesis of the iron exporter protein ferroportin was delayed [26]. Effect that may explain at least in part, organelle damage in the aging cell that occurs after natural oxidants depletion (**Figure 2B**).

A diet enriched in calories and lipids increases free fatty acids (FA) in plasma obligating cells to protect themselves from lipotoxicity or death by either oxidizing FA's or sequestering them as triacylglycerol (TAG) within lipid droplets (LD) [13]. PGC-1, an exercise-induced transcriptional coactivator may play an important role in coordinating intra-muscular LD-signaling with mitochondrial remodeling. TAG within lipid droplets are the major form of energy storage in the body (muscle, liver, fat tissue) and a reservoir of membrane lipid component. TAG synthesis is initiated by glycerol-3-phosphatase acetyltransferases (GPAT) at the mitochondrial and sarcoplasmic reticulum membranes and it is completed at the sarcoplasmic reticulum by the sn-1-acyl-glycerol-3-phosphatase acyltransferase (AGPAT), phosphatidic acid phosphatase (PAP) and sn-1,2-diacylglycerol acyltransferase (DGAT) [13]. Synthetized LD-TAG are localized preferentially in proximity to mitochondrial membranes named "contact zones". Once TAG's are released, they are mainly used in the mitochondria for ATP synthesis via oxidative phosphorylation from the ß-oxidation path. The "athlete paradox" states that the accumulation of TAG in the trained and insulin sensitive cells is in greater proportion than the TAG accumulation in cells from diabetic subjects with insulin resistance. This observation supports the hypothesis of mitochondrial dysfunction as a factor of TAG accumulation from a sustained lipid charge.

The protein family of perilipins (Plin) is associated with LD's and their scaffolding may affect the interaction between TAG and the mitochondria [13]. The Plin family consists of Plin1 to 5; the most common PAT (perilipin/ADRP/TIP47) interacts with LD in different proportions. In the liver, down-regulation of Plin2 promotes a reduction of hepatic steatosis and increases insulin sensitivity, albeit a reduction in both Plin2 and Plin3 is associated with insulin resistance [13]. In the heart, a Plin5 deficiency causes increased lipid oxidation, increased ROS production and decreased cardiac function. In heart and skeletal muscle TAG and FA are the main metabolic source of energy through the ß-oxidation pathway, suggesting a very tightly regulated process from cell storage to mitochondrial metabolic use. While TAG may come from LD, FA's are mainly transported in plasma as albumin-bound or as part of the very low density lipid-protein (VLDL) complex. Different transmembrane transporter systems are involved in their translocation to the inner cell compartment where the long chain fatty acid (LCFA) forms thioesters with coenzyme A (CoA). LCFA-CoA can form TAG for storage as LD, or can enter the outer mitochondrial membrane where CPT1 catalyzes the reaction of LCFA-CoA to LC-acylcarnitine. The former compound can actively cross the inner mitochondrial membrane with the exchange of carnitine for acylcarnitine. CACT is highly expressed in tissues with predominant ß-oxidation metabolism.

2.1. In Health

The metabolism of FA in the mitochondrial matrix is sequentially catalyzed through a ß-oxidation process by four enzyme families: acyl-CoA dehydrogenase, enoyl-CoA hydratase, 3-hydroxyacyl-CoA dehydrogenase and 3-ketoacyl-CoA thiolase. While acyl-carnitine is converted back to acyl-CoA to enter the TCA cycle, dehydrogenases activity shows different affinity for short, medium, long and very long FA's [13]. Every cycle of ß-oxidation renders acyl-CoA and shortens the FA chain by 2 carbons providing the equivalents of electron donors NADH and $FADH_2$ which is the driving force for the synthesis of ATP. Although the ß-oxidation pathway is an effective way of ATP production, an overload of FA may play the role of un-coupler that exercises an inhibitory effect on the respiratory chain through a proton-phoric effect on the inner mitochondrial membrane. This effect results from the implicit effect of FA on mitochondrial membrane porosity by opening of the permeability transition pores, which results in the subsequent loss of electrical gradient and arrest of the respiratory chain [13]. The above concept favors the hypotheses of mitochondrial dysfunction from FA overload as the primary step of the insulin resistance state in obese patients. Other authors have found no mitochondrial respiratory changes in the steatotic liver but in mitochondria from skeletal muscle from a rodent model of high fat diet induced obesity [27]. Authors have proposed mitochondrial changes are due to an adaptation of the mitochondria to the high lipid charge rather than a defect per se in its function. No explanation was provided by the authors regarding the increase in ROS and inflammatory changes observed. Others suggested a protected effect from caloric lipid surplus against the development of metabolic dysfunction, as long as cells maintained functional adipocyte storage with low levels of tissue inflammation [28]. Once adipose accumulation saturates cell capacity, fatty excess spills over into other tissues leading to LD accumulation with subsequent lipid oxidation and an inflammatory response which precedes the metabolic syndrome manifestations [28]. The Delete in Breast Cancer-1 (DBC-1) protein is an important regulator of fat accumulation and storage in fat tissue which exercises its action by inhibition of SIRT1. In the DBC-/KO mice exposed to HFD, it was observed high plasma levels of FA with no liver steatosis, lower expression of senescence cells and increased storage of FA in the adipocytes with no development of insulin resistance [28]. Thus, DBC-1 protected liver and adipocytes from senescence by preservation of the fat compartment function with liver sparing and insulin sensitivity. Interestingly, a comparison has been made between this rodent model and the so called "healthy obese subjects" where there is fat accumulation but no signs of metabolic syndrome or systemic inflammation.

2.1.1. Metabolism and inflammation

Obesity depresses the anti-inflammatory effects of the heat shock proteins (HSP70) pathway, an inhibition that may contribute to the progression from NAFLD to NASH [29]. Excess of lipids and fuels trigger a low grade inflammatory response in both fat and liver tissues that correlates with the impaired insulin responsiveness. TBARS, a simple but fair estimate of lipoperoxidation/malondialdehyde (systemic oxidative stress) produced throughout the body was shown to be elevated in plasma from NASH patients when compared to normal subjects and its levels were correlated with insulin-resistance status [29]. The former response involved activation of the c-Jun NH2-terminal kinases (JNK's), endoplasmic reticulum (ER) stress, unfolded proteins response (UPR), and the ceramide pathway by blocking nuclear factor κB (NF-κB) expression at different levels [29]. In liver tissue, HSP70 downregulates TNF-α and inducible nitric oxide synthase (NOS2), genes that increase the inflammatory response in rodents. In addition, HSP70 in humans induces apoptosis and increases the concentration of cyclopentenone prostaglandins, a potent local inhibitor of inflammation. In human liver and fat tissues, the suppression of HSP70 was strongly correlated with the upregulation of JNK1 and JNK2 [29]. The authors hypothesized that the senescence-like state in fat cells have evolved in obese individuals as an adaptation to the metabolic overutilization of fat cells, supporting the observation that hepatocyte senescence predicts NAFLD progression to NASH and to cirrhosis. Patients with different grades of ESLD from NASH or HCV had significantly decreased levels of glutathione reduced and increased levels of glutathione oxidized in plasma when compared to healthy controls [30]. Therefore, a continuous increase in the cell oxidative stress consumes the antioxidant protective mechanisms and increases the spillage of oxidative molecules. Increased oxidative compounds accumulation may induce a progressive larger number of liver cells into senescence which in turn will enlarge the SASP component worsening the inflammatory environment with further increase of stressors into the liver mieleu by triggering an activation of local and systemic immune-regulators (**Figure 3**).

In old mice, hyperglycemia increased chromatin remodeling and polyploidy levels; changes observed as well in non-obese diabetic mice [31]. Genes involved in glycemic control and metabolism are also involved in inflammation such as Ppargc1a (PGC-1α). It acts on the histone deacetylase SIRT1 as a metabolic sensor in hepatocytes and increases gene activation involved in the gluconeogenesis pathway [31]. Furthermore, PGC-1α also plays a role in lipid metabolism [31]. Through the thyroid receptor pathway, it induces the expression of Srb1 (Scavenger receptor B member 1), enhances the uptake of cholesterol esters from high density lipoproteins (HDL) in the liver and inhibits the expression of Srebp-1 (sterol regulatory element-binding transcription factor-1) down-regulating fatty acid synthesis [31]. As SASP builds up due to an increasing number of cells entering senescence, an increasing insulin resistance state starts to develop with its manifestation, hyperglycemia which further favors replicative cell arrest.

The fat compartment has emerged not only as an energy reservoir but as an endocrine organ capable of modulating metabolic states where the adiponectin/leptin ratio determines an anti or pro-inflammatory response. Leptin is a 167-aminoacid hormone expressed predominantly in adipocytes. Its signaling is an important determinant of food intake, adiposity and energy expenditure [32]. In the *ob/ob* mouse, a homozygous mutation in the gene that encodes leptin is associated with increased appetite, obesity and an insulin-resistant state. When leptin was provided to the ob/ob animal, there was a dramatic improvement in glucose homeostasis and energy metabolism. Although leptin related glucose homeostasis is largely conserved in rodents and humans, most subjects with insulin-resistant diabetes have a hyperleptinemic state with a central resistance to leptin [32]. Adiponectin is a protein hormone of 244 amino acids synthesized as a monomer of 28–30 kDa and assembled in various molecular weights: low, medium and high molecular weight (LMW, MMW and HMW) oligomers [33, 34]. HMW oligomers are the major relevant forms in terms of physiological activities of adiponectin while, low amounts of HMW oligomers represent an independent risk factor for several metabolic pathologies such as obesity-related diseases. Adiponectin plays a pivotal role in energy metabolism being an insulin-sensitizing hormone and it is involved in a wide variety of physiological cellular processes including inflammation, immunity and vascular

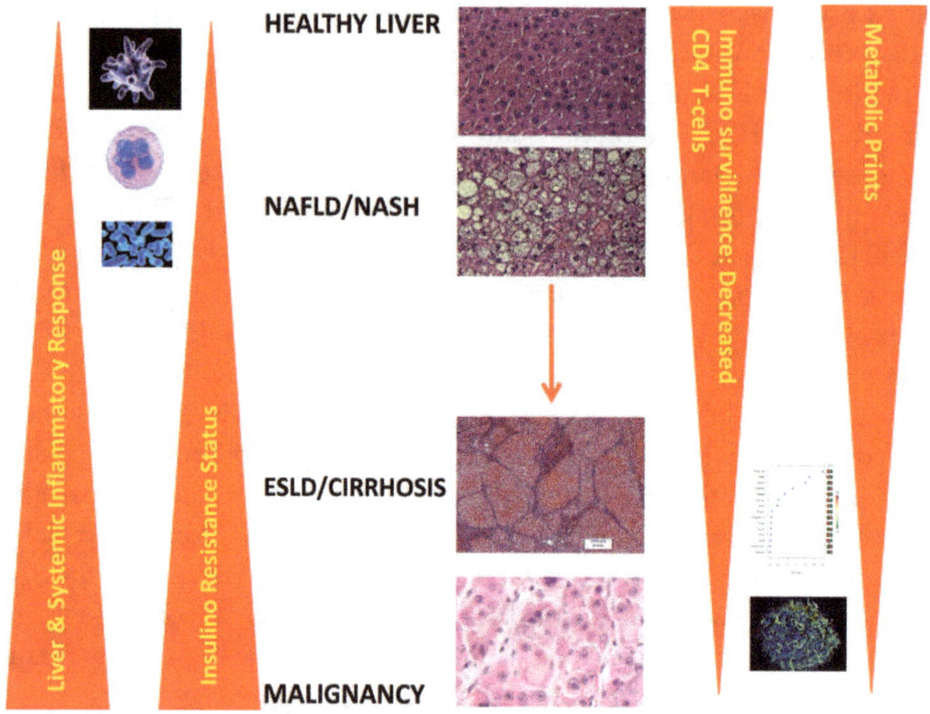

Figure 3. *Local and systemic responses that occur in the progression of NAFLD to NASH and ESLD associated HCC and their metabolomic print.* The liver local progression from NAFLD to NASH is associated with a local inflammatory response that eventually involves several other organs evolving into a systemic reaction. The systemic inflammatory response is associated with the development of an insulin resistance status and the metabolic syndrome phenotype: HTN, central obesity, DMType II and NASH. The continuous liver lipotoxicity decreases mitochondria function and decreases ATP production as well as enhances the secretion of lipid intermediates which are toxic to CD4 T lymphocytes. All together enhances a regenerative stimulus of senescence cells with mitochondrial dysfunction generating at some point a metabolic swap of ATP production to the cytosol, which may be associated with a mitochondrial generated apoptotic switch and in an environment of progressive fibrosis and therefore low oxygen and nutrients delivery favoring the survival of the already highly mutated cells which in turn have escaped physiological cell cycle control and immuno-recognition assuring cell clone growth. Metabolic disturbances precede variations in cell cycle and genetic expression creating metabolic signatures of liver status in health and disease.

physiology. Adiponectin acts through three major physiologically different and distinctly expressed receptors: AdipoR1, AdipoR2 and T-cadherin. Adipo receptors mediate pleiotropic adiponectin actions through signaling mechanisms involving AMPK, ERK1/2, AKT and P38. In addition, Polymerase I and transcription release factor (PTRF) regulates adipocyte differentiation, perhaps fat cell senescence and thus may determine fat compartment expandability, condition that under continuous HFD exposure increase the spill-over of FFA to the liver in combination to a pro-inflammatory adipokine repertoire [35].

2.1.2. *Signaling of energy expenditure and metabolism*

Rapamycin has an effect in cell life span with significant changes in the liver transcriptome, effects that are more pronounced when animals are exposed to caloric restriction [36, 37]. In a rodent model, rapamycin prevented senescent changes with significant differences by gender but with some common genetic pathways, mainly in the preservation of mitochondrial function. Those pathways included protein ubiquitination, NRF2-mediated oxidative stress response and glucocorticoid and OGF-1 signaling [36, 37]. Cell culture studies, indicated that treatment with rapamycin decreased mitochondrial membrane potential, decreased O_2

consumption, and increased ATP production [36, 37]. Other effects from transcriptome pathways include a decrease in proteasome activity in parallel with an increase in cell autophagy, suggesting protein quality improvement processes and increased resistance to oxidative cell stress effects associated with reduced cell aging.

A highly conserved signaling pathway in all eukaryotic cells is the Target of Rapamycin (TOR), which plays a central role as regulator of cell growth and metabolism. The mammalian TOR complex (mTOR) encompasses two structurally and distinct proteins. While the mTORC1 is associated with anabolic processes such as protein synthesis, lipid synthesis, nutrient uptake and inhibition of catabolic processes including autophagy, mTORC2 is an insensitive to rapamycin regulation protein. mTOR2 becomes activated by a family of kinases like the serum/glucocorticoid kinase (SGK) and protein kinase C (PKC). mTORC1 is upregulated by growth factors, cellular energy status and is inhibited by the macrolide rapamycin [36–38]. Protein synthesis is one of the most energy demanding cell functions; a favorable redox status activates mTORC1 which in turn exercises its actions down-stream through the ribosomal protein 6 kinase (S6K) and the eukaryotic translation initiation factor 4E binding protein (4R-BP) [36–38]. Due to the high demand of ATP, mitochondrial function regulation is of paramount importance on mTOR signaling pathways. Moreover, mitochondrial dysregulation and continuous mTOR activation may play a metabolic central role in the transformation and survival of cancer cells. Mutated cells with malignant potential may shift their bioenergetic state from ATP mitochondrial production to cytosol ATP production through the tricarboxylic acid (TCA) cycle. A connection between mTORC2 and mitochondrial function and cancer appears to be dependent through the HK2 pathway [38]. Nevertheless, recently mTORC2 has been linked to cytoskeleton regulation through the actin remodeling pathway, which has been suggested to have an effect on insulin sensitivity/resistance balance [36, 37]. Whole energy expenditure was affected by the mTORC1 signaling pathway, as demonstrated in the tissue specific knockout mice where a down-regulation of signaling pathways on adipose tissue also impacts on thermogenesis and systemic sensitivity to insulin [38]. In addition, mTORC2 signaling pathway, in the same animal model was a crucial regulator of liver and pancreas metabolism affecting animal growth and insulin homeostasis. mTORC 1 and 2 signaling in the liver affects systemic glucose and insulin homeostasis mainly due to their effects on Akt and hepatic glucose uptake. Interestingly, liver tumors in the tissue specific raptor knockout mice, showed a shift from glucose to glutamine as the main fuel source, making tumor cells glutamine addictive with high expression of mTORC1 and FGF-21. Rapamycin treatment may be beneficial as it may inhibit growth on glutamine addictive tumors. Some liver transplant programs switch their immunosuppression protocol from tacrolimus to rapamycin in patients with high risk for HCC recurrence after transplantation. However and on retrospective studies, its effect on long term overall survival on patients after liver transplantation for HCC, have had conflicting results [39, 40].

The functional relationship between poly-unsaturated lipid metabolism, inflammation and cancer development has been discussed in multiple avenues. Cyclooxygenases (COX's) and lipoxygenases (LOX's) are enzymatic families that metabolize poly-unsaturated fatty acids. COX is present in two isoforms (COX-1 and COX-2) that produce prostaglandins (PG's) and thromboxanes, respectively [41]. LOXs constitute a family of dioxygenases that insert O_2 into poly-unsaturated fatty acids with regional specificity [41]. These metabolites are biologically active hydroperoxyeicosatetraenoic acids that upon reduction forms hydro-eicosatetranoic acids (HETE's), while the metabolism of linoleic acids preferentially results in hydroxyl-octadecadienoic acids (HODE's), metabolites known to modulate inflammation and carcinogenesis [41]. An excess of poly-unsaturated fatty acids could enhance a higher production of HETE's and/or HODE's with an override of pathways that enhances cancer development. Hepatic COX-2 overexpression induces spontaneous HCC formation in vitro and in mice through Akt, SKT33 and mTOR signaling cascades [42]. In the healthy liver, the inhibitor of the prostaglandin degrading enzyme 15-PGDH potentiates liver regeneration after partial hepatectomy when compared to control and sham animals [43]. Thus, prostaglandin active derivatives have the potential not only to modulate local inflammatory responses but to promote cell regeneration in the healthy cell and potentially reversal of cell arrest in the senescent cell.

2.2. Metabolism in the liver graft

Evidence seems to indicate a peculiar aging pattern for liver grafts after transplantation. Biological age of the graft does not correspond to its behavior when transplanted to a different environment of a younger recipient [44]. One of the most important intracellular protease systems is represented by the proteasome, the central catalytic unit of the ubiquitin-proteasome system (UPS). No difference in the accumulation of oxidized proteins and polyubiquitin conjugates with maintenance of their proteolytic activity was found in liver grafts after transplantation from younger donors to older recipient when compared to liver grafts from older donors placed into younger recipients. Furthermore, there was an increase of the ß5i/α4 ratio, suggesting a shift towards proteasomes containing immune-subunits [44]. Thus, it appears older liver grafts transplanted in younger recipients switched their biological metabolism to resemble the recipient's metabolic age. However, the pattern of liver cell senescence may differ. Liver biopsies, as judged by the senescent markers telomerase and SMP-30 from older transplanted livers showed histological damage in asymptomatic patients with up to 43% and 64% at 5 and 10 years, respectively [45].

In the warm ischemic/reperfusion liver model, glycogen synthase kinase 3 (GSK-3) inhibition ameliorated liver injury upon reperfusion through an energy-dependent mitochondrial mechanism [46]. GSK-3 is a serine/threonine kinase regulated by inactivation through serine phosphorylation. GSK-3 inhibition down regulates the opening of mitochondrial permeability transition pore (MPTP) site, preventing leakage of mitochondrial respiratory chain proteins; a key step in the activation of caspase dependent apoptosis and therefore mitochondrial-dependent cell termination. This effect was present in young animals but abrogated in old animals, and a partial response was re-established in the older group by glucose infusion with hepatic glycogen build up storage [46]. Authors speculated that during reperfusion glycogen degradation provides mitochondrial fuel in forms of glutamate and α-ketoglutarate maintaining enough energy levels that preserve mitochondrial membrane integrity or mitohormesis lowering ROS production, factors needed to decrease MPTP susceptibility. Former approach in the human was entertained, where liver graft glycogen replenishment was performed during the donor phase and evaluated upon reperfusion [47, 48]. Metabolic benefit with improved organ graft function was observed only in borderline grafts and the ones with high fat content. Nevertheless, the concept of metabolic replenishment with further graft function improvement may be refined by strategies of ex-vivo euthermic graft perfusion prior implantation [49–56].

2.3. The chronically diseased liver

Hepatocyte senescence expression has been shown to be present in up to 80% of the cells in advanced liver disease [57]. The effects of insulin in the liver cell are mediated through two main cellular pathways: the phosphatidylinositol 3-kinase (PI3K)-Akt and the Ras-MAP kinase (MAPK) pathways. While both pathways are active in the regulation of cellular growth, proliferation and differentiation the PI3K-Akt mediates the metabolic actions of insulin. Those actions include activation of mTOR1 and its S6 kinase and the inactivation of glycogen synthase kinase-3 (GSK3) as well as its AS160 with nuclear exclusion of the Forkhead box protein (Fox01) [57]. In culture, HepG2 cell lines showed a signaling defect downstream of the Akt pathway with an impact upon insulin mediated Fox01 cytosol sequestration and AS160 phosphorylation; a cascade that translated into insulin resistance of older cells when compared to younger cells. Nevertheless, maintenance of the senescent state requires an active role in the transcriptional activity of Fox01 as cell cycle inhibitor, even in the presence of growth factors. Thus, it appears gluconeogenesis and insulin resistance are unwanted but unavoidable effects of Fox01 gene, which is involved in cell cycle arrest, detoxification of oxygen species, DNA repair and gluconeogenesis [57].

FA overload can damage the respiratory chain in the mitochondrion through a dual role: as an un-coupler and as an inhibitor [13]. Impairment of the key respiratory state 4 → 3 can occur via inhibition of ATP-synthase thereby producing an increase production of ROS irrespective of ADP concentration. The concept of redox-optimized ROS balance (R-ORB) postulates that ROS efflux from the mitochondrion will attain a minimum at intermediate values of oxidation, when VO_2 reaches a maximum following ADP stimulation. Under state 3 respiration, GSH and thioredoxin systems are essential for minimizing ROS release from the mitochondria [13]. Moreover, mitochondria from cells with chronic liver disease under oxidant challenge displayed a two-fold increase in H_2O_2 emission when compared to controls along with a 50% decrease in GSH [13]. Since 90% of GSH in plasma is excreted by the liver, glutathione sp. could serve as a surrogate of cell/mitochondrial stress and their ratio in plasma may reflect overall liver redox balance [24]. In animal models of liver malignancy, with or without cirrhosis glutathione sp. (glutathione reduced-GSH, glutathione oxidized-GSSG and ophthalmate) predicted the growth of malignant cells on normal livers as early as 14 days after malignant cells implantation and differentiated animals with cirrhosis by tumor status (HCC+ vs. HCC−) [58, 59]. Furthermore, glutathione sp. in plasma were part of the metabolic signature that discriminated healthy controls and subjects after liver transplantation with normal graft function from subjects with chronic liver disease (**Figure 3**). In addition, metabolic prints graded patient's degree of end stage liver disease which correlated with the MELD score, and they were able to separate patients with cirrhosis by tumor status, i.e. HCC+ vs. HCC− [30].

Others argued mitochondrial dysfunction by FA's respiratory chain uncoupling is incompatible with thermo-regulatory principles that governs mitochondrial respiratory chain through energy demand: intracellular lipids will accumulate whenever FA's supply exceeds the energy needs of the cell [13]. While TAG-LD in cells from a trained individual increases as the source of energy, in the diabetic obese subject TAG-LD are the result of accumulation with the subsequent potential overproduction of lipid derived toxins in the form of LCFA-CoA, diacylglycerides (DAG) and ceramide, metabolites responsible, at least in part for the development of insulin cell resistance [13]. The former theory is attractive in the heart and skeletal muscle. In contractile cells, optimal excitation-contraction coupling requires an optimal energy and O_2 supply which in turn affects the Ca^{2+} handling at the sarcoplasm reticulum (SR) release channels (ryanodine receptors), the SR Ca^{2+} pumps and the sarcolemmal Na^+/Ca^{++} exchanger. The heart at rest beats in average 100,000 times per day catalyzing about 6 kg of ATP to ADP. The mitochondrion provides the ATP needed for contraction (≈66%) and the ATP needed for ion transporting (≈33%) essential for the cardiac electrical activity. Thus, the link among lipid supply and mitochondrial function, insulin sensitivity/resistance and ion pump exchange is established for optimal cardiac function or dysfunction in the obese individual [13]. Perhaps, there is no argument lipid oxidation confers a metabolic advantage during starvation and exercise, but its role as the fuel of election during food abundance against metabolic disease deserves further studies.

In liver, cellular senescence is associated with a pro-fibrogenic environment and the relation between advanced liver fibrosis and shortening of the cell telomere appears to be consistent [11, 60]. Telomeres are repetitive DNA sequences (TTAGGG) associated with the specialized protein shelterin. They are located at the chromosomal end acting as a cap that stabilizes and protect the chromosome from erosion and miss-identification as DNA breaks. During normal cell division, telomeres shorten due to the "end replicating problem": the inability of DNA polymerases to fully replicate the 3′ end of chromosomes [61]. Germline cells overcome this problem by expressing telomerase, a reverse transcriptase that maintains telomere length by synthetizing new DNA sequences at the end of the chromosome [60]. The telomerase complex includes a reverse transcriptase (TERT) and the RNA component (TERC) [61]. In other somatic cells, continuous cell division results in telomere shortening which in turn start signaling cell arrest mechanisms, i.e. senescence or apoptosis. Failure of cell arrest signaling, as in a silence p53 state sparks further cell proliferation with chromosomal end-to-end fusions and instability. In addition, exhaustion of liver regenerative paths and invested mechanisms of telomere repair could be overcome under continuous and chronic cell injury with subsequent acceleration of cell senescence and aging. Some studies had shown that telomere biology is involved in HCC initiation and its progression [60]. Therefore, telomere shortening is a physiological marker of cell aging signaling and/or cell arrest preventing further cell division; failure of cell arrest may end in chromosomal instability and subsequent mutations favoring tumor development [11, 61]. In fact, the strength of the DNA damage response (DDR) in the normal cell depends ultimately to the degree of p53 gene regulation: a higher p53 response is associated with apoptosis, a lower response is associated with cell senescence and a silence p53 response may favor tumor development and growth [62]. In addition, a sirtuin (SIRT7) showed an in vivo hyperacetylation of p53 and the SIRT7 knockout mice suffered among other maladies steatotic liver disease. Sirtuins were initially identified in yeast as the Silent Information Regulator (SIR). In mammals, SIRT protein family comprises seven distinct members involved in cellular survival, senescence and tumorigenesis [62]. The SIRT7 knockout mice showed a 2.5 fold increase in the liver triglyceride content and an increased accumulation of hepatocyte inflammatory markers [62]. Findings that were associated with liver cells mitochondrial dysfunction through a deacetylate GABPß1 mitochondrial protein pathway and with the development of HCC through maintaining a deacetylated state of H3K18 at promoters sites of many tumor suppressor genes [62].

Lipodystrophic syndromes are rare and heterogeneous diseases, genetic or acquired, where partial atrophy is associated with a phenotype consistent with insulin-resistant diabetes, dyslipidemia and NAFLD. Although the genetic cause of these syndromes are largely unknown, most of the monogenic diseases have in common primary alterations in the fat tissue consistent with disturbances of the adipogenesis process or defects in the formation, maintenance and/or regulation of the lipid droplet [63]. Acquired syndromes are seen mainly after HIV therapy with anti-retroviral agents as zidovudine and stavudine (tNRTI's). Agents known to render mitochondrial toxicity with metabolic disturbances similar to the metabolic syndrome seen in obesity. This metabolic adverse effects include premature aging associated with impaired prelamin-A maturation [63]. Lamin-A alterations could produce fragile nuclear envelopes, alter chromatin organization, increase oxidative stress and promote premature senescence at the cellular level. The metabolic disturbances observed in genetic or acquired lipodystrophic syndromes support the hypothesis of a primary fat compartment dysfunction as the source of metabolic disturbances, similar to the ones detected in obesity.

Chronic liver disease is associated with an increased translocation of intestinal bacteria contributory to the liver inflammatory response and may promote the development of HCC [12]. Liposaccharide (LPS) produced by Gram (−) bacteria hosted in intestines from obese humans and rodents was associated with the transition of NAFLD to NASH and consequently to its progression to cirrhosis and HCC. LPS is recognized by the Toll like receptor 4 (TLR4) which is expressed upon cell activation on migrating and local macrophages (Kupffer cells). TLR4 is central for the secretion of TNF-ß and IL-6, cytokines present in the chronic inflammatory environment that precedes the detection of malignancy [12]. Further support to the role of LPS was found by interventions such as gut sterilization, removal of LPS or inactivation of TLR4; maneuvers that diminished tumor growth in chronically injured livers [12]. In experimental models, dietary or genetic obesity alterations on the gut microbiota increased levels of metabolites like deoxycholic acid (DCA) that in turn damages DNA. The enterohepatic circulation may further enhance the concentration of such metabolites by both encouraging the senescent-associated secretory phenotype response and favoring a tumor-promoting environment.

3. Cellular senescence

3.1. Hepatocytes

Historical views of liver cell replication supports the physiological properties of the hepatocytes to restore function as response to parenchymal loss [64]. However, massive or unending injury may overcome regenerative processes or may promote a dysfunctional repair process leading to progressive liver fibrosis, development of portal hypertension and eventually liver failure. Senescent status was induced in HepG2 cells by exposure to H_2O_2. Its consequences and metabolic activity were interrogated [18] and morphological changes were noted with respect to SA-ß-GAL and SAF's expression, cell cycle arrest as well as the upregulation of p53, p21 and p16 genes. Regarding cytokine expression, IL-8 was upregulated while IL-6 was downregulated. Disturbances in glucose and lipid metabolism were evident with upregulation of growth hormone/IGF1 (SOCS2) and glycolysis (PGM2LT). Nonetheless, the downregulation of glucogenolysis and gluconeogenesis (G6PC) were more prominent. The unsaturation of fatty acids was hyperactive (FADS3) with parallel hypo activity of lipoprotein and hepatic lipase activity through the Apo-lipoprotein (APC3) system. APC3 also limits the uptake of chylomicrons by the liver cell. Other fatty acid downregulated proteins included SORL1 (involved in the uptake of LDL), ACSM2B (a medium-chain fatty-acid-CoA ligase) and PHGDH indirectly involved in amino-acid synthesis [18]. In addition, senescent cells secreted a variety of bioactive molecules including pro-inflammatory cytokines and chemokines that may influence extracellular matrix and the micro-environment but as well modulate the immune response with the promotion of macrophage migration leading to further increase in the inflammatory mielue [65]. Monocyte chemotactic protein (MCP-1) could provide a signal for monocyte recruitment into the liver followed by activation of Kupffer cells with the upregulation of death ligands. The expression of Fas ligand, TNF-α, and TNF-related apoptosis inducing ligand (TRAIL) further aggravates lipo-apoptosis [66]. In addition the FFA palmitate increases the expression of TRAIL and abrogation of the TRAIL receptor expression suppresses the inflammation induced by nutrient excess in mice [66].

Prior assumptions on cellular senescence determined that cell cycle arrest was a mechanism to protect the cell towards tumorigenesis. Nevertheless, it has been shown that the cell in cycle arrest can produce pro-inflammatory mediators, the senescence-associated secretory phenotype that promotes tumor growth [67]. During chronic liver disease, senescent machinery becomes "hijacked" perhaps triggering proliferation and transformation of hepatocytes, thus, promoting metabolic adaptation which may enhance tumor grafting and growth [68, 69]. The above metabolic paths could at least in part, be mediated by the over expression of the phosphatase and tensin homolog (PTEN) described in T-leukemia but later shown in liver tumors to inhibit the pentose phosphatase pathway (PPP) by binding to glucose-6-phophodiesterase (G6PD). With no active G6DP dimer, cells favor glycolysis with the production of lactate even in the presence of oxygen [70].

Aging and senescent liver cells have different genetic paths that may converge to similar metabolic traits. Aging liver cells have a proliferative response after injury associated with the repression of C/EBPα, Farnesoid X Receptor (FXR), telomere reverse transcriptase (TERT), and a decrease in the Wnt signaling pathway [71, 72]. A physiological Wnt signaling pathway involves a soluble ligand that binds to the Frizzled receptor (Fzd) and the LRP5/6 co-receptor on the plasma membrane; this interaction activates the cytoplasmic Disheveled protein which inhibits the ß-catenin (Ctnnb1) destruction complex (APC, GSK3ß, and Axin) by preventing Ctnnb1 phosphorylation and its subsequent destruction. Stable ß-catenin (intact Wnt signaling) translocates to the nucleus to form a complex with Lef and Tcf transcription factors that target genes as c-Myc and Cyclin D1. In cell culture and a mice model of HCC, tumor growth was ablated by the suppression of N-Myc downregulated gene 1 (NDRG1) expression; it promoted HCC cells to go into cell arrest [73]. The induction of senescence on malignant cells was accomplished by upregulation of the tumor suppressor genes p53, p21 and p16 in addition to decreased phosphorylated Rb. Senescent liver cells response to injury included transcription of Nf-kB, Myb, Nkx2-1, Nr5a2 and Ep300 factors; proteins known to be involved in inflammation, cell differentiation, lipid metabolism and chromatin remodeling. In addition, the chronic inflammatory phenotype of senescent cells induces telomere dysfunction and accelerates liver cell aging [74]. Thus, decreased physiological cell signaling that occurs with aging plus stress induced cell senescence may add to the lipid toxic microenvironment by promoting a vicious circle that overrules redundant mechanisms that prevent uncontrolled cell division. Mechanisms that imply an apoptosis "switch" from a pro-apoptotic to an anti-apoptotic status. Nonetheless, it is no clear the role of mitochondrial Bcl-2 proteins family and their expression may determine cellular fate [75].

Cellular events that follows are the activation/repression of factors involved in cell proliferation. In the liver cell, the known transcriptional shift includes activation of FOXO3, FOXII, E2F1, c-jun, C/EBPß, Myb, USF and neutralization of inhibitors of cell proliferation such as Rb family and C/EBP family of proteins [76]. In C/EBP-S193A mice, failure to stop liver regeneration after surgery correlated with the epigenetic repression of C/EBPß, p53, FXR, SIRT1, PGC1α and TERT. The repression was performed by a protein formed by C/EBPß-HDCAC1 complex which also inhibit the promoters of enzymes for glucose synthesis PEPCK and G6P [76]. The response of cell cycle engaged hepatocytes and cell cycle arrested hepatocytes (senescent cell) to injury is different and it may awake an unregulated cell growth on quiescent stem liver cells [76, 77]. Oval shaped liver cells may differentiate into cholangiocytes with a distinct metabolism and perhaps pathway towards malignancy [15, 16]. Although cholangiocytes are metabolically very active cells involved in the secretion and resorption of water and soluble bile components, they are not directly involved in the metabolism and/or regulation of biliary lipid species (cholesterol, bile acids and phosphatidyl-choline vesicles) [78, 79].

3.2. Hepatic stellate cells (HSC) & portal myofibroblasts (MF)

HSC are quiescent cells that express typical markers of both neural cells and adipocytes (glial fibrillary acid protein-GFAP, peroxisome proliferator-activated receptor gamma-PPAϒ, and adiponectin receptors). They are activated by cytokines, growth factors, ROS, damaged cells and apoptotic bodies [64]. In health, MF are located adjacent to bile duct epithelia and are the first responder to biliary injuries. Upon activation HSC's acquire a MF phenotype, cells that upon phagocytosis of LD and/or apoptotic bodies from damaged cells get additional energy and became Fas-ligand and TNF-α unresponsive to apoptosis; mechanism in use for increase collagen synthesis and deposition [64]. Furthermore, activation of the adenosine receptor A_{2A} increases HSC proliferation and inhibits death and senescence by down regulation of p53 and Rb through the cAMP-PKA/Rac1/p38 MAPK pathway [80]. Activated MF's express CCN1/CYR61, an important regulator of inflammation and wound healing. Cystein-rich 61-protein (CCN1/CYR61) is a matrix-cellular protein that induces senescence at later stages of wound healing by promoting tissue remodeling through fibrogenic cell apoptosis and attenuation of TGF-ß signaling [81]. HSC and MF senescent fibrogenic cells no longer proliferate, thereby reducing the load of ECM deposition. In addition, senescent fibrogenic cells express an increase in the secretion of metalloproteinases (MTP's) leading to matrix degradation. Apoptotic fragments from HSC and MF are cleared by natural killer cells promoting wound healing, the best characterized mechanism of fibrogenesis resolution [64, 81]. NF-κB is a key regulator for HSC survival and proliferation by maintaining the expression of Mcl-2. Inhibition of NF-κB increases HSC apoptosis by up-regulation of the JNK pathway. Thus, the activation as well as the induction of senescence/apoptosis of HSC/MF are normal wound healing mechanisms that promote the establishment of normal organ architecture and function with clear paths of initiation and resolution.

During chronic cell injury, such as in a state of high caloric intake enriched with lipids, an increase and progressive pool of biologically active HSC's may become prominent [11]. An incremental chronic state of fibrogenesis alters hepatic architecture leading to a concomitant increase in portal flow resistance, portal hypertension and the development of collateral circulation. In addition, HSC's produce a microenvironment with altered extracellular matrix (ECM) that provides biochemical and mechanical cues to the growth and establishment of tumor cells [67]. Nevertheless, since 90% of the HCC's flourish in a highly progressive fibrotic ECM, the question raises if it is the changes on the microenvironment that further promotes metabolic transformation with an "apoptotic switch" and tumor development. Interestingly, progressive liver fibrogenic ECM becomes enriched with vascular growth factor (VGF) receptor promoting angiogenesis, paving the way for the much needed arterial high O_2 supply for HCC expansion [67].

The different components of the ECM, cellular and non-cellular interact directly and indirectly with malignant cells therefore changing the phenotype of the evolving cells that in turn produces feedback signals to further adapt the microenvironment to the needs of the malignant cell. The link between the actin cytoskeleton and the microenvironment provides an input of intracellular contractile forces capable of regulating signaling pathways fundamental to the definition of cell phenotype, mechanism that constitute the ECM "out-side-in" code to the cell. In response, the anchored cells expressed adhesions molecules and secreted proteins that signals HSC and other ECM regulators increasing anchoring sites in response to the "in-side-out" signaling [67]. Therefore, the metabolic transformation of the already stressed parenchymal cells help to choose a path different to senescence and necrosis but to a path of unregulated regeneration, thus escaping apoptosis. A path that needs an ECM differentiation to assure cell survival in a non-efficient energy redox status.

3.3. Sinusoidal endothelial cells (SEC)

SEC's are specialized endothelial cells that lie flat in the liver sinusoids along and in direct contact with the hepatocytes. Through their membranes and specialized pores or fenestra passes high concentrations of metabolites, proteins and other blood compounds, traffic which is regulated by the size of the fenestra. SEC's play a critical role in immune-activation, rolling of T cells, macrophages and PMN migration. Liver sinusoidal endothelial cells may be affected with age and obesity. SEC from old individuals have impaired and reduced expression of VEGF likely due to impaired nuclear transport of P-STST3 and P-CREB transcription factors [82, 83]. In a rodent model of sepsis, endothelial nitrogen oxide synthase (eNOS) deficient mice and aging mice had the same mortality and mitochondrial dysfunction upon the isolation of SEC mitochondrion [84]. In obesity and during early fibrogenesis, SEC lose their fenestra, decreasing the exchange of metabolites and increase the secretion of several basement membrane components (type IV collagen, perlecan, entactin and laminin) [64]. Authors concluded that an endothelial base-line dysfunction in the aging animal is manifested by a weakened antioxidant response and inappropriate energy production from mitochondrial dysfunction due to a tipped-balance of the SEC oxi-redox systems when exposed to additional stress. This is seen in the obese towards a state of energy depletion and cellular death, apoptosis or activation of a pro-coagulant/pro-fibrogenic phase. The changes of SEC's with aging may limit O_2 delivery and availability to liver cells with its potential effects on mitochondrial function, a pro-fibrogenesis state and the promotion of insulin resistance status. Changes exaggerated in obesity, implying obesity may promote accelerated SEC aging processes. Interestingly, endothelial cellular senescence was inhibited in vitro and in the rodent by the activation of the liver x receptor (LXR), a nuclear receptor involved in the control of hepatic lipid and cholesterol metabolism [85]. Furthermore, LXR has been shown to play an important role in glucose metabolism, cytokine production and anti-inflammatory response.

Three types of SEC's co-exist in the normal liver sinusoid: mature SEC, SEC progenitors and bone marrow-derived SEC progenitors [86]. Mature SEC are gatekeepers of fibrogenesis by maintaining HSC in their inactivated state. SEC's regulate sinusoidal blood flow through their action on HSC and thus keep a low portal pressure [86]. In addition, mature SEC's have the largest endocytic capacity in the body fulfilling their dual cell clearance capacity (from the arterial/systemic and portal/gut systems). The liver endocytic function has been implicated in a liver-renal axis where the lack of SEC-stabilin-2 receptors inhibit the clearance of toxic molecules that manifest with mild liver fibrosis without liver dysfunction but with renal glomerular fibrosis. Not only do SEC's have many glycoproteins that serve as receptors for bacterial epitopes but as receptors for immune-modulation and pro-coagulant activity. The above mentioned SEC functions are at least partially lost at the time of sinusoid capillarization [86]. SEC capillarization is characterized by the disappearance of the fenestrae, development of a basement membrane and the appearance of characteristic markers. This phenomenon happens in chronic liver injury and it precedes activation of HSC and sequestration of macrophages. The angiogenesis process that follows is mediated by VEGF, an angiocrine response that drives neo-vessel formation in direct proportion to the degree of the sinusoidal pressure gradient. Furthermore, SEC pseudo-capillarization refers to changes that occur in endothelial cells associated with aging and senescence. It is manifested by a decrease of up to 50% of their fenestrae, development of a patchy basement membrane and partial SEC dysfunction [86]. Chronic exposure of high fat diet may accelerate aging/senescence of SEC, endothelial dysfunction with recruitment of systemic immune cells and activation of Kupffer cells inducing HSC into a fibrogenic state followed by an angiocrine response that decreases hepatic blood flow, O_2 delivery, and clearance of toxic molecules. As metabolic stress of neighbor hepatic cells already in mitochondrial distress due to fat accumulation progresses, a constant and growing inflammatory mielue enhances tumor development, immune-recognition failure and malignant cell expansion.

Interestingly, aging endothelial cells from the fat compartment of mice was associated with adipose dysfunction manifested by ectopic (liver) fat deposition and adipose tissue fibrosis, increased adipose mitochondrial oxygen flux, altered lipid utilization, increased tissue oxidative stress and lower gene expression in visceral fat [87]. Nevertheless, and most important, these findings were associated with reduce fat tissue vascularity, reduced angiogenic capacity and endothelial dependent dilation with reduced nitric oxide (NO) bioavailability [87]. Limited oxygen mitochondrial availability contributes to the pro-oxidative older adipose tissue phenotype that can further impair both insulin action and vascular function, a key element in local and systemic insulin-resistant related metabolic syndromes. Changes that are exaggerated in obesity, implying obesity may promote accelerated aging processes in many organs.

3.4. Resident liver immunocells

The anatomical location of the liver and its dual blood supply ensures an optimal exposure of antigens to the hepatic resident immune cells not only from nutrients and GI microbiota but from systemic compartments, such as the adipose compartment. Kupffer cells in concert with NK, CD4+ T-cells, and local antigen presenting cells modulates the liver immune status. Kupffer cells constitutes 80% of the tissue fixed macrophages and 20% of the non-parenchymal cell population of a normal liver [9]. Their characteristic macrophage activity is polarized mainly in portal tracts where the antigen dynamics is higher from food and bacteria. Innate macrophages have the potential to initiate an inflammatory response of different proportions by upregulating adhesion molecules such as ICAM-1, and cytokines as TNF-α, IL-1, IL-6, MIP1α, TGF-ß and RANTES. Activation that can only lead to antigen presenting, cell to cell communication and amplification and enrichment of the microenvironment with ROS promoting subsequent parenchymal cell apoptosis/necrosis. Natural Killer (NK) and CD8+ T cells developed a specific signature in livers with NASH from mice under HFD [88]. The depletion of CD8+ T cells protected murine from NASH progression but not from weight gain. In addition, NK T-cells in the liver expresses markers that recognize lipid antigen CD1d [9]. Liver NK cells undergo Thymus clonal double deletion but are positive for CD3 and CD56 and they were thought to be CD1d independent. Nevertheless, hepatic antigen-presenting cells may introduce microbial glycolipid antigens to NK cells, stimulating secretion of Th1 or Th2 cytokines which subsequently initiates an adaptive response. Hepatic NK cells have as well the ability to secrete osteopontin and sonic hedgehog, molecules known to promote the transition from NAFLD to NASH [9].

The most accepted hypothesis, continuous cell parenchymal damage and necrosis adds to a chronic inflammatory environment a dysregulation of the cell cycle regenerative process rendering tandem mutations and thus malignant cells was challenged [89]. On the NEMO knockout mouse, authors were able to develop HCC through a death receptor-independent FADD signaling pathway. Nevertheless, it wasn't until recently that the link between a metabolic hostile microenvironment, immune-recognition failure and HCC presence was established [90]. The enrichment of linoleic acid in the cirrhotic microenvironment of NASH patients promotes disruption of mitochondrial function in a greater proportion than other fatty acids as palmitic acid. Since CD4(+) T lymphocytes have a larger mitochondrial load than CD8(+) T lymphocytes, they not only generate more mitochondrial derived ROS but CD4(+) cells may undergo larger selective loss of mitochondrial function and viability. Therefore, disruption of mitochondrial function by linoleic acid mediates selective loss of intrahepatic CD4(+) T lymphocytes, status associated with HCC presence. Local metabolic changes could alter the immune response to a one that favors malignant cell expansion.

In the obesogenic environment, aberrant activation of immune cells has emerged as key features of the metabolic syndrome. The interaction between the adipose compartment and the liver tissue has been hypothesized as a critical interface for nutrient sensing and metabolic control [9]. In the rodent model, neutrophils infiltrate the adipose compartment as early as 3 days after starting a high fat diet, however its role as well as the role of basophils and eosinophil cells has not yet been clarified. Mast cells, which has been observed in increasing number have been implicated in the secretion of IL-6 and IFN-ϒ [9]. Moreover, leptin, a hormone secreted specifically by adipocytes has been found to be increased during high fat diets and upregulated the expression of leptin receptors on NK T-cells. This regulation is time sensitive, and chronic leptin stimulation change NK cells from an inflammatory like response to a damped one, favoring at long term, in the liver and perhaps in other organs a susceptibility to low recognition of no self-cells, impaired anti-tumor surveillance and a flourishing nest of cancer. The former hypothesis finds support in the obese mice, where it was observed a switch from the normal Th1 immunoresponse to the Th17 immunorepertoire, phenotype that deteriorates autoimmunity [9].

3.5. Extracellular matrix (ECM)

The extracellular matrix (ECM) is formed by a non-cellular component in tissues and organs composed primarily of water, proteins and proteoglycans. Components created an intricate scaffold where organ cells get structural support with a dynamic and continuous traffic of water, ions, metabolites, proteins and cells on passant to maintain organ physiology. As such, ECM interactions with organ cell components regulate cell differentiation, adhesion, proliferation, migration and survival [64]. The collagen family is the major fibrillar proteins of the ECM and the body (approx. 30% of the total protein contain) [64]. There are three main classes of collagen, fibril-forming which include types I, II, III, XI, XXIV and XXVII the most common varieties and their role is mainly mechanical by conferring tensile strength to both tissue and organs. Fibril-associated collagens with interrupted triple helix (FACIT's) includes type IX, XII, XIV, XIX, XX, XXI and XXII; this subclass of proteins do not form fibrils themselves but bind to the surface of pre-existing collagen favoring fibril enlargement. Finally, type III collagen serves as anchoring collagen between the epithelial cells and the lamina reticularis constituting the basement membrane where type IV collagen is most abundant. Non-collagenous proteins include fibronectin, tenascin, laminins, fibrillins and matrix-cellular proteins. While the former peptides play a major role in cell differentiation, cell growth, adhesion and migration, matrix-cellular proteins, i.e. thrombospondin-1 and 2, osteonectin, osteopontin and cyr-61/connective tissue growth factor (CTGF) serve mainly as a vehicle for cell signaling. Proteoglycans are carbohydrate enriched proteins which retain large quantities of water regulating the smooth trafficking of molecules to and from the cell with numerous signaling active sites for growth factors.

The ECM continuous remodeling is a complex process that integrates proteins and cellular components from local and distal environments [64]. The degradation of ECM proteins are closely controlled by matrix metalloproteinases (MMP's), a superfamily of zinc-dependent endopeptidases highly regulated by specific inhibitors such as the tissue inhibitor of metalloproteinases (TIMP's). In the liver, cellular component involved in collagen synthesis and deposition included HSC, MF and vascular smooth muscle cells [64]. In chronic liver injury, an override mechanism of collagen deposition regulation promotes massive ECM expansion. The characteristic features of abnormal liver fibrogenesis as a consequence of continuous liver injury and activation of collagen secreting cells include damage to the epithelial/endothelial barrier, recruitment of inflammatory cells, secretion of cytokines and other inflammatory mediators, further generation of ROS, progressive deposition of collagen with expansion of ECM and worsening organ fibrosis and subsequent metabolic changes of portal hypertension.

4. Mitochondrial senescence

The mitochondria, a double membrane cell organelle varies in number and its presence is linearly associated with the metabolic activity of the organ and its required energy requirements in form of ATP. Within the mitochondrial matrix a series of biochemical reactions occur. Acetyl-choline primer is reduced through the tricarboxylic acid cycle converting glycolysis-derived pyruvate into NADH and succinate. The former compounds couple another set of reactions at the inner membrane border where the electron transport chain (ETC) is present to boil an oxidative phosphorylation process. The ETC is composed of five enzymatic complexes (I to V; NADH-CoQ, succinate-CoQ, CoQ-cytochrome reductases, cytochrome c oxidase and ATP synthase, respectively) where NADH is the substrate of ETC-C1 and succinate the substrate of ETC-CII [10]. After oxidation, electrons are transferred from Complex I to CII to CIII and finally to Complex

IV where oxygen is reduced to form H_2O. The electron transport process is coupled to a proton pumping process creating a proton gradient between the mitochondrial membranes, gradient that is dissipated by Complex V (ATP synthase) through ATP synthesis. A control mechanism is created by the "proton leak", mechanism that generates heat instead of ATP [10]. Much of the leak is a catalytic reaction generated by the uncoupling proteins (UCP's) which play an important role in reducing proton gradient, heat and ROS [10]. Mitochondrial aging and senescence are linked to reduced ATP production and increase ROS production, i.e. superoxide (O^{2-}), hydrogen peroxide (H_2O_2) and hydroxyl radical (OH^-) which are mostly produced because electron leakage at the level of CI and CIII [17]. Mitochondria function benefit from the role of estrogen in plasma through its binding to the nuclear estrogen receptor that enhances a signaling to prevent oxidant stress and also inhibits the renin-angiotensin-aldosterone system [10]. Thus, sex differences in mitochondrial function may explain the disparity in overall survival between men and women, differences that may be taken into account during animal models studies.

The reasons why the mitochondrion conserves a cell independent genome are not clear, but it is intuitive to imply self-energy regulatory processes are united through a fine tune mechanism between energy expenditure (ATP use) and energy production (ATP synthesis) at every organelle level. It may provide an overall advantage for survival of the cell, the organ and entire biological living system. The gradual ROS response theory of aging argues a protective role of ROS in early life, when cell oxidative damage and ROS production are low; however, later in life ROS reaches a level where its beneficial effects (as the one observed in dietary restriction and/or exercise) are overcome by its detrimental effects elicited by a higher cell oxidative stress (as the one observed in high fat diet and sedentary habits) [17]. The effects that are amplified include loss of genomic controls (p53), microRNA dysregulation, loss of function of telomerase reverse transcriptase (TERT) and a lower immune-surveillance status. Although the role of p53 in the mitochondrion is not completely clear, p53 binds to the Peroxisome proliferator-activated receptor Gamma-Coactivator 1 alpha and Beta (PGC-1α and ß) fomenting their inhibition of expression and therefore downregulated oxidative function. In addition, p53 target p16 and p21, factors that triggers G1-phase cycle arrest by inhibiting cell cycle regulatory kinases Cdk4 and Cdk2 [17]. The third known effect of p53 at the mitochondrion level is to promote cell apoptosis by increasing mitochondrial membrane permeability with leakage of cytochrome proteins, a direct activator of the caspase cascade. The function of TERT is highly affected by levels of ROS production and its protective patterns are only observed with low ROS levels. The role of microRNA in the mitochondrial environment remains to be elucidated.

The Mitochondrial Free Radicals Theory of Aging (MFRTA) has been the most popular theory to explain the cell aging process where increasing production of mitochondrial ROS with lower ATP production are the main factors responsible for cell aging and corresponding mitochondrial ultrastructure changes [17, 91]. As mentioned, leakage of electrons at the level of CI and CIII transfer are larger with age and the higher potential for DNA damage. 8-oxo-7.8-dihydro-2'deoxyguanosine (8-oxodG) is one of the most abundant DNA mutations caused by oxidative conversion to guanosine. Furthermore, its accumulation follows an inverse and exponential curve against life expectancy in several mammals [17]. Recently, it was described that humans with longer longevity have a higher content of mitochondrial DNA (mtDNA) per cell in different organs, and support the notion of ethnic background on mtDNA influence and life span. The frequency of mtDNA mutations occurs at different rate depending on the organ. Skeletal and cardiac muscles, liver and kidney are more affected by somatic mtDNA mutations compared to other organs such as the skin and lung [17]. Furthermore, the clonal expansion of mtDNA mutations occurs via a phenomenon called genetic drift, a random propagation and expansion of DNA mutations occurring at each DNA replication. The drift of mutations may be more important in metabolically more active organs that require more energy expenditure and therefore more ATP synthesis. The expansion of mtDNA mutations may be enhanced not only by its duplication and drift but also by a lower state of DNA damage repair mechanisms [17]. The Base Excision Repair (BER) process is impaired in senescence and aging due to a loss of function to BER associated proteins CSA and CSB. Thus, the increase production of ROS creates a vicious loop of mtDNA mutations than in turn favor an increase production of ROS perpetuating and enhanced organelle dysfunction by defective reparative mechanisms. A naturally occurring thymidine to cytidine mutation in the mitochondrial stressors $tRNA^{ILE}$ gene is associated with phenotypes of hypertension, hypercholesterolemia and hypomagnesemia [10]. Furthermore, the DNA A3243G mutation causes impaired insulin secretion and polymorphisms in the promoter of the UCP2 protein, alterations associated with increased incidence of obesity, reduced insulin secretion and DMII [10].

Mitochondrial function may be impaired in chronic high fat diet challenge as a result of a decrease in ß-lipid oxidation. Indirect evidence showed an accumulation of diacylglycerol and fatty-Acyl-CoA which in turn activates stress-related serine/threonine kinase activity and inhibit glucose transport [10]. Oxidative stress contributes further to impaired insulin signaling increasing UCP2 activity which in turn enhances "proton leak" with uncoupling of the glucose metabolism pathway and decreased ATP production. A progressive higher lipid peroxidation may favor further oxidative stress with DNA damage and low DNA repair by affecting members of the Bcl-2 family, triggering an influx of Ca^{2+} with subsequent opening of the mitochondrial permeability transition pore, cytochrome-c leakage to the cytosol and activation of the caspace-3 complex. Cell self-digestion and nuclear DNA fragmentation overcomes with the typical cell fragments morphology [10]. Alternatively, DNA damage and telomerase shortening results in mutations that may affect mitochondrial function to a level of organelle survival but inefficient ATP production assuring the "apoptosis switch" and diverting biochemical reactions to a cytosolic site for ATP production. The later assumption may find some support in the observations that tumor development and early growth is favored in low O_2 delivery zones and that tumor development is associate with increase lactate production, the Warburg effect [30, 69].

5. Future directions

Prevention of metabolic syndrome and its health consequences is primordial. A healthy diet that is balanced not only in calories but also in its components, specially fats and carbohydrates would avoid fat storage spillage from a saturated fat body compartment. In addition, a substantial use of lean mass through directed exercise will decrease further cell, organ and body aging. In the brain, the melacortin forms a network of neural food sensing connecting signals of metabolic rate with neurological sites that regulates food intake behaviors and energy expenditure homeostasis. Central administration of α-MSH reduces food intake and may also increase energy expenditure resulting in weight loss [92]. Metabolic disturbances in the liver renders liver cell changes that progress from NAFLD to NASH to cirrhosis and malignancy. A non-invasive plasma based monitoring of such changes on disease progression and treatment response as well as for tumor screening may be possible by metabolomic liver prints in the near future [30].

There have been a myriad or reports on compounds that not only prevent but reverse cell aging and some even malignant development in the animal model [25, 93–102]. Curcumin, the major bioactive compound of turmeric spice, through its antioxidant and anti-inflammatory properties has been claimed to retard tumorigenesis and diabetes and to modulate lipid metabolism [103]. Furthermore, curcumin prevents the development of atherosclerosis and NASH, perhaps by the upregulation of a fatty acid binding protein present in adipocytes (aP2) but also found in macrophages (FABP-4). This protein is a cytosolic protein present in adipocytes and macrophages which modulates the trafficking of lipids/cholesterol processes and activation of inflammatory mechanisms through CD36 upregulation and reduced expression of NF-kß thus, decreasing cytokine secretion [103]. Prior studies showed that high fat diet and obesity promoted liver tumorigenesis by inducing chronic inflammation through the IL6/STAT3 pathway and, STAT3 activated tumors has been showed to be more aggressive in humans. Lycopene attenuated HCC occurrences in the animal model through downregulation of the STAT3 signaling [95]. The aqueous extract of *Ligustrum lucidum* fruit induced apoptosis through the activation of the caspase cascade and cellular senescence by upregulation of p21 and downregulation of RB phosphorylation [102].

Other molecules with promising cell aging and tumor repression properties included the COX-2 and a Na/K/ATP signaling mechanisms. Inhibition of 15-hydroxyprostaglandin dehydrogenase (15-PGDH), a prostaglandin-degrading enzyme, potentiates tissue regeneration in multiple organs in mice [43]. During a chemical screen, a low molecular compound was identified capable of selectively inhibiting 15-PGDH with the subsequent increase of PGE2 levels in bone marrow and other organs, accelerating hematopoietic recovery in mice receiving bone marrow transplant and tissue regeneration in the colon and liver. It also promoted tissue regeneration in mouse models of colon and liver injury. Selective COX-2 products may have rescued telomere dysfunction, cell senescence and tissue regenerative potential [74]. However, its mechanism and signal transduction remains to be determined. pNaKtide is a synthetic peptide that conserves the active sequence for the ligand-binding capacity to the ß-subunit of the transmembrane Na/K-ATPase. Although the Na/K-ATPase mainly exercise its function as an ion exchanger pump vital for cell survival, recently it was shown to elicit nuclear signaling that regulates mitochondrial function and cell energy production through a Src/ERK pathway [104–112]. Furthermore, pNaKtide prevents the development of atherosclerosis and fatty liver disease in the HFD mice model with significant amelioration of ROS. In addition, it downregulates collagen synthesis and inhibit growth of human cancer cells in vitro. Translation of promising compounds to the treatment of patients with NAFLD/NASH is expected in the near future to further prevent the consequences of advanced liver fibrosis and HCC development.

Abbreviations

4R-BP	Factor 4E binding protein
ADP	Adenosine diphosphate
AGPAT	sn-1-acyl-glycerol-3-phosphatase acyltransferase

ATP	Adenosine triphosphate
CACT	Carnitine-acylcarnitine transferase
DBC-1	Delete in Breast Cancer-1
DGAT	sn-1,2-diacylglycerol acyltransferase
DM	Diabetes mellitus
ECM	Extracellular matrix
ER	Endoplasmic reticulum
FA	Fatty acids
Fox01	Fork head box protein
GBD	Global Burden of Disease
GPAT	Glycerol-3-phosphatase acetyltransferases
GSH	Reduced glutathione
GSK-3	Glycogen synthase kinase 3
HBV	Hepatitis B virus infection
HCV	Hepatitis C virus infection
HSC	Hepatic stellate cells
HSP70	Heat shock proteins
HTN	Hypertension
IL-1ß	Interleukin-1 beta
IL-6	Interleukin-6
INF-α	Interferon alpha
JNK's	c-Jan NH2-terminal kinases
LD	Lipid droplet
MAPK	Ras-MAP kinase
MF	Portal myofibroblast
MMP	Matrix metalloproteinases
MPTP	Mitochondrial permeability transition pore
NAFLD	Non-alcoholic fatty liver disease
NASH	Non-alcoholic fatty steatohepatitis
NF-κB	Nuclear factor κB
NO	Nitric oxide
PAP	Phosphatidic acid phosphatase

PI3K	Phosphatidylinositol 3-kinase
PKC	Protein kinase C
ROS	Radical oxygen species
SA-ß-GAL	ß-galactosidase
SAH	Senescence associated heterochromatic foci
SASP	Senescence associated secretary phenotype
SEC	Sinusoidal endothelial cells
SGK	Serum/glucocorticoid kinase
SMase	Neural Smase
TAG	Triacylglycerol
TCA	Tricarboxylic cycle
TIMP	Tissue inhibitor of metalloproteinases
TNF-α	Tumor necrosis alpha
TOR	Target of Rapamycin
UPR	Unfolded proteins response

Author details

Matthew Schade[1†], Jacqueline A Sanabria[1†], Milad Modarresi[1], Bryan Gillon[1], Zach Hunter[1], Jacqueline Fannin[1], Amrita Mallick[1], Henri Brunengraber[2] and Juan Sanabria[1,2*]

*Address all correspondence to: sanabriaj@marshall.edu

1 Department of Surgery and the Marshall Institute for Interdisciplinary Research, Marshall University Joan Edwards School of Medicine, Huntington, WV, United States

2 Department of Nutrition Proteomic & Metabolomic Core Facility at Case Western Reserve University, Cleveland, OH, United States

† Authors contributed equally and should be considered as first authors

References

[1] Collaborators GBDRF, Forouzanfar MH, Alexander L, Anderson HR, Bachman VF, Biryukov S, et al. Global, regional, and national comparative risk assessment of 79 behavioural, environmental and occupational, and metabolic risks or clusters of risks in 188 countries, 1990-2013: A systematic analysis for the Global Burden of Disease Study 2013. Lancet. 2015;**386**(10010):2287-2323

[2] DALYs GBD, Collaborators H, Murray CJ, Barber RM, Foreman KJ, Abbasoglu Ozgoren A, et al. Global, regional, and national disability-adjusted life years (DALYs) for 306 diseases and injuries and healthy life expectancy (HALE) for 188 countries, 1990-2013: Quantifying the epidemiological transition. Lancet. 2015;**386**(10009):2145-2191

[3] Global Burden of Disease Cancer Collaborators, Fitzmaurice C, Allen C, Barber RM, Barregard L, Bhutta ZA, et al. Global, regional, and national cancer incidence, mortality, years of life lost, years lived with disability, and disability-adjusted life-years for 32 cancer groups, 1990 to 2015: A systematic analysis for the Global Burden of Disease Study. JAMA Oncology. 2017;**3**(4):524-548

[4] Global Burden of Disease Cancer Collaborators, Fitzmaurice C, Dicker D, Pain A, Hamavid H, Moradi-Lakeh M, et al. The global burden of cancer 2013. JAMA Oncology. 2015;**1**(4):505-527

[5] Global Burden of Disease Pediatrics C, Kyu HH, Pinho C, Wagner JA, Brown JC, Bertozzi-Villa A, et al. Global and national burden of diseases and injuries among children and adolescents between 1990 and 2013: Findings from the Global Burden of Disease 2013 Study. JAMA Pediatrics. 2016;**170**(3):267-287

[6] Khachatryan V, Sirunyan AM, Tumasyan A, Adam W, Bergauer T, Dragicevic M, et al. Search for dark matter, extra dimensions, and unparticles in monojet events in proton-proton collisions at [Formula: see text][Formula: see text]. The European Physical Journal. C, Particles and Fields. 2015;**75**(5):235

[7] Stanaway JD, Flaxman AD, Naghavi M, Fitzmaurice C, Vos T, Abubakar I, et al. The global burden of viral hepatitis from 1990 to 2013: Findings from the Global Burden of Disease Study 2013. Lancet. 2016;**388**(10049):1081-1088

[8] GBD 2015 Obesity and Overweight Collaborators. Obesity and overweight and their health impact 1990-2015 in 195 countries. The New England Journal of Medicine. 2017:**377**;13-27. https://www.ncbi.nlm.nih.gov/pubmed/28604169

[9] Eheim A, Medrikova D, Herzig S. Immune cells and metabolic dysfunction. Seminars in Immunopathology. 2014;**36**(1):13-25

[10] Jia G, Aroor AR, Sowers JR. Estrogen and mitochondria function in cardiorenal metabolic syndrome. Progress in Molecular Biology and Translational Science. 2014;**127**:229-249

[11] Dongiovanni P, Romeo S, Valenti L. Hepatocellular carcinoma in nonalcoholic fatty liver: Role of environmental and genetic factors. World Journal of Gastroenterology. 2014; **20**(36):12945-12955

[12] Karagozian R, Derdak Z, Baffy G. Obesity-associated mechanisms of hepatocarcinogenesis. Metabolism. 2014;**63**(5):607-617

[13] Aon MA, Bhatt N, Cortassa SC. Mitochondrial and cellular mechanisms for managing lipid excess. Frontiers in Physiology. 2014;**5**:282

[14] Huppert SS, Campbell KM. Emerging advancements in liver regeneration and organogenesis as tools for liver replacement. Current Opinion in Organ Transplantation. 2016;**21**(6):581-587

[15] Alison MR, Lin WR. Regenerating the liver: Not so simple after all? FIOOO Research, F1000 Faculty Rev-1818. 2016;5-15. DOI: 10.12688/f1000research.8827.1. eCollection 2016

[16] Lisman T, Porte RJ. Mechanisms of platelet-mediated liver regeneration. Blood. 2016; **128**(5):625-629

[17] Lauri A, Pompilio G, Capogrossi MC. The mitochondrial genome in aging and senescence. Ageing Research Reviews. 2014;**18**:1-15

[18] Aravinthan A, Shannon N, Heaney J, Hoare M, Marshall A, Alexander GJ. The senescent hepatocyte gene signature in chronic liver disease. Experimental Gerontology. 2014; **60**:37-45

[19] Carr SK, Chen JH, Cooper WN, Constancia M, Yeo GS, Ozanne SE. Maternal diet amplifies the hepatic aging trajectory of Cidea in male mice and leads to the development of fatty liver. The FASEB Journal. 2014;**28**(5):2191-2201

[20] Chen J, King K, Zhang JX. Effect of caloric restriction on hepatic sinusoidal system and stellate cells in mice. Journal of Aging Research. 2014;**2014**:670890

[21] Bozhkov AI, Nikitchenko YV. Thermogenesis and longevity in mammals. Thyroxin model of accelerated aging. Experimental Gerontology. 2014;**60**:173-182

[22] Uebi T, Umeda M, Imai T. Estrogen induces estrogen receptor alpha expression and hepatocyte proliferation in the livers of male mice. Genes to Cells. 2015;**20**(3):217-223

[23] Cechella JL, Leite MR, Dobrachinski F, da Rocha JT, Carvalho NR, Duarte MM, et al. Moderate swimming exercise and caffeine supplementation reduce the levels of inflammatory cytokines without causing oxidative stress in tissues of middle-aged rats. Amino Acids. 2014;**46**(5):1187-1195

[24] Kombu RS, Zhang GF, Abbas R, Mieyal JJ, Anderson VE, Kelleher JK, et al. Dynamics of glutathione and ophthalmate traced with 2H-enriched body water in rats and humans. American Journal of Physiology. Endocrinology and Metabolism. 2009;**297**(1): E260-E269

[25] Deevska G, Sunkara M, Karakashian C, Peppers B, Morris AJ, Nikolova-Karakashian MN. Effect of procysteine on aging-associated changes in hepatic GSH and SMase: Evidence for transcriptional regulation of smpd3. Journal of Lipid Research. 2014;**55**(10):2041-2052

[26] Bloomer SA, Han O, Kregel KC, Brown KE. Altered expression of iron regulatory proteins with aging is associated with transient hepatic iron accumulation after environmental heat stress. Blood Cells, Molecules & Diseases. 2014;**52**(1):19-26

[27] Franko A, von Kleist-Retzow JC, Neschen S, Wu M, Schommers P, Bose M, et al. Liver adapts mitochondrial function to insulin resistant and diabetic states in mice. Journal of Hepatology. 2014;**60**(4):816-823

[28] Escande C, Nin V, Pirtskhalava T, Chini CC, Tchkonia T, Kirkland JL, et al. Deleted in breast cancer 1 limits adipose tissue fat accumulation and plays a key role in the development of metabolic syndrome phenotype. Diabetes. 2015;**64**(1):12-22

[29] Di Naso FC, Porto RR, Fillmann HS, Maggioni L, Padoin AV, Ramos RJ, et al. Obesity depresses the anti-inflammatory HSP70 pathway, contributing to NAFLD progression. Obesity (Silver Spring). 2015;**23**(1):120-129

[30] Sanabria JR, Kombu RS, Zhang GF, Sandlers Y, Ai J, Ibarra RA, et al. Glutathione species and metabolomic prints in subjects with liver disease as biological markers for the detection of hepatocellular carcinoma. HPB. 2016;**18**(12):979-990

[31] Ghiraldini FG, Silveira AB, Kleinjan DA, Gilbert N, Mello ML. Genomic profiling of type-1 adult diabetic and aged normoglycemic mouse liver. BMC Endocrine Disorders. 2014;**14**:19

[32] D'Souza AM, Asadi A, Johnson JD, Covey SD, Kieffer TJ. Leptin deficiency in rats results in hyperinsulinemia and impaired glucose homeostasis. Endocrinology. 2014;**155**(4): 1268-1279

[33] Bianco A, Nigro E, Monaco ML, Matera MG, Scudiero O, Mazzarella G, et al. The burden of obesity in asthma and COPD: Role of adiponectin. Pulmonary Pharmacology & Therapeutics. 2017;**43**:20-25

[34] Gairolla J, Kler R, Modi M, Khurana D. Leptin and adiponectin: Pathophysiological role and possible therapeutic target of inflammation in ischemic stroke. Reviews in the Neurosciences. 2017;**28**(3):295-306

[35] Perez-Diaz S, Johnson LA, DeKroon RM, Moreno-Navarrete JM, Alzate O, Fernandez-Real JM, et al. Polymerase I and transcript release factor (PTRF) regulates adipocyte differentiation and determines adipose tissue expandability. The FASEB Journal. 2014;**28**(8): 3769-3779

[36] Fok WC, Bokov A, Gelfond J, Yu Z, Zhang Y, Doderer M, et al. Combined treatment of rapamycin and dietary restriction has a larger effect on the transcriptome and metabolome of liver. Aging Cell. 2014;**13**(2):311-319

[37] Fok WC, Chen Y, Bokov A, Zhang Y, Salmon AB, Diaz V, et al. Mice fed rapamycin have an increase in lifespan associated with major changes in the liver transcriptome. PLoS One. 2014;**9**(1):e83988

[38] Albert V, Hall MN. mTOR signaling in cellular and organismal energetics. Current Opinion in Cell Biology. 2015;**33**:55-66

[39] Gunsar F. Liver transplantation for hepatocellular carcinoma beyond the Milan criteria. Experimental and Clinical Transplantation. 2017;**15**(Suppl 2):59-64

[40] Lee HW, Suh KS. Advancements of liver transplantation for hepatocellular carcinoma in Korea. Japanese Journal of Clinical Oncology. 2017;**47**(2):93-100

[41] Cabral M, Martin-Venegas R, Moreno JJ. Differential cell growth/apoptosis behavior of 13-hydroxyoctadecadienoic acid enantiomers in a colorectal cancer cell line. American Journal of Physiology. Gastrointestinal and Liver Physiology. 2014;**307**(6):G664-G671

[42] Chen H, Cai W, Chu ES, Tang J, Wong CC, Wong SH, et al. Hepatic cyclooxygenase-2 overexpression induced spontaneous hepatocellular carcinoma formation in mice. Oncogene. 2017:1-12

[43] Zhang Y, Desai A, Yang SY, Bae KB, Antczak MI, Fink SP, et al. TISSUE REGENERATION: Inhibition of the prostaglandin-degrading enzyme 15-PGDH potentiates tissue regeneration. Science. 2015;**348**(6240):aaa2340. https://www.ncbi.nlm.nih.gov/pubmed/26068857

[44] Bellavista E, Martucci M, Vasuri F, Santoro A, Mishto M, Kloss A, et al. Lifelong maintenance of composition, function and cellular/subcellular distribution of proteasomes in human liver. Mechanisms of Ageing and Development. 2014;**141-142**:26-34

[45] Hodgson R, Christophi C. What determines ageing of the transplanted liver? HPB. The Official Journal of the International Hepato Pancreato Biliary Association. 2015;**17**(3): 222-225

[46] Fu H, Xu H, Chen H, Li Y, Li W, Zhu Q, et al. Inhibition of glycogen synthase kinase 3 ameliorates liver ischemia/reperfusion injury via an energy-dependent mitochondrial mechanism. Journal of Hepatology. 2014;**61**(4):816-824

[47] Cywes R, Greig PD, Morgan GR, Sanabria JR, Clavien PA, Harvey PR, et al. Rapid donor liver nutritional enhancement in a large animal model. Hepatology. 1992;**16**(5):1271-1279

[48] Cywes R, Greig PD, Sanabria JR, Clavien PA, Levy GA, Harvey PR, et al. Effect of intraportal glucose infusion on hepatic glycogen content and degradation, and outcome of liver transplantation. Annals of Surgery. 1992;**216**(3):235-246; discussion 46-7

[49] Bellomo R, Marino B, Starkey G, Fink M, Wang BZ, Eastwood GM, et al. Extended normothermic extracorporeal perfusion of isolated human liver after warm ischaemia: A preliminary report. Critical Care and Resuscitation. 2014;**16**(3):197-201

[50] Bral M, Gala-Lopez B, Bigam D, Kneteman N, Malcolm A, Livingstone S, et al. Preliminary single-center Canadian experience of human normothermic ex vivo liver perfusion: Results of a clinical trial. American Journal of Transplantation. 2017;**17**(4):1071-1080

[51] Goldaracena N, Barbas AS, Selzner M. Normothermic and subnormothermic ex-vivo liver perfusion in liver transplantation. Current Opinion in Organ Transplantation. 2016;**21**(3):315-321

[52] Ikeda T, Yanaga K, Lebeau G, Higashi H, Kakizoe S, Starzl TE. Hemodynamic and biochemical changes during normothermic and hypothermic sanguinous perfusion of the porcine hepatic graft. Transplantation. 1990;**50**(4):564-567

[53] Nassar A, Liu Q, Farias K, D'Amico G, Tom C, Grady P, et al. Ex vivo normothermic machine perfusion is safe, simple, and reliable: Results from a large animal model. Surgical Innovation. 2015;**22**(1):61-69

[54] Ravikumar R, Jassem W, Mergental H, Heaton N, Mirza D, Perera MT, et al. Liver transplantation after ex vivo normothermic machine preservation: A Phase 1 (first-in-man) clinical trial. American Journal of Transplantation. 2016;**16**(6):1779-1787. https://www.ncbi.nlm.nih.gov/pubmed/26752191

[55] Selzner M, Goldaracena N, Echeverri J, Kaths JM, Linares I, Selzner N, et al. Normothermic ex vivo liver perfusion using steen solution as perfusate for human liver transplantation: First North American results. Liver Transplantation. 2016;**22**(11):1501-1508

[56] Vogel T, Brockmann JG, Friend PJ. Ex-vivo normothermic liver perfusion: An update. Current Opinion in Organ Transplantation. 2010;**15**(2):167-172

[57] Aravinthan A, Challis B, Shannon N, Hoare M, Heaney J, Alexander GJ. Selective insulin resistance in hepatocyte senescence. Experimental Cell Research. 2015;**331**(1):38-45

[58] Abbas R, Kombu RS, Ibarra RA, Goyal KK, Brunengraber H, Sanabria JR. The dynamics of glutathione species and ophthalmate concentrations in plasma from the VX2 rabbit model of secondary liver tumors. HPB Surgery. 2011;**2011**:709052

[59] Andres Ibarra R, Abbas R, Kombu RS, Zhang GF, Jacobs G, Lee Z, et al. Disturbances in the glutathione/ophthalmate redox buffer system in the woodchuck model of hepatitis virus-induced hepatocellular carcinoma. HPB Surgery. 2011;**2011**:789323

[60] Carulli L, Anzivino C. Telomere and telomerase in chronic liver disease and hepatocarcinoma. World Journal of Gastroenterology. 2014;**20**(20):6287-6292

[61] Dlouha D, Maluskova J, Kralova Lesna I, Lanska V, Hubacek JA. Comparison of the relative telomere length measured in leukocytes and eleven different human tissues. Physiological Research. 2014;**63**(Suppl 3):S343-S350

[62] Kiran S, Oddi V, Ramakrishna G. Sirtuin 7 promotes cellular survival following genomic stress by attenuation of DNA damage, SAPK activation and p53 response. Experimental Cell Research. 2015;**331**(1):123-141

[63] Guenantin AC, Briand N, Bidault G, Afonso P, Bereziat V, Vatier C, et al. Nuclear envelope-related lipodystrophies. Seminars in Cell & Developmental Biology. 2014;**29**:148-157

[64] Arriazu E, Ruiz de Galarreta M, Cubero FJ, Varela-Rey M, Perez de Obanos MP, Leung TM, et al. Extracellular matrix and liver disease. Antioxidants & Redox Signaling. 2014; **21**(7):1078-1097

[65] Irvine KM, Skoien R, Bokil NJ, Melino M, Thomas GP, Loo D, et al. Senescent human hepatocytes express a unique secretory phenotype and promote macrophage migration. World Journal of Gastroenterology. 2014;**20**(47):17851-17862

[66] Idrissova L, Malhi H, Werneburg NW, LeBrasseur NK, Bronk SF, Fingas C, et al. TRAIL receptor deletion in mice suppresses the inflammation of nutrient excess. Journal of Hepatology. 2015;**62**(5):1156-1163

[67] Carloni V, Luong TV, Rombouts K. Hepatic stellate cells and extracellular matrix in hepatocellular carcinoma: More complicated than ever. Liver International. 2014;**34**(6):834-843

[68] Abbas R, Adam SJ, Okadal S, Groar H, Anderson J, Sanabria J. Development of a swine model of secondary liver tumor from a genetically induced swine fibroblast cell line. HPB. 2008;**10**(3):204-210

[69] Ibarra R, Dazard JE, Sandlers Y, Rehman F, Abbas R, Kombu R, et al. Metabolomic analysis of liver tissue from the VX2 rabbit model of secondary liver tumors. HPB Surgery. 2014;**2014**:310372

[70] Hong X, Song R, Song H, Zheng T, Wang J, Liang Y, et al. PTEN antagonises Tcl1/hnRNPK-mediated G6PD pre-mRNA splicing which contributes to hepatocarcinogenesis. Gut. 2014;**63**(10):1635-1647

[71] Hong IH, Lewis K, Iakova P, Jin J, Sullivan E, Jawanmardi N, et al. Age-associated change of C/EBP family proteins causes severe liver injury and acceleration of liver proliferation after CCl_4 treatments. The Journal of Biological Chemistry. 2014;**289**(2):1106-1118

[72] Hofmann JW, McBryan T, Adams PD, Sedivy JM. The effects of aging on the expression of Wnt pathway genes in mouse tissues. Age (Dordrecht, Netherlands). 2014;**36**(3):9618

[73] Lu WJ, Chua MS, So SK. Suppressing N-Myc downstream regulated gene 1 reactivates senescence signaling and inhibits tumor growth in hepatocellular carcinoma. Carcinogenesis. 2014;**35**(4):915-922

[74] Jurk D, Wilson C, Passos JF, Oakley F, Correia-Melo C, Greaves L, et al. Chronic inflammation induces telomere dysfunction and accelerates ageing in mice. Nature Communications. 2014;**2**:4172

[75] Lopez-Dominguez JA, Khraiwesh H, Gonzalez-Reyes JA, Lopez-Lluch G, Navas P, Ramsey JJ, et al. Dietary fat and aging modulate apoptotic signaling in liver of calorie-restricted mice. The Journals of Gerontology. Series A, Biological Sciences and Medical Sciences. 2015;**70**(4):399-409

[76] Jin J, Hong IH, Lewis K, Iakova P, Breaux M, Jiang Y, et al. Cooperation of C/EBP family proteins and chromatin remodeling proteins is essential for termination of liver regeneration. Hepatology. 2015;**61**(1):315-325

[77] Sadri AR, Jeschke MG, Amini-Nik S. Advances in liver regeneration: Revisiting hepatic stem/progenitor cells and their origin. Stem Cells International. 2016;**2016**:7920897

[78] Sanabria JR, Gordon ER, Harvey PR, Goresky CA, Strasberg SM. Accumulation of unconjugated bilirubin in cholesterol pellets implanted in swine gallbladders. Gastroenterology. 1996;**110**(2):607-613

[79] Sanabria JR, Upadhya A, Mullen B, Harvey PR, Strasberg SM. Effect of deoxycholate on immunoglobulin G concentration in bile: Studies in humans and pigs. Hepatology. 1995;**21**(1):215-222

[80] Ahsan MK, Mehal WZ. Activation of adenosine receptor A2A increases HSC proliferation and inhibits death and senescence by down-regulation of p53 and Rb. Frontiers in Pharmacology. 2014;**5**:69

[81] Borkham-Kamphorst E, Schaffrath C, Van de Leur E, Haas U, Tihaa L, Meurer SK, et al. The anti-fibrotic effects of CCN1/CYR61 in primary portal myofibroblasts are mediated through induction of reactive oxygen species resulting in cellular senescence, apoptosis and attenuated TGF-beta signaling. Biochimica et Biophysica Acta. 2014;**1843**(5):902-914

[82] Ahluwalia A, Jones MK, Szabo S, Tarnawski AS. Aging impairs transcriptional regulation of vascular endothelial growth factor in human microvascular endothelial cells: Implications for angiogenesis and cell survival. Journal of Physiology and Pharmacology. 2014;**65**(2):209-215

[83] Ahluwalia A, Jones MK, Tarnawski AS. Key role of endothelial importin-alpha in VEGF expression and gastric angiogenesis: Novel insight into aging gastropathy. American Journal of Physiology. Gastrointestinal and Liver Physiology. 2014;**306**(4):G338-G345

[84] Coletta C, Modis K, Olah G, Brunyanszki A, Herzig DS, Sherwood ER, et al. Endothelial dysfunction is a potential contributor to multiple organ failure and mortality in aged mice subjected to septic shock: Preclinical studies in a murine model of cecal ligation and puncture. Critical Care. 2014;**18**(5):511

[85] Hayashi T, Kotani H, Yamaguchi T, Taguchi K, Iida M, Ina K, et al. Endothelial cellular senescence is inhibited by liver X receptor activation with an additional mechanism for its atheroprotection in diabetes. Proceedings of the National Academy of Sciences of the United States of America. 2014;**111**(3):1168-1173

[86] Poisson J, Lemoinne S, Boulanger C, Durand F, Moreau R, Valla D, et al. Liver sinusoidal endothelial cells: Physiology and role in liver diseases. Journal of Hepatology. 2017; **66**(1):212-227

[87] Donato AJ, Henson GD, Hart CR, Layec G, Trinity JD, Bramwell RC, et al. The impact of ageing on adipose structure, function and vasculature in the B6D2F1 mouse: Evidence of significant multisystem dysfunction. The Journal of Physiology. 2014;**592**(18):4083-4096

[88] Bhattacharjee J, Kirby M, Softic S, Miles L, Salazar-Gonzalez R-M, Shivakumar P, et al. Hepatic natural killer T-cell and CD8+ T-cell signatures in mice with nonalcoholic steatohepatitis. Hepatology Communications. 2017;**1**(4):299-310

[89] Ehlken H, Krishna-Subramanian S, Ochoa-Callejero L, Kondylis V, Nadi NE, Straub BK, et al. Death receptor-independent FADD signalling triggers hepatitis and hepatocellular carcinoma in mice with liver parenchymal cell-specific NEMO knockout. Cell Death and Differentiation. 2014;**21**(11):1721-1732

[90] Ma C, Kesarwala AH, Eggert T, Medina-Echeverz J, Kleiner DE, Jin P, et al. NAFLD causes selective CD4(+) T lymphocyte loss and promotes hepatocarcinogenesis. Nature. 2016;**531**(7593):253-257

[91] Khraiwesh H, Lopez-Dominguez JA, Fernandez del Rio L, Gutierrez-Casado E, Lopez-Lluch G, Navas P, et al. Mitochondrial ultrastructure and markers of dynamics in hepatocytes from aged, calorie restricted mice fed with different dietary fats. Experimental Gerontology. 2014;**56**:77-88

[92] Girardet C, Begriche K, Ptitsyn A, Koza RA, Butler AA. Unravelling the mysterious roles of melanocortin-3 receptors in metabolic homeostasis and obesity using mouse genetics. International Journal of Obesity Supplements. 2014;**4**(Suppl 1):S37-S44

[93] Ahn M, Park JS, Chae S, Kim S, Moon C, Hyun JW, et al. Hepatoprotective effects of *Lycium chinense* Miller fruit and its constituent betaine in CCl_4-induced hepatic damage in rats. Acta Histochemica. 2014;**116**(6):1104-1112

[94] Bae KH, Min AK, Kim JG, Lee IK, Park KG. Alpha lipoic acid induces hepatic fibroblast growth factor 21 expression via up-regulation of CREBH. Biochemical and Biophysical Research Communications. 2014;**455**(3-4):212-217

[95] Ip BC, Liu C, Ausman LM, von Lintig J, Wang XD. Lycopene attenuated hepatic tumorigenesis via differential mechanisms depending on carotenoid cleavage enzyme in mice. Cancer Prevention Research (Philadelphia, Pa.). 2014;**7**(12):1219-1227

[96] Jiang Y, Huang W, Wang J, Xu Z, He J, Lin X, et al. Metformin plays a dual role in MIN6 pancreatic beta cell function through AMPK-dependent autophagy. International Journal of Biological Sciences. 2014;**10**(3):268-277

[97] Momchilova A, Petkova D, Staneva G, Markovska T, Pankov R, Skrobanska R, et al. Resveratrol alters the lipid composition, metabolism and peroxide level in senescent rat hepatocytes. Chemico-Biological Interactions. 2014;**207**:74-80

[98] Park KH, Kim JM, Cho KH. Elaidic acid (EA) generates dysfunctional high-density lipoproteins and consumption of EA exacerbates hyperlipidemia and fatty liver change in zebrafish. Molecular Nutrition & Food Research. 2014;**58**(7):1537-1545

[99] Spartano NL, Lamon-Fava S, Matthan NR, Obin MS, Greenberg AS, Lichtenstein AH. Linoleic acid suppresses cholesterol efflux and ATP-binding cassette transporters in murine bone marrow-derived macrophages. Lipids. 2014;**49**(5):415-422

[100] Yao WL, Ko BS, Liu TA, Liang SM, Liu CC, Lu YJ, et al. Cordycepin suppresses integrin/FAK signaling and epithelial-mesenchymal transition in hepatocellular carcinoma. Anti-Cancer Agents in Medicinal Chemistry. 2014;**14**(1):29-34

[101] Zhang J, Wang M, Zhang Z, Luo Z, Liu F, Liu J. Celecoxib derivative OSU-03012 inhibits the proliferation and activation of hepatic stellate cells by inducing cell senescence. Molecular Medicine Reports. 2015;**11**(4):3021-3026

[102] Hu B, Du Q, Deng S, An HM, Pan CF, Shen KP, et al. *Ligustrum lucidum* Ait. fruit extract induces apoptosis and cell senescence in human hepatocellular carcinoma cells through upregulation of p21. Oncology Reports. 2014;**32**(3):1037-1042

[103] Hasan ST, Zingg JM, Kwan P, Noble T, Smith D, Meydani M. Curcumin modulation of high fat diet-induced atherosclerosis and steatohepatosis in LDL receptor deficient mice. Atherosclerosis. 2014;**232**(1):40-51

[104] Drummond CA, Hill MC, Shi H, Fan X, Xie JX, Haller ST, et al. Na/K-ATPase signaling regulates collagen synthesis through microRNA-29b-3p in cardiac fibroblasts. Physiological Genomics. 2016;**48**(3):220-229

[105] Hangaard L, Bouzinova EV, Staehr C, Dam VS, Kim S, Xie Z, et al. Na-K-ATPase regulates intercellular communication in the vascular wall via cSrc kinase-dependent connexin43 phosphorylation. American Journal of Physiology. Cell Physiology. 2017;**312**(4):C385-CC97

[106] Li Z, Cai T, Tian J, Xie JX, Zhao X, Liu L, et al. NaKtide, a Na/K-ATPase-derived peptide Src inhibitor, antagonizes ouabain-activated signal transduction in cultured cells. The Journal of Biological Chemistry. 2009;**284**(31):21066-21076

[107] Li Z, Zhang Z, Xie JX, Li X, Tian J, Cai T, et al. Na/K-ATPase mimetic pNaKtide peptide inhibits the growth of human cancer cells. The Journal of Biological Chemistry. 2011;**286**(37):32394-32403

[108] Liu J, Tian J, Chaudhry M, Maxwell K, Yan Y, Wang X, et al. Attenuation of Na/K-ATPase mediated oxidant amplification with pNaKtide ameliorates experimental uremic cardiomyopathy. Scientific Reports. 2016;**6**:34592

[109] Sodhi K, Maxwell K, Yan Y, Liu J, Chaudhry MA, Getty M, et al. pNaKtide inhibits Na/K-ATPase reactive oxygen species amplification and attenuates adipogenesis. Science Advances. 2015;**1**(9):e1500781

[110] Sodhi K, Srikanthan K, Goguet-Rubio P, Nichols A, Mallick A, Nawab A, et al. pNaKtide attenuates steatohepatitis and atherosclerosis by blocking Na/K-ATPase/ROS amplification in C57Bl6 and ApoE knockout mice fed a western diet. Scientific Reports. 2017;**7**(1):193. https://www.ncbi.nlm.nih.gov/pubmed/28298638

[111] Srikanthan K, Shapiro JI, Sodhi K. The role of Na/K-ATPase signaling in oxidative stress related to obesity and cardiovascular disease. Molecules. 2016;(9): 21-34. https://www.ncbi.nlm.nih.gov/pubmed/27598118

[112] Wang Y, Ye Q, Liu C, Xie JX, Yan Y, Lai F, et al. Involvement of Na/K-ATPase in hydrogen peroxide-induced activation of the Src/ERK pathway in LLC-PK1 cells. Free Radical Biology & Medicine. 2014;**71**:415-426

8

Oncogenic Secretory Clusterin: A Promising Therapeutic Target for Hepatocellular Carcinoma

Min Yao, Wenjie Zheng, Li Wang, Miao Fang,
Dengfu Yao and Zhizheng Dong

Abstract

Oncogenic secretory clusterin (sCLU) is a stress-induced molecular chaperone that confers proliferative and survival advantages to hepatocellular carcinoma (HCC), plays a crucial role in cell proliferation, multiple drug resistance, metastasis, and tumor progression. However, the targeted effects and molecular mechanisms of sCLU for malignant tumor are still unknown. This chapter aims to review some progression of oncogenic sCLU as a promising therapeutic target for HCC. An English-language literature search was conducted using bibliographic databases on some valuable articles in focused review questions to analyze the interventions and findings of included studies using a conceptual framework. The positive rate of hepatic sCLU expression in cancerous tissues was significantly higher more than that in their surrounding non-cancerous ones at gene transcription level or at protein level, with increasing according to tumor-node-metastasis (TNM) staging. Abnormal expression of oncogenic sCLU associated with poor differentiation degree and TNM stage of HCC also has been considered as a valuable diagnostic or independent prognostic biomarker for HCC. Furthermore, silencing sCLU at mRNA level by specific shRNA or inhibition by OGX-011 suppressed the colony formation and proliferation of tumor cells with apoptosis increasing, cell cycle arrested, alterations of cell migration and invasion behaviors, decreasing phosphorylation level of Akt and GSK-3β in vitro, and significantly suppressing the xenograft tumor growth with decreasing expression of β-catenin, p-GSK3β, and cyclinD1 in vivo. The oncogenic sCLU expression was closely associated with tumor progression, and it should be a novel potential molecular-targeted therapy for HCC.

Keywords: hepatocellular carcinoma, secretory clusterin, targeted therapy

1. Introduction

Hepatocellular carcinoma (HCC) is the third leading cause of cancer-related death worldwide [1]. Growing understanding of the multiple pathogenic factors including hepatitis B or C virus (HBV or HCV) infection, toxic, lipid accumulation, aflatoxin B1 intake, and so on with complex molecular mechanisms underlying HCC reveal that hepatocarcinogenesis is a multistep process including lots of activated or suppressed oncogenes or anticancer genes [2–4]. Some techniques for HCC therapy have experienced great progress. However, the prognosis of HCC patients is still very poor due to the high rates of tumor recurrence and metastasis. Effective therapy of HCC is dependent on early specific diagnosis, therefore, to provide optimal treatment for patients, more precise and effective markers are urgently needed in all phases of management from early detection to staging, treatment monitoring, and prognosis [5–7]. Numerous studies have shown the clinical utility of novel blood-based markers, such as circulating tumor cells, key signal molecules, long non-coding RNA, and microRNA with great potential for HCC [8, 9].

Molecular chaperones are proteins that response to cellular stresses including genotoxic agents, nutrient starvation, and heat shock, with cellular stresses-induced protein misfolding, aggregation, and denaturation [10, 11]. To date, only few specific markers such as hepatoma-specific γ-glutamyl transferase [12, 13], oncofetal antigen glypican-3 (GPC-3) [14, 15], hepatoma-specific alpha-fetoprotein (HS-AFP or AFP-L3) [16], member 3a of Wingless-type MMTV integration site family (Wnt3a) [17, 18], and molecular chaperones like heat shock proteins (Hsp27 or Hsp90) [19] and clusterin have been developed as valuable biomarkers for primary hepatocellular carcinoma (PHC) diagnosis and surveillance. The clusterin (CLU) that was first detected in HCC tissues by Tobe et al., who found that SP40-40 gene in hepatoma cells was located in human chromosome 8, also designated as apolipoprotein J (APOJ), SP-40, sulfated glycoprotein 2 (SGP2), and testosterone-repressed prostate message 2 (TRPM2) [20]. Following the detection of their complete cDNA cloning, sequencing and comparison, secretory CLU (sCLU) is found to be the mature isoform of cytoplasm endoplasmic reticulum (ER)-Golgi CLU, which is over-expressed in a wide variety of tumors with oncogenicity [21, 22]. Recently, the mechanisms of abnormal sCLU expression and its targeted effects for HCC have been explored [23, 24]. This article summarizes some progression of sCLU as a promising target for HCC gene therapy.

2. Gene structure and functions of sCLU

Human CLU gene is a single-copy gene on chromosome 8p21-p12 including 9 exons and 8 introns, encoding an mRNA of 2877 bp and translating to a polypeptide with 449 amino acids (a.a.) [25]. The secretory glycoprotein (1st a.a.) is a signal sequence of hydrophobic leader, and targets the ER protein. CLU gene encodes two isoforms with distinct functions as a result of alternative splicing and post-translational modifications: cytoplasm sCLU (75–80 kDa) and nuclear CLU (nCLU, 55 kDa), which is mainly located in the nucleus. The sCLU molecule is a highly conserved heterodimeric disulfide-linked 449 amino acid polypeptide that represents the major product of CLU gene. The ER-Golgi sCLU is considered to influence immune regulation, transformation, tissue remodeling, lipid transport, membrane recycling, complements cascade, DNA repair, cell adhesion, and cell-cell interactions, indicated that sCLU is widely distributed in tissues and body fluids involved in various physiological processes [11, 26, 27].

Multiple reports have shown that the cytoplasm sCLU is cytoprotective and anti-apoptotic [28, 29], whereas nCLU protein is proapoptotic. Abnormal oncogenic sCLU expression was reported to correlate closely with HCC progression, such as inducing epithelial-mesenchymal transition (EMT) [30], formation of multiple drug resistance (MDR) [31], distal metastasis of tumor cells, and malignant transformation of hepatocytes, interaction with oncogenes or suppressor genes, and related signal pathways (**Figure 1**) [32, 33]. Because of ischemic or hypoxic microenvironment existence in cancerous tissues, the sCLU are often adaptively over-expressed and closely related with increased tumorigenicity, metastatic potential, and MDR to chemotherapy. As a stress-induced chaperone that inhibits protein misfolding and aggregation in a manner similar to small heat shock proteins (HSPs) [34, 35], its promoter

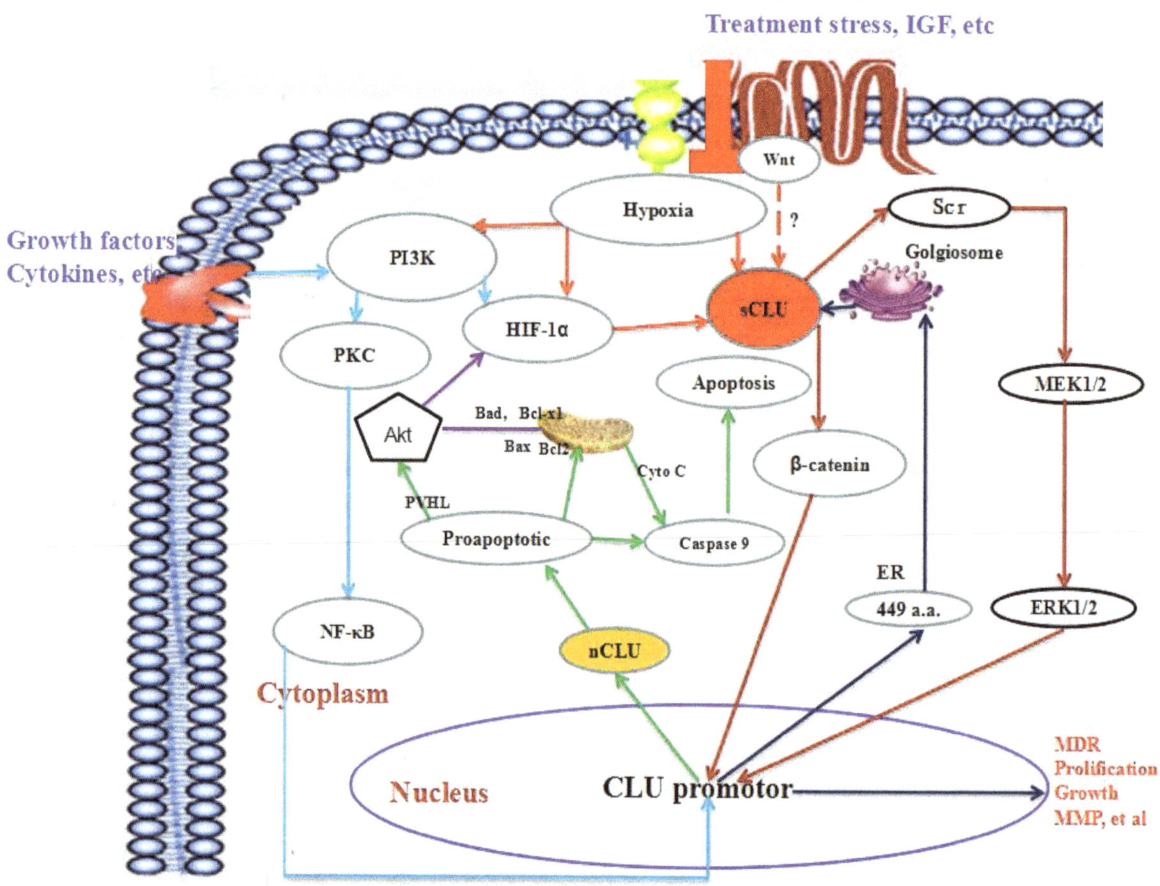

Figure 1. Potential mechanisms of hepatic sCLU in hepatocellular carcinoma. Cyto C, cytochrome c; ER, endoplasmic reticulum; Gene Reg., gene regulation; HIF-1α, hypoxia inducible factor-1α; IGF, insulin-like factor; MDR, multiple drug resistance; MMP, matrix metalloproteinase; nCLU, nuclear clusterin; NF-κB, nuclear factor-κB; PKC, protein kinase C; PI3K, phosphatidylinositol 3-kinase; Scr, sarcoma gene; sCLU, secretory clusterin.

region contains an element recognized by heat shock factor 1 (HSF-1) [36]. Cytoplasm sCLU-inhibited apoptosis by interacting with activated Bax, and protects HCC cells from ER stress-induced apoptosis through a physical interaction with glucose-regulated prptein78 (GRP78) [29, 37].

Hepatic sCLU has been confirmed that it was physically associated with eukaryotic translation initiation factor 3 subunit I (EIF3I), and might protect EIF3I protein from degradation. A positive correlation was founded between sCLU and EIF3I, and both of their functions might be as a cooperative unit in HCC. The levels of sCLU and EIF3I expression were investigated in HCC using tissue microarray (TMA) and the patients with high EIF3I level exhibited poor prognosis. After silenced EIF3I, Akt phosphorylation was significantly inhibited. The EIF3I-Akt complex could prevent PP2A-mediated dephosphorylation, which in turn led to a constitutive Akt signal activation, suggesting that the CLU-EIF3I complex might prevent EIF3I degradation, and then contribute to Akt upregulation [33, 38].

3. Biological behaviors of sCLU expression in cancerous tissues

Although great efforts have been made to explore molecular mechanism of HCC invasion and metastasis in the past decade [39–41], the mechanism of HCC remains incompletely understood. The alterations of sCLU expression at messenger RNA (mRNA) or protein level were investigated in HCC- and their non-tumorous tissues (NT) with self-control [42]. The overall level of sCLU mRNA in the HCC group was 75% up-regulated, 7.5% down-regulated, and 17.5% non-changed. Although no significant difference of the sCLU mRNA level at staging I was found between NT and HCC, they were drastically up-regulated expression from staging II to IV. The staining of sCLU mainly presented in the cytoplasm at protein level in HCC and their NT tissues were analyzed by tissue microarray (TMA) with immunohistochemistry (IHC). Its incidence in the HCC group (73.3%), with 37.5, 68 and 88.9% at staging I, II and III & IV, was significantly higher than that in the NT group (23.3%), respectively. The levels of sCLU protein consistent with their mRNA expression were gradually upregulation with increasing HCC staging [42, 43], indicated that high sCLU should be a valuable biomarker to distinguish malignant from benign liver nodular lesions [44].

The sCLU as a functional homolog of HSPs is a stress-induced chaperone that confers proliferative and closely associates with poor prognosis of HCC. Recurrence and metastasis are the most causes of poor prognosis of HCC. Clinicopathological features of sCLU revealed that its high expression was significantly linked to poor differentiation and advanced TNM stage [45]. There was a trend toward a poorer overall survival in HCC with high sCLU expression. Besides, survival time of HCC with high TNM stage was significantly shorter than that of cases with low stage. Moreover, in the subset of HCC patients with III and IV stage, high sCLU expression was prone to result in a shorter survival time (**Table 1**). There is a closely positive correlation between abnormal sCLU expression and HCC. High sCLU expression has more invasive phenotype for HCC [46]. The upregulation of sCLU is associated with HCC progression by contributing to angiogenesis, chemoresistance, cells survival, and metastasis.

Group		n	Pos. n (%)	χ^2 value	*P* value
AFP (μg /L)	≤50	37	31 (83.78)	1.733	0.118
	>50	38	27 (71.05)		
Portal vein invasion	With	7	6 (85.71)	0.309	0.578
	Without	68	52 (76.47)		
HBsAg	Negative	46	36 (78.26)	0.058	0.809
	Positive	29	22 (75.86)		
Tumor size	≤5 cm	45	33 (73.33)	1.027	0.311
	>5 cm	30	25 (83.33)		
Liver cirrhosis	With	57	45 (78.95)	0.353	0.552
	Without	18	13 (72.22)		
Lymph node metastasis	With	23	22 (95.65)	6.351	0.012*
	Without	52	36 (69.23)		
Differentiation	Well & moderate	58	43 (74.14)	1.491	0.222
	Poor	17	15 (88.24)		
Gross classification	Unifocal	62	46 (74.19)	1.744	0.187
	Multifocal	13	12 (92.31)		
TNM	I & II	45	30 (66.67)	7.683	0.021*
	III & IV	30	28 (93.33)		
Child degree	A	44	30 (68.18)	5.086	0.024*
	B&C	31	29 (90.32)		
5 years' survival	No	51	43 (84.31)	4.430	0.035*
	Yes	24	15 (62.50)		

Pos. n (%), positive number (%). *P<0.05

Table 1. Clinicopathological features of hepatic sCLU expression in HCC.

Growing evidences showed that sCLU with molecular chaperones played an important role in MDR formation, cells proliferation, metastasis of HCC [47]. Furthermore, univariate and multivariate analyses indicated that sCLU might be an independent prognostic indicator, in line with the factor of lymph node metastasis.

4. Circulating sCLU as diagnostic marker

The observations were in accordance with the early literature showing that upregulation of sCLU-positive expression might be associated with poor clinical outcome in HCC patients [21, 48]. According to previous clinical studies, average serum sCLU level was significantly higher in the HCC group more than that in any of groups with cirrhosis, chronic hepatitis, or healthy control (**Table 2**). The area under receiver operating characteristic (ROC) curve and diagnostic sensitivity were 0.75 and 74.7% in serum sCLU, and 0.74 and 58.7% in serum AFP, respectively. The incidence of both combining detection rose up to 90.7% for HCC diagnosis (**Table 3**). High-circulating sCLU levels were observed in HCC patients, consistent with a recent study using a three-step serum proteome analysis, which showed that serum sCLU levels in HCC were significantly higher than those in benign liver diseases [42].

CLU is related to reverse cholesterol transport, platelet degranulation and human immune response pathways [49]. Protein-protein interaction analysis and pathway assessment showed a closed molecular relationship between cirrhosis and HCC [50]. Serum samples collected from HCCLM3-R metastatic HCC tumor model at specific stages of metastasis (1., 3 and 6 weeks) were subjected to iTRAQ labeling followed by 2DLC-ESI-MS/MS analysis. Circulating sCLU was significantly up-regulated during cancer progression and metastasis. The expression of sCLU was significantly higher in metastatic HCC cells and samples from HCC patients. Serum sCLU was highly increased with tumor size, tumor number, lymph node infiltration (**Table 4**) [42], and showed that the ROC area under curve value was 0.95 in sCLU more than that (0.85) in AFP. If 128 μg/mL as a cutoff value, the sensitivity or specificity of serum sCLU level for predicting HCC was 90 or 87%, respectively. The data indicated that circulating sCLU is a promising molecular marker of diagnosis or predicting metastasis for HCC [22, 51, 52].

Group	n	Mean ± SD	Positive n (%)	χ^2 value	*P* value
sCLU		**μg/mL**			
HCC	75	119.21 ± 16.67	56 (74.67)		
LC	30	97.78 ± 19.06	8 (26.67)**	20.744	<0.001
CH	30	106.30 ± 19.22	12 (40.00)**	11.285	<0.001
NC	36	89.96 ± 7.27	0 (0.00)**	54.249	<0.001
AFP		**ng/mL**			
HCC	75	2177.32 ± 3757.99	44 (58.67)		
LC	30	126.84 ± 244.76	10 (33.33)*	5.505	0.019
CH	30	30.27 ± 50.09	5 (16.67)**	15.188	<0.001
NC	36	7.1 ± 3.50	1 (2.78)**	31.520	<0.001

Serum sCLU values >104.0 μg/mL or AFP values >50 ng/mL were considered positive.

sCLU, secretory clusterin; LC, liver cirrhosis; CH, chronic hepatitis; NC, normal control; and AFP, α-fetoprotein.

*$P < 0.05$, compared with HCC group.

**$P < 0.01$, compared with HCC group.

Table 2. Serum sCLU or AFP levels among patients with chronic liver diseases and comparative analysis of both diagnostic values for HCC.

	sCLU level > 104.2 μg/mL (%)	AFP level > 50 ng/mL (%)	Both (%)
Sensitivity (%)	74.67	58.67	90.67
Specificity (%)	66.67	75.00	60.00
Accuracy (%)	71.11	65.93	77.03
Positive predictive value (%)	73.68	74.58	73.91
Negative predictive value (%)	67.80	59.21	83.72

AFP, α-fetoprotein; sCLU, secretory clusterin.

Table 3. Assessment diagnostic validity of serum sCLU or AFP level for HCC.

Group	n	Average (μg/mL)	*t* value	*P* value	Positive, n (%)	χ^2 value	*P* value
Age (years)							
≤60	47	118.09 ± 16.45	0.751	0.455	33 (70.21)	1.320	0.251
>60	28	121.09 ± 17.16			23 (82.14)		
AFP (μg/L)							
≤50	31	120.15 ± 17.12	0.405	0.686	24 (77.42)	0.212	0.645
>50	44	118.55 ± 16.50			32 (72.73)		
Portal vein invasion							
With	28	119.34 ± 14.52	0.050	0.960	22 (78.57)	0.360	0.548
Without	47	119.14 ± 17.97			34 (72.34)		
Tumor size							
≤5 cm	34	114.63 ± 18.10	2.221	0.029[a]	21 (61.76)	5.473	0.019
>5 cm	41	123.00 ± 14.52			35 (85.37)		
Lymph node metastasis							
Without	44	114.84 ± 15.21	2.826	0.006[b]	29 (65.91)	4.316	0.038
With	31	125.40 ± 16.91			27 (87.10)		
Differentiation							
Well & moderate	57	117.43 ± 16.34	1.662	0.101	42 (73.68)	0.121	0.728
Poor	18	124.84 ± 16.90			14 (77.78)		
Gross classification							
Unifocal	36	114.02 ± 18.57	2.698	0.009[c]	23 (63.89)	4.251	0.039
Multifocal	39	124.00 ± 13.20			33 (84.62)		

Group	n	Average (μg/mL)	*t* value	*P* value	Positive, n (%)	χ^2 value	*P* value
TNM stage							
I & II	31	113.93 ± 14.36	2.375	0.02[d]	20 (64.52)	2.878	0.09
III & IV	44	122.93 ± 17.31			36 (81.82)		
Child classification							
A	55	117.60 ± 14.56	1.395	0.167	40 (72.73)	0.410	0.522
B&C	20	123.63 ± 21.23			16 (80.00)		

AFP, α-fetoprotein; TNM, tumor node metastasis.
[a]With the tumor size ≥5 cm group.
[b]The lymph node metastasis group.
[c]With the multifocal group.
[d]With TNM III & IV group.

Table 4. Clinicopathologic features of serum sCLU expression in HCC patients (Mean ± SD).

5. Application prospect of targeting CLU gene

5.1. Antisense oligonucleotide (ASO) therapy

ASO is a useful technique to inhibit specific-targeted CLU genes, with a small synthetic natural nucleic acid analogue, that can complementary to CLU mRNA that induce degradation or inhibit translation into protein [52]. It is considered to be a potent inhibitor of sCLU expression in vitro, in vivo, and in human clinical trials, with no apparent effect on the expression of nCLU. Custirsen (OGX-011, 5′-CAGCAGCA GAGTCTTCATCAT-3′, 50 nM) is a novel 2′-methoxy-ethyl-modified phosphorothioate ASO, which is a 21-nucleoside complement to target the translation initiation site of CLU gene exon II mRNA translation initiation site with one CpG motif [53]. Hence, OGX-011 plays the role of chemosensitization by influencing the anti-apoptotic protein sCLU instead of the proapoptotic protein nCLU. Xiu et al. have reviewed the current state of research on clusterin, to predict future research directions and to analyze the potential of the clinical application of custirsen in HCC [54]. However, the median overall survival of HCC cases were ms 23.4 mo in the group of the OGX-011 combining anti-cancer drugs (docetaxel/prednisone) and ms 22.2 mo in the other group of cases with docetaxel/prednisone alone. No significant difference was found between two groups. Some potential key factors might contribute to its results, and still want to do more clinical trials to be ongoing [55].

5.2. Reversal MDR by specific shRNA-targeted sCLU

Resistance of tumor cells to chemotherapy continues to be a major clinical obstacle to extend the survival rate of patients with HCC. Recently, one of the major strategies for liver cancer is surgical resection with adjuvant anti-HCC drug chemotherapy [10]. However, the HCC patients always tend to acquire MDR during tumor progression. MDR-related P-glycoprotein (P-gp), encoded by MDR1 gene is positively linked closely with chronic liver diseases, because of its drug efflux via ATP-binding cassette (ABC) family transporters, which can decrease intracellular concentration of anti-HCC drugs. Targeting sCLU to sensitize cancer cells to chemotherapy has become an attractive new strategy for cancer treatment. Previous studies found sCLU expressed in line with P-gp via immunohistochemical staining. The sCLU expression was analyzed in human hepatoma cells and chemoresistant counter-part HepG2/ADM cells. After transfection of shRNA-1 (5′-GTAAGTACGTC AATAAGGA-3′) into HepG2/ADM cells, the inhibition of CLU expression was 73.68% at mRNA level with obvious enhancement in chemosensitivity, and increasing apoptosis induced by doxorubicin [56]. Knockdown CLU also significantly decreased the drug efflux pump activity through the depression of MDR1/P-gp. Moreover, silencing CLU led to downregulation of β-catenin, suggesting that downregulation of CLU might be a key point to reverse MDR of HepG2/ADM cells [57].

5.3. Blockade-related pathway

5.3.1. PI3K/Akt/NF-κB pathway

Previous data revealed that CLU promoted cell survival through the PI3K/Akt pathway and induced MMP-9 expression via ERK1/2 and PI3K/Akt/NF-κB pathways [32]. CLU could increase p-Akt and MMP13 expression. A positive correlation between CLU expression and p-Akt level was observed in cohort of HCC tissues. Where CLU knockdown using OGX-011 significantly decreased p-Akt and MMP13 levels and suppressed HCC metastasis in two metastatic models through inhibiting EIF3I/Akt/MMP13 signaling. The related signaling molecule blockade of the PI3K-Akt pathway could significantly inhibited MMP13 expression in human HepG2-CLU or HCCLM3 cells [38, 58]. Decreased level of CLU accompanied with downregulation of MMP13 and p-Akt was observed in tumors derived from HCCLM3-shCLU group, revealed that p-Akt level was significantly correlated with poor prognosis and indicated that CLU may play a crucial role in HCC metastasis [38].

5.3.2. Wnt/β-catenin pathway

Wnt canonical pathway is often constitutively active in neoplastic cells, although, normally β-catenin is negatively regulated by GSK-3β that phosphorylates β-catenin to drive it for proteosomal degradation [30, 59]. Previous data emphasized sCLU modification after being exposed to Wnt/β-catenin inhibitor, and expressions of the crucial β-catenin and GSK-3β genes were detected in cases of sCLU depletion. The data indicated that sCLU suppression might lead to the inhibition of Wnt/β-catenin pathway in reverse. Hence, sCLU might play an important role in chemoresistance of HepG2/ADM cells together with Wnt/β-catenin signaling molecules [31, 56].

5.3.3. IGF-1/IGF-1R/Src/Mek/Erk pathway

Hepatic sCLU is a general genotoxic stress-induced, prosurvival gene product implicated in cancer [36, 37]. The regulatory signal transduction processes that control sCLU expression, the induction of sCLU is delayed, peaking 72 h after low doses of ionizing radiation, and is dependent on up-regulating IGF-1 and phosphorylation-dependent IGF-1R activation [23, 27] that stimulates the downstream Src-Mek-Erk signal transduction cascade to ultimately

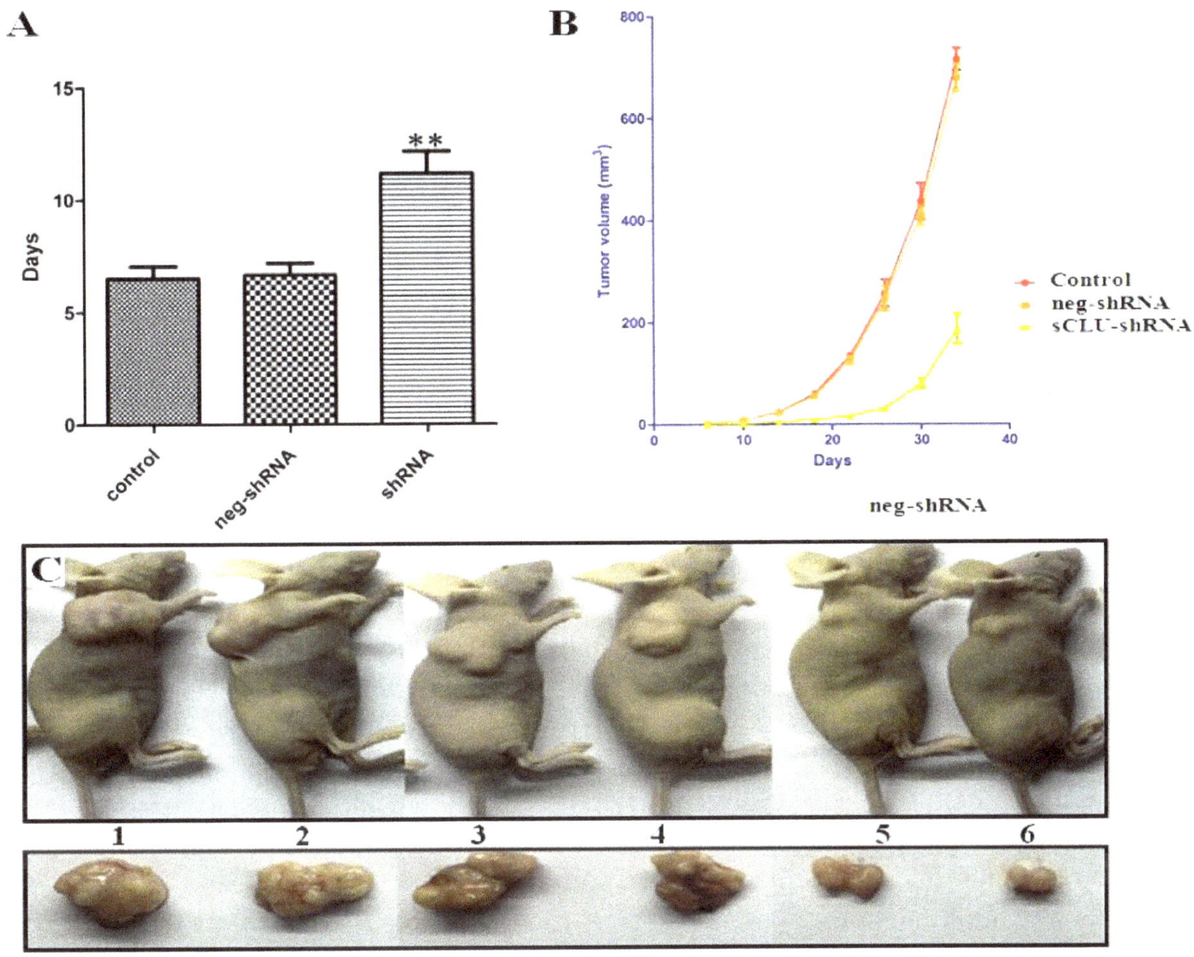

Figure 2. Inhibition of sCLU gene transcription by specific shRNA-1 on effects of forming time, growth curve and size of orthotopic xenograft tumors. The control, neg-shRNA, or sCLU-shRNA groups were injected with the plasmid contained specific shRNA-1 into nude mice. (A) The forming time of the orthotopic xenograft tumors from each group. (B) The growth curves of the xenograft tumors from each group. And the tumor volumes were measured at the indicated time point. (C) The representative photographs of the nude mice and corresponding dissected tumors from each group. 1 and 2, the xenografts in the control group; 3 and 4, the xenografts in the neg-shRNA group; 5 and 6, the xenografts in the sCLU-shRNA group. The data are presented as the mean ± SD. Compared with the control group, $^{**}P < 0.01$.

transactivate the early growth response-1 (Egr-1) transcription factor. Thus, the ionizing radiation exposure causes stress-induced IGF-1R-Src-Mek-Erk-Egr-1 activation that regulates the sCLU prosurvival cascade pathway for radiation resistance in HCC therapy [60].

5.4. Suppressed HCC growth in vivo by silencing sCLU

The inhibition of sCLU gene transcription by specific shRNA-1 on effects of forming time, growth curve, and size of orthotopic xenograft tumors after sacrifice of the mice at the 34th day with injection are shown in **Figure 2**. The mean weight of the xenograft tumors in the shRNA-1 group was significantly less than that of the control or NC-shRNA group, respectively. The curves of xenograft tumor growth indicated that tumor sizes in the shRNA-1 group with lower mRNA level were significantly smaller less than those of the control or NC-shRNA group [31, 46]. Consistently, the sCLU protein expression in the shRNA-1 group was also lower than that in the control or the NC-shRNA group; and the sCLU staining in the control or NC-shRNA group was stronger than that in the shRNA-1 group by immunohistochemistry [46]. Specific shRNA-mediated downregulation of sCLU resulted in a reduced migratory capacity in HCC cell lines, as well as a reduction in pulmonary metastasis *in vivo* [38]. Overexpression of sCLU in HepG2 cell line showed increased cell migratory ability. In addition, sCLU also plays an important role in the regulation of TGF-β1-smad3 signaling pathway, suggested that oncogenic sCLU might promote HCC metastasis via the induction of EMT process and could be a promising candidate target for HCC therapy [32, 61–63].

6. Conclusions

In conclusion, the upregulation of sCLU expression at early staging of HCC is considered to promote tumor development, which may be related to the phosphorylation of AKT/GSK-3β. An increasing number of reports have provided evidence that sCLU level could be a novel biomarker for HCC diagnosis and prognosis, and there will be of great significance for the individualized treatment in HCC patients. The sCLU regulating signaling pathways could be critical to unraveling the solution for MDR in HCC. Therefore, silencing sCLU gene transcription and inhibiting sCLU expression by specific Custirsen inhibition have provided a new mechanism insight into molecular-targeted therapy for HCC in injected- or orthotopic model, indicated that sCLU gene would be a potential molecular-targeted for HCC therapy. Further study found that sCLU contributed to HCC migration and EMT *in vitro*, and metastasis *in vivo*. Although additional preclinical and clinical trials are necessary to explore the sCLU role in HCC, targeting the oncogenic sCLU could validate the approach as a systemic therapy to increase chemotherapy sensitivity.

Acknowledgements

This work was supported by grants-in-aid from Projects of the National Natural Science Foundation (81673241, 81702419), the Jiangsu Health Plans (2014-YY-028 and BE2016698), the Jiangsu Graduate Innovation Plan (KYCX17_1934), the Nantong Science Foundation of Health and Family Planning Commission (WQ2016083), and the International Science & Technology Cooperation Program (2013DFA32150) of China.

Abbreviations

AFP alpha-fetoprotein

HCC hepatocellular carcinoma

IHC immunohistochemistry

MDR multiple drug resistance

miRNA	microRNA
sCLU	secretory clusterin
shRNA	short hairpin RNA
TMA	tissue microarray
VEGF	vascular endothelial growth factor
Wnt	Wnt/β-catenin signaling pathway

Author details

Min Yao[1,2†], Wenjie Zheng[2†], Li Wang[1], Miao Fang[2†], Dengfu Yao[2*] and Zhizheng Dong[3]

*Address all correspondence to: yaodf@ahnmc.com

1 Medical School of Nantong University, Affiliated Hospital of Nantong University, Nantong, Jiangsu Province, China

2 Institute of Clinical Oncology, Affiliated Hospital of Nantong University, Nantong, Jiangsu Province, China

3 Department of Diagnostics, Affiliated Hospital of Nantong University, Nantong, Jiangsu Province, China

† These authors contributed equally to this work.

References

[1] Jayachandran M. An updated portrait of pathogenesis, molecular markers and signaling pathways of hepatocellular carcinoma. Current Pharmaceutical Design. 2017. **23**(16):2356-2365 [PMID: 28356044]

[2] Kirstein MM, Vogel A. The pathogenesis of hepatocellular carcinoma. Digestive Diseases. 2014;**32**(5):545-553 [PMID: 25034287]

[3] Nuño Solinís R, Arratibel Ugarte P, Rojo A, Sanchez Gonzalez Y. Value of treating all stages of chronic hepatitis C: A comprehensive review of clinical and economic evidence. Infectious Disease and Therapy. 2016;**5**(5):491-508 [PMID: 27783223]

[4] Bellentani S. The epidemiology of non-alcoholic fatty liver disease. Liver International. 2017;**37**(S1):81-84 [PMID: 24843434

[5] Bang CS, Song IH. Impact of antiviral therapy on hepatocellular carcinoma and mortality in patients with chronic hepatitis C: Systematic review and meta-analysis. BMC Gastroenterology. 2017;**17**(1):46-65 [PMID: 28376711]

[6] Hollebecque A, Malka D, Ferte C, Ducreux M, Boige V. Systemic treatment of advanced hepatocellular carcinoma: From disillusions to new horizons. European Journal of Cancer. 2015;**51**(3):327-339 [PMID: 25559615]

[7] Choi SH, Park JY. Regulation of the hypoxic tumor environment in hepatocellular carcinoma using RNA interference. Cancer Cell International. 2017;**17**(1):3-11 [PMID: 28053598]

[8] Bruix J, Reig M, Sherman M. Evidence-based diagnosis, staging, and treatment of patients with hepatocellular carcinoma. Gastroenterology. 2016;**150**(4):835-853 [PMID: 26795574]

[9] Juárez-Hernández E, Motola-Kuba D, Chávez-Tapia NC, Uribe M, Barbero Becerra V. Biomarkers in hepatocellular carcinoma: An overview. Expert Review of Gastroenterology & Hepatology. 2017;**11**(6):549-558 [PMID: 28347162]

[10] Zoubeidi A, Chi K, Gleave M. Targeting the cytoprotective chaperone, clusterin, for treatment of advanced cancer. Clinical Cancer Research. 2010;**16**(4):1088-1093 [PMID: 20145158]

[11] Trougakos IP, Djeu JY, Gonos ES, Boothman DA. Advances and challenges in basic and translational research on clusterin. Cancer Research. 2009;**69**(2):403-406 [PMID: 19147550]

[12] Yao DF, Huang ZW, Chen SZ, Huang JF, Lu JX, Xiao MB, Meng XY. Diagnosis of hepatocellular carcinoma by quantitative detection of hepatoma-specific bands of serum gamma-glutamyl transferase. American Journal of Clinical Pathology. 1998;**110**(6):743-749 [PMID: 9844586]

[13] Yao DF, Jiang DR, Huang ZW, Lu JX, Tao QY, Yu ZJ, Meng XY. Abnormal expression of hepatoma specific γ-glutamyl transferase and alteration of γ-glutamyl transferase gene methylation status in patients with hepatocellular carcinoma. Cancer. 2000;**88**(4):761-769 [PMID: 10679644]

[14] Yao M, Wang L, Fang M, Zheng W, Dong Z, Yao D. Advances in the study of oncofetal antigen glypican-3 expression in HBV-related hepatocellular carcinoma. Bioscience Trends. 2016;**10**(5):337-343 [PMID: 27795482]

[15] Wang L, Pan L, Yao M, Cai Y, Dong Z, Yao D. Expression of oncofetal antigen glypican-3 associates significantly with poor prognosis in HBV-related hepatocellular carcinoma. Oncotarget. 2016;**7**(27):42150-42158 [PMID: 27286460]

[16] Wu W, Yao DF, Yuan YM, Fan JW, Lu XF, Li XH, Qiu LW, Zong L, Wu XH. Combined serum hepatoma-specific alpha-fetoprotein and circulating alpha-fetoprotein-mRNA in diagnosis of hepatocellular carcinoma. Hepatobiliary & Pancreatic Diseases International. 2006;**5**(4):538-544 [PMID: 17085339]

[17] Pan LH, Yao M, Zheng WJ, Gu JJ, Yang XL, Qiu LW, Cai Y, Wu W, Yao DF. Abnormality of Wnt3a expression as novel specific biomarker for diagnosis and differentiation of hepatocellular carcinoma. Tumour Biology. 2016;**37**:5561-5568 [PMID: 26577850]

[18] Pan LH, Yao M, Cai Y, Gu JJ, Yang XL, Wang L, Yao DF. Oncogenic Wnt3a expression as an estimable prognostic marker for hepatocellular carcinoma. World Journal of Gastroenterology. 2016;**22**:3829-3837 [PMID: 27076768]

[19] Malhi H, Kaufman RJ. Endoplasmic reticulum stress in liver disease. Journal of Hepatology. 2011;**54**:795-809 [PMID: 21145844]

[20] Tobe T, Minoshima S, Yamase S, Choi NH, Tomita M, Shimizu N. Assignment of a human serum glycoprotein SP-40,40 gene (CLI) to chromosome 8. Cytogenetics and Cell Genetics. 1991;**57**:193-195 [PMID: 1660393]

[21] Bertuzzi M, Marelli C, Bagnati R, Colombi A, Fanelli R, Saieva C, Ceroti M, Bendineli B, Caini S, Airoldi L, Palli D. Plasma clusterin as a candidate pre-diagnosis marker of colorectal cancer risk in the florence cohort of the European prospective investigation into cancer and nutrition: A pilot study. BMC Cancer. 2015;**15**(1):56-67 [PMID: 25884309]

[22] Nafee AM, Pasha HF, Abd EL, Aal SM, Mostafa NA. Clinical significance of serum clusterin as a biomarker for evaluating diagnosis and metastasis potential of viral-related hepatocellular carcinoma. Clinical Biochemistry. 2012;**45**(13-14):1070-1074 [PMID: 22580393

[23] Luo X, Suzuki M, Ghandhi SA, Amundson SA, Boothman DA. ATM regulates insulin-like growth factor 1-secretory clusterin (IGF-1-sCLU) expression that protects cells against senescence. PLoS One. 2014;**9**(6):e99983 [PMID: 24937130]

[24] Essabbani A, Garcia L, Zonetti MJ, Fisco T, Pucci S, Chiocchia G. Exon-skipping strategy by ratio modulation between cytoprotective versus pro-apoptotic clusterin forms increased sensitivity of LNCaP to cell death. PLoS One. 2013;**8**(2):e54920 [PMID: 23418433]

[25] Novinec M, Lenarčič B, Baici A. Clusterin is a specific stabilizer and liberator of extracellular cathepsin K. FEBS Letters. 2012;**586**(7):1062-1066 [PMID: 22569264]

[26] Liao FT, Lee YJ, Ko JL, Tsai CC, Tseng CJ, Sheu GT. Hepatitis delta virus epigenetically enhances clusterin expression via histone acetylation in human hepatocellular carcinoma cells. The Journal of General Virology. 2009;**90**(Pt 5):1124-1134 [PMID:19264665]

[27] Goetz EM, Shankar B, Zou Y, Morales JC, Luo X, Araki S, Bachoo R, Mayo LD, Boothman DA. ATM-dependent IGF-1 induction regulates secretory clusterin expression after DNA damage and in genetic instability. Oncogene. 2011;**30**(35):3745-3754 [PMID:21460853]

[28] Wang X, Luo L, Dong D, Yu Q, Zhao K. Clusterin plays an important role in clear renal cell cancer metastasis. Urologia Internationalis. 2014;**92**(1):95-103 [PMID:24008723]

[29] Zhang H, Kim JK, Edwards CA, Xu Z, Taichman R, Wang CY. Clusterin inhibits apoptosis by interacting with activated Bax. Nature Cell Biology. 2005;**7**(9):909-915 [PMID: 16113678]

[30] Wang C, Jiang K, Kang X, Gao D, Sun C, Li Y, Sun C, Zhang S, Liu X, Wu W, Yang P, Guo K, Liu Y. Tumor-derived secretory clusterin induces epithelial-mesenchymal transition and facilitates hepatocellular carcinoma metastasis. The International Journal of Biochemistry & Cell Biology. 2012;**44**(12):2308-2320 [PMID: 23010347]

[31] Zheng WJ, Sai WL, Yao M, Cai Y, Pan LH, Gu JJ, Wu W, Yao DF. Down-regulated clusterin expression enhances sensitivity of hepatoma cells to anti-cancer drugs. Zhonghua Gan Zang Bing Za Zhi. 2015;**23**(11):844-848 [PMID: 26743245]

[32] Shim YJ, Kang BH, Jeon HS, Park IS, Lee KU, Lee IK, Park GH, Lee KM, Schedin P, Min BH. Clusterin induces matrix metalloproteinase-9 expression via ERK1/2 and PI3K/Akt/NF-kappaB pathways in monocytes/macrophages. Journal of Leukocyte Biology. 2011;**90**(4):761-769 [PMID: 21742938]

[33] Ammar H, Closset JL. Clusterin activates survival through the phosphatidylinositol 3-kinase/ Akt pathway. The Journal of Biological Chemistry. 2008;**283**(19):12851-12861 [PMID: 18321852]

[34] Wang C, Zhang Y, Guo K, Wang N, Jin H, Liu Y, Qin W. Heat shock proteins in hepatocellular carcinoma: Molecular mechanism and therapeutic potential. International Journal of Cancer. 2016;**138**(8):1824-1834 [PMID: 26853533]

[35] Lamoureux F, Thomas C, Yin MJ, Fazli L, Zoubeidi A, Gleave ME. Suppression of heat shock protein 27 using OGX-427 induces endoplasmic reticulum stress and potentiates heat shock protein 90 inhibitors to delay castrate-resistant prostate cancer. European Urology. 2014;**66**(1):145-155 [PMID: 24411988]

[36] Loison F, Debure L, Nizard P, le Goff P, Michel D, le Drean Y. Up-regulation of the clusterin gene after proteotoxic stress: Implication of HSF1-HSF2 heterocomplexes. The Biochemical Journal. 2006;**395**(1):223-231 [PMID: 16336210]

[37] Wang C, Jiang K, Gao D, Kang X, Sun C, Zhang Q, Li Y, Sun L, Zhang S, Guo K, Liu Y. Clusterin protects hepatocellular carcinoma cells from endoplasmic reticulum stress induced apoptosis through GRP78. PLoS One. 2013;**8**(2):e55981 [PMID: 23457489]

[38] Wang C, Jin G, Jin H, Wang N, Luo Q, Zhang Y, Gao D, Jiang K, Gu D, Shen Q, Huo X, Hu F, Ge T, Zhao F, Chu W, Shu H, Yao M, Cong W, Qin W. Clusterin facilitates metastasis by EIF3I/Akt/MMP13 signaling in hepatocellular carcinoma. Oncotarget. 2015;**6**(5):2903-2916 [PMID: 25609201]

[39] Maluccio M, Covey A. Recent progress in understanding, diagnosing, and treating hepatocellular carcinoma. CA: A Cancer Journal for Clinicians. 2012;**62**(6):394-399 [PMID: 23070690]

[40] Qu Z, Yuan CH, Yin CQ, Quan Q, Chen H, Wang FB. Meta-analysis of the prognostic value of abnormally expressed lncRNAs in hepatocellular carcinoma. OncoTargets and Therapy. 2016;**9**(8):5143-5152 [PMID: 27574455]

[41] Wang Y, Zeng LI, Chen W. HBV X gene point mutations are associated with the risk of hepatocellular carcinoma: A systematic review and meta-analysis. Molecular and Clinical Oncology. 2016;**4**(6):1045-1051 [PMID: 27284442]

[42] Zheng W, Yao M, Sai W, Qian Q, Pan L, Qiu L, Huang J, Wu W, Yao D. Diagnostic and prognostic significance of secretory clusterin expression in patients with hepatocellular carcinoma. Tumour Biology. 2016;**37**(1):999-1008 [PMID: 26264614]

[43] Kang YK, Hong SW, Lee H, Kim WH. Overexpression of clusterin in human hepatocellular carcinoma. Human Pathology. 2004;**35**(11):1340-1346 [PMID: 15668890]

[44] Lai JP, Chen ZM, Lok T, Chan OT, Himmelfarb E, Zhai Q, Lin F, Wang HL. Immunohistochemical stains of proliferating cell nuclear antigen, insulin-like growth factor 2 and clusterin help distinguish malignant from benign liver nodular lesions. Journal of Clinical Pathology. 2014;**67**(6):464-469 [PMID: 24407433]

[45] Lau SH, Sham JS, Xie D, Tzang CH, Tang D, Ma N, Hu L, Wang Y, Wen JM, Xiao G, Zhang WM, Lau GK, Yang M, Guan XY. Clusterin plays an important role in hepatocellular carcinoma metastasis. Oncogene. 2006;**25**(8):1242-1250 [PMID: 16247463]

[46] Zheng W, Yao M, Qian Q, Sai W, Qiu L, Yang J, Wu W, Dong Z, Yao D. Oncogenic secretory clusterin in hepatocellular carcinoma: Expression at early staging and emerging molecular target. Oncotarget. 2017;**8**(32):52321-52323 [PMID: 28881732]

[47] Klokov D, Leskov K, Araki S, Zou Y, Goetz EM, Luo X, Willson D, Boothman DA. Low dose IR-induced IGF-1-sCLU expression: A p53-repressed expression cascade that interferes with TGFbeta1 signaling to confer a pro-survival by stander effect. Oncogene. 2013;**32**(4):479-490 [PMID: 22391565]

[48] Kimura A, Sogawa K, Satoh M, Kodera Y, Yokosuka O, Tomonaga T, Nomura F. The application of a three-step serum proteome analysis for the discovery and identification of novel biomarkers of hepatocellular carcinoma. International Journal of Proteomics. 2012;**2012**:623190 [PMID: 22957256]

[49] Wang Y, Liu YH, Mai SJ, He LJ, Liao YJ, Deng HX, Guan XY, Zeng YX, Kung HF, Xie D. Evaluation of serum clusterin as a surveillance tool for human hepatocellular carcinoma with hepatitis B virus related cirrhosis. Journal of Gastroenterology and Hepatology. 2010;**25**(6):1123-1128 [PMID: 20594228]

[50] Ehsani Ardakani MJ, Safaei A, Arefi Oskouie A, Haghparast H, Haghazali M, Mohaghegh Shalmani H, Peyvandi H, Naderi N, Zali MR. Evaluation of liver cirrhosis and hepatocellular carcinoma using Protein-Protein Interaction Networks. Gastroenterology and Hepatology From Bed to Bench. 2016;**9**(Suppl1):S14-S22 [PMID: 28224023

[51] Comunale MA, Wang M, Rodemich-Betesh L, Hafner J, Lamontagne A, Klein A, Marrero J, Di Bisceglie AM, Gish R, Block T, Mehta A. Novel changes in glycosylation of serum Apo-J in patients with hepatocellular carcinoma. Cancer Epidemiology, Biomarkers & Prevention. 2011;**20**(6):1222-1229 [PMID: 21467232]

[52] Chen D, Wang Y, Zhang K, Jiao X, Yan B, Liang J. Antisense oligonucleotide against clusterin regulates human hepatocellular carcinoma invasion through transcriptional regulation of matrix metalloproteinase-2 and E-cadherin. International Journal of Molecular Sciences. 2012;**13**(8):10594-10607 [PMID: 22949882]

[53] Lamoureux F, Thomas C, Yin MJ, Kuruma H, Beraldi E, Fazli L, Zoubeidi A, Gleave ME. Clusterin inhibition using OGX-011 synergistically enhances Hsp90 inhibitor activity by suppressing the heat shock response in castrate-resistant prostate cancer. Cancer Research. 2011;**71**(17):5838-5849 [PMID: 21737488]

[54] Xiu P, Dong XF, Li XP, Li J. Clusterin: Review of research progress and looking ahead to direction in hepatocellular carcinoma. World Journal of Gastroenterology. 2015;**21**(27):8262-8270 [PMID: 26217078]

[55] Sad F, Hotte S, North S, Eigl B, Chi K, Czaykowski P, Wood L, Pollak M, Berry S, Lattouf JB, Mukherjee SD, Gleave M, Winquist E. Randomized phase II trial of Custirsen (OGX-011) in combination with docetaxel or mitoxantrone as second-line therapy in patients with metastatic castrate-resistant prostate cancer progressing after first-line docetaxel: CUOG trial P-06c. Clinical Cancer Research. 2011;**17**(17):5765-5773 [PMID: 21788353]

[56] Zheng W, Sai W, Yao M, Gu H, Yao Y, Qian Q, Yao D. Silencing clusterin gene transcription on effects of multidrug resistance reversing of human hepatoma HepG2/ADM cells. Tumour Biology. 2015;**36**(5):3995-4003 [PMID: 25600802]

[57] Xiu P, Xu Z, Liu F, Li Z, Li T, Zou F, Sun X, Li J. Downregulating sCLU enhances the sensitivity of hepatocellular carcinoma cells to gemcitabine by activating the intrinsic apoptosis pathway. Digestive Diseases and Sciences. 2014;**59**(8):1798-1809 [PMID: 24671452]

[58] Wang YW, Lin KT, Chen SC, Gu DL, Chen CF, Tu PH, Jou YS. Over-expressed-eIF3I interacted and activated oncogenic Akt1 is a theranostic target in human hepatocellular carcinoma. Hepatology. 2013;**58**(1):239-250 [PMID: 23460382]

[59] Yao M, Wang L, Qiu L, Qian Q, Yao D. Encouraging microRNA-based therapeutic strategies for hepatocellular carcinoma. Anticancer Agents Medicinal Chemistry. 2015;**15**:453-460 [PMID: 25511513]

[60] Criswell T, Beman M, Araki S, Leskov K, Cataldo E, Mayo LD, Boothman DA. Delayed activation of insulin-like growth factor-1 receptor/Src/MAPK/Egr-1 signaling regulates clusterin expression, a pro-survival factor. The Journal of Biological Chemistry. 2005;**280**(14):14212-14221 [PMID: 15689620]

[61] Shiota M, Zardan A, Takeuchi A, Kumano M, Beraldi E, Naito S, Zoubeidi A, Gleave ME. Clusterin mediates TGF-beta-induced epithelial-mesenchymal transition and metastasis via Twist1 in prostate cancer cells. Cancer Research. 2012;**72**(20):5261-5272 [PMID: 22896337]

[62] Nannuru KC, Futakuchi M, Varney ML, Vincent TM, Marcusson EG, Singh RK. Matrix metalloproteinase (MMP)-13 regulates mammary tumor-induced osteolysis by activating MMP9 and transforming growth factor-beta signaling at the tumor-bone interface. Cancer Research. 2010;**70**(9):3494-3504 [PMID: 20406980]

[63] Kalyan A, Nimeiri H, Kulik L. Systemic therapy of hepatocellular carcinoma: Current and promising. Clinics in Liver Disease. 2015;**19**(2):421-432 [PMID: 25921671]

9

Diagnostic Algorithm of Hepatocellular Carcinoma: Classics and Innovations in Radiology and Pathology

Dzeina Mezale, Ilze Strumfa, Andrejs Vanags,
Arturs Kalva, Dainis Balodis, Boriss Strumfs,
Ilze Fridrihsone, Arnis Abolins and Janis Gardovskis

Abstract

In the global cancer statistics, hepatocellular carcinoma (HCC) ranges sixth by incidence and second by oncological mortality. The risk factors comprise hepatitis B and C virus infection, non-alcoholic steatohepatitis, as well as long-lasting peroral exposure to alcohol or aflatoxins. Liver cirrhosis is the most important single predisposing factor. Ultrasonography once per 6 months is recommended for surveillance in cirrhotic patients. Computed tomography (CT) and magnetic resonance imaging (MRI) represent the gold standard of non-invasive diagnostics while core biopsy and/or immunohistochemistry (IHC) are indicated for controversial and non-cirrhotic HCC cases. Molecular classification is under development. At present, classics of HCC diagnostics is based on evaluation of risk factors, surveillance in cirrhotic patients, preference for CT or MRI-confirmed non-invasive diagnosis and biopsy proof in equivocal cases. Diffusion-weighted imaging and hepatobiliary phase contrasting represent significant recent developments in MRI. Contrast-enhanced ultrasonography is recommended by some but not all guidelines. Positron emission tomography is advocated before liver transplantation to detect extrahepatic metastases but has limited role in the initial diagnostic evaluation of liver nodule. Innovations are expected in the field of molecular diagnostics, including IHC panels and novel antigens, e.g. clathrin and bile salt export pump protein, and development of molecular classification.

Keywords: hepatocellular carcinoma, HCC, diagnosis, imaging, CT, MRI, contrast-enhanced ultrasound, CEUS, positron emission tomography, PET, liver biopsy, immunohistochemistry

1. Introduction

Hepatocellular carcinoma (HCC) is a primary malignant liver tumour exhibiting hepatocellular differentiation [1]. It is well known for the strong association with preceding chronic liver disease and liver cirrhosis [2]. However, nowadays an increasing proportion of HCCs develops in non-fibrotic liver or on the background of mild fibrosis [3, 4]. The changing patterns of presentation influence the diagnostic approach both because of alterations in risk groups that could be targeted by surveillance and limits of non-invasive diagnostics in non-cirrhotic cases. In addition, the differential diagnostics of liver nodule differs in regard to the presence or absence of background liver cirrhosis. In cirrhotic liver, 59–94% (depending on size) of new mass lesions are malignant [5]. Thus, in patients with liver cirrhosis or preceding chronic liver disease, new nodule favours the diagnosis of HCC, as metastases and benign liver tumours are uncommon in cirrhotic liver [6, 7]. Hence, any mass lesion in cirrhotic liver must be considered HCC until proven otherwise [7].

In the global cancer statistics, HCC represents a frequent and aggressive tumour although different geographic regions face various burden of it. Worldwide, liver cancer is estimated to range sixth by incidence and second by oncological mortality causing 5.6% of global cancer incidence and 9.1% of mortality [8]. HCC is the most frequent primary liver cancer (>90%) being significantly more widespread than cholangiocarcinomas, hepatoblastomas and other primary liver malignancies [1]. Number of death cases per year (recently assessed by Ferlay et al. for the year 2012 as 745,000) is virtually identical to the incidence throughout the world (782,000; the same source) underlining the unfavourable course. The high ratio of mortality to incidence (0.95) reflects the dismal prognosis. As the geographical patterns of incidence and mortality closely follow each other [8], liver cancer is still an unsolved problem in the whole world.

According to the data provided by Surveillance, Epidemiology and End Results (SEER) Program of the National Cancer Institute, the 5-year survival for liver cancer is 16.6%, ranging from 30.5% in localised stage to 10.7% in regional stage and 3.1% in distant stage [2]. Different but similarly discouraging estimates have been reported, including 1-, 5- and 10-year survival of 31.3, 5.1 and 0.8%. The median survival is 6 months. However, significantly better outcome can be reached in early cases. Thus, median survival reaches 107 months in patients receiving liver transplantation for early HCC [9].

The incidence of liver cancer is high in Eastern and Southeastern Asia, followed by Northern and Western Africa [8]. China, Mongolia and Japan experience high occurrence [10]. In Europe, the highest age-standardised incidence rate of liver cancer is observed in Southern Europe [8] including Italy and France [10]. Although more developed regions generally show lower incidence of liver cancer (except Japan, France and Italy), its incidence is growing in many countries [8, 10]. Thus, although the total cancer incidence in the United States of America (USA) decreased in males and remained stable in females over time period 2003–2012, liver cancer incidence rates increased in both genders: 3.7% yearly in males and 3.0% in females. According to the National Program of Cancer Registries and SEER database, liver cancer incidence rate (2008–2012) in USA has increased by 2.3% per year [2]. The incidence rate of histologically proved HCC in USA has increased from 1.4/100,000 persons per year between 1976 and 1980 to 2.4/100,000 persons per year between 1991 and 1995 [11] followed by further growth of HCC incidence rate reaching 6.2/100,000 persons per year in 2011 as shown by SEER-based analysis [9].

Similarly, although death rates attributable to other frequent cancers, including lung, breast, colorectal and prostate cancers, are declining in USA, mortality from liver cancer has increased by 2.8% per year (2003–2012) in males and by 2.2% per year in females. The growing mortality from liver cancer in USA contrasts with the general decline in cancer mortality reaching 1.5% per year. Among all cancers, HCC is the fastest growing cause of death in the USA [2] and poses a significant economic burden on healthcare [10].

The spectrum of risk factors in HCC (see **Table 1**) explains the geographic heterogeneity. Awareness of these factors is important to understand the incidence and the associated needs for diagnostics and treatment. Worldwide, men have a higher incidence than women; gender ratio ranges around 3:1 both in global epidemiological studies of liver cancer [8] and more targeted analysis of HCC [9]. Incidence starts to increase at the sixth decade of life [2].

Liver cirrhosis of any aetiology represents the single largest risk factor of HCC and is found in 70–90% of cases. Worldwide, hepatitis B virus (HBV) infection accounts for more than 50% of HCC cases. In comparison to non-infected individuals, the relative risk of HCC is increased 100-fold in HBV-infected persons, and the risk further increases if HBV-infected patient develops cirrhosis, has longer duration of infection and higher virus burden in blood. The yearly risk of HCC in HBV-infected patients is 2% [18]. In East Asia and sub-Saharan Africa, HBV is the most common risk factor for HCC [12].

Hepatitis C virus (HCV) infection is implicated in 25–31% of patients [13, 19]. Although the presence of HCV infection holds 17-fold risk of HCC in comparison with non-infected persons [13], risk is significantly higher in cirrhotic patients. Thus, surveillance is limited to those having

Risk factor	Risk assessment	References
Hepatitis B virus infection	100-fold higher	[13]
Hepatitis C virus infection	17-fold higher	[13]
Alcohol consumption	2.2 times higher in people who consume at least 50 g of alcohol per day	[15]
Non-alcoholic fatty liver disease	More than 4 times higher	[16]
Aflatoxin exposure	Of the 550,000–600,000 new HCC cases worldwide each year, about 25,200–155,000 may be attributable to aflatoxin exposure	[14]
Primary biliary cirrhosis	Incidence of HCC is 3–5% per year	[12]
Primary sclerosing cholangitis (PSC)	The risk of HCC for PSC patients with cirrhosis is up to 2% per year	[17]
Hemochromatosis	Approximately 20-fold higher	[12]

Table 1. Risk factors of hepatocellular carcinoma [12–17].

HCV-associated cirrhosis or advanced fibrosis [12]. Annually, HCC develops in 2–8% of HCV-infected patients [13]. In North America, Latin America, Europe and Japan, HCV infection, together with alcohol abuse, represent the main risk factors [3, 13]. In Europe and Japan where HCV infection spread earlier than in the United States, HCC incidence has almost reached a plateau, while in the United States it is still increasing. HCV infection may have a synergistic effect with other risk factors, such as non-alcoholic fatty liver disease [3].

Globally, 15% of HCC cases can be attributed to alcohol-induced liver damage and non-alcoholic steatohepatitis [19], although the estimates range between 4 and 22% [20]. Non-alcoholic fatty liver disease (NAFLD) is the major hepatic manifestation of metabolic disturbances including obesity, type 2 diabetes mellitus, dyslipidaemia and metabolic syndrome [4]. As prevalence of these conditions is increasing, NAFLD has become the most common liver disorder in industrialised countries [21]. In NAFLD, HCC incidence reaches 44 (range, 29–66) per 100,000 person-years [22] contrasting with the general incidence of 6 per 100,000 in USA population [20]. The proportion of HCC related to NAFLD and non-alcoholic steatohepatitis (NASH) is increasing worldwide, especially in Western countries [20]. Although previously it was considered that HCC risk was limited to patients with liver cirrhosis, nowadays a significant fraction of NASH-associated HCC is found in non-cirrhotic liver or liver showing mild fibrosis [4].

Aflatoxins are a group of mycotoxins produced by *Aspergillus* fungi *(A. flavus; A. parasiticus)*, which can contaminate food products such as grains, rice, cassava, soybeans, corn and peanuts, stored in hot climate and high moisture. Aflatoxins are major risk factors of HCC in sub-Saharan Africa and Eastern Asia [23]. Chronic exposure to aflatoxin results in DNA damage, including mutation of the tumour suppressor gene *TP53* in hepatocytes [13]. In people subjected to aflatoxin ingestion and chronic HBV infection, HCC risk is 30- to 60-fold higher, *versus* HBV-uninfected people exposed to aflatoxin alone. Synergistic action is observed also between aflatoxin and HCV [14, 23, 24].

Planning the surveillance for individual patient, the presence of known risk factors must be considered and the relative risk must be taken into account. Organising surveillance measures in the society, population-attributable fraction (PAF) is also important. PAF depends both on relative risk and population prevalence of the corresponding risk factor. Thus, in USA, the risk increase of HCC is highest in HCV infection (odds ratio (OR), 39.9), followed by HBV infection (OR, 11.2), alcohol-induced liver disease (OR, 4.1) and diabetes mellitus and/or obesity (OR, 2.3). However, considering the prevalence of these conditions, diabetes and/or obesity are associated with the highest population attributable fraction (36.6%), followed by alcohol (23.5%), HCV (22.4%) and HBV (6.3%) as reported by Welzel et al. [25]. PAFs differ by the population. Worldwide, 54% of HCC occur in HBV-infected patients, 31% can be attributed to HCV and 15% to alcohol and NASH [19].

Considering the serious prognosis, early diagnosis is crucial, however, not always easy. Thus, correctly interpreted radiological findings, combined with biopsy when necessary, and appropriate immunohistochemical examination of biopsied tissues have diagnostic value. The molecular portrait of the tumour as well as easily available markers of the systemic inflammatory response, such as neutrophil-to-lymphocyte ratio or platelet-to-lymphocyte ratio, are recently reported to have prognostic and predictive value in HCC.

The aim of the present chapter is to highlight the current approach and innovations for diagnostic evaluation of a liver nodule, suspected to be hepatocellular carcinoma. Non-invasive radiologic assessment represents the gold standard in certain patients. In contrast, difficult cases need biopsy evaluation, supplemented by immunohistochemistry, and may remain controversial even then.

2. Radiology

Radiological imaging and functional evaluation are significant in screening and diagnostics of HCC [26]. The gold standard techniques comprise ultrasonography (US), computed tomography (CT) and magnetic resonance imaging (MRI). A major advance in the diagnostics of HCC was reached in 2001, when non-invasive criteria were developed and accepted by the European Association for the Study of the Liver (EASL) to diagnose HCC in cirrhotic liver [27]. In addition to the presence of liver mass, radiologic studies of HCC evaluate the typical vascularity. HCC receives enhanced arterial blood supply reflected histologically by unpaired arteries. The blood supply via portal vein decreases in comparison with surrounding parenchyma. However, in early stages of development, HCC can be hypovascular if the portal flow has already decreased but the arterial supply has not yet fully developed.

According to the guidelines, ultrasonography is advocated for screening and surveillance of patients having high risk to develop HCC due to HBV or HCV infection, cirrhosis or other known risk factors [28]. The specificity is mostly higher than 90%, ranging 45–94% [5, 27]. The reported sensitivity ranges widely from 33 to 96%, at least partially because of differences in the equipment and qualification of radiologists [18]. The sensitivity decreases in advanced chronic liver disease because of the coarse cirrhotic nodularity seen both grossly and by US [5]. In a large group of 200 patients undergoing US and liver transplantation, the sensitivity for HCC diagnostics was 29.6% in regard to patients and only 20.5% counting the tumours themselves. Even a large tumour exceeding the diameter of 5 cm was missed [29].

The typical US presentation of HCC is a hypoechoic nodule although iso- or hyperechogenicity is possible as is nodule-in-nodule appearance [7]. Small HCCs (less than 2 cm in the greatest diameter) are mostly hypoechoic with or without posterior enhancement. Hyperechoic appearance is seen in 17% of small HCCs and can be associated with fat accumulation. Larger HCCs are heterogeneous reflecting necrosis (hypoechoic), calcifications and fibrosis. If hypoechoic halo (seen in 50% of HCC) and posterior enhancement is evident, these findings increase the specificity of diagnosis [5, 7, 18]. HCC in dysplastic nodule might seem hyperechoic within a larger hypoechoic area. If a nodule is identified on US, either CT or MRI is indicated for masses larger than 20 cm, while both methods are advocated for pathologic foci measuring 10–20 mm. If either CT or MRI confirms HCC, the diagnosis is reliable. Biopsy is indicated only for lesions that remain controversial after both imaging modalities. Nodules measuring less than 10 mm are followed up by US every 4 months [18].

By Doppler US, HCC is characterised by so-called basket pattern reflecting rich arterial vascularisation. Benign cirrhotic nodules feature either low vascularity or arterial vessels with low frequency (high in HCC: >1 kHz) and normal resistive index (elevated in HCC: >0.71). However, the typical Doppler pattern is seen only in 50% of small HCC [7].

A significant innovation in ultrasonography is the application of contrast enhancement by stabilised gaseous microbubbles. Consequently, three phases can be assessed analogously to CT and MRI: arterial phase (beginning 20 seconds after injection and lasting for 30–45 seconds); portal venous phase (starting at 30–45 seconds and lasting for 2–3 minutes) and late phase (4–6 minutes). Some contrast agents display additional post-vascular phase characterised by contrast uptake in Kupffer cells (10–60 minutes). To avoid overlap with late phase, the post-vascular phase must be assessed not earlier than 10 minutes after contrast injection. The typical pattern of HCC upon contrast-enhanced ultrasound (CEUS) examination is arterial hyperenhancement followed by washout in the late phase. The evaluation of washout is important in order to exclude arterial hyperenhancement in hemangioma or dysplastic cirrhotic nodule. However, well-differentiated HCC can remain isoechoic in portal venous or late phase; such pattern is suspicious for HCC, but CT or MRI is mandatory [7]. The benefits of CEUS include the easy procedure and high safety as the technique is not associated with ionising radiation or renal toxicity. Pitfalls include false positives in cholangiocarcinoma [30]. The lack of specificity is associated with the intravascular location of microbubbles in contrast to CT or MRI contrast agents that reach the extravascular extracellular space. At present, CEUS has been excluded from diagnostic guidelines provided by the European Association for the Study of the Liver (EASL) and the American Association for the Study of the Liver Diseases (AASLD) but is advocated by Asian Pacific and Japanese guidelines [27].

US can be applied to recognise benign or secondary liver tumours. Sensitivity of US to detect liver metastases varies between 40 and 80%, again depending on experience of radiologist and available US equipment. Metastases can be hypovascular, e.g., gastric or colorectal carcinoma, or hypervascular as malignant melanoma or sarcoma [18].

If US or CEUS discloses a suspicious nodule, in-depth evaluation by CT or MRI is indicated [31] based on the risk of malignancy. Nodules smaller than 1 cm are mostly benign. Risk of HCC is 66% in nodules measuring 10–20 mm, 80% in nodules 20–30 mm in size and 92–95% in nodules larger than 3 cm [7]. Both methods (CT and MRI) are advocated for lesions measuring 10–20 mm while one is sufficient for larger nodules (>20 mm). The diagnosis of HCC is confirmed by the typical pattern of arterial hypervascularity and late washout [27].

For CT, dynamic multidetector row, multiphase contrast-enhanced computed tomography approach is recommended [27, 32] as the diagnosis is based on dynamic evaluation of blood flow. However, contrasting is not possible in all patients in order to avoid anaphylactic reactions, acute renal failure or hyperthyroidism [33]. To disclose HCC, CT must be evaluated in three phases (late arterial, portal venous and equilibrium) in addition to the first unenhanced image. HCC classically is hypervascular, characterised by high contrast in the arterial phase, followed by washout in portal and/or equilibrium phases [27]. Portal venous phase can be useful in some cases of HCC when the tumour is otherwise not visible in CT. Portal venous phase is generally less informative for HCC because the tumour shows rarefaction similar as liver parenchyma. This phase is most useful for detecting hypovascular metastases, e.g., from colorectal carcinoma [34].

Examination of hypovascular or hypervascular liver metastases with multidetector CT is similar to CEUS. Hypovascular metastasis presents as rounded and uniformly hypoattenuating mass in portal venous phase and peripheral rim in arterial phase. Hypervascular metastasis is characterised by homogeneous late arterial enhancement. Inhomogeneous enhancement can develop in necrosis or haemorrhage [35].

MRI has excellent results for detection and characteristics of HCC. By meta-analysis, MRI was characterised by sensitivity of 88% and specificity of 94%, exceeding the characteristics of multidetector CT [36]. Contrasting usually is applied in liver MRI, most frequently by gadolinium compounds. The gadolinium-based contrast agents can be classified as extracellular *versus* hepatobiliary. Extracellular agents are small molecules that can reach interstitium moving out from vascular space. In turn, hepatobiliary contrast agents move even further becoming absorbed by hepatocytes [37, 38].

Classic MRI protocol for HCC includes a 3D T1-weighed fat saturated sequence with intravenous contrast. The first phase is called late arterial phase. It is seen 25–30 seconds after injection of contrast. This phase is followed by portal venous phase, at 65–70 seconds. In this phase, there is a dense contrast enhancement in portal vein, and hepatic veins also become highlighted. Finally, delayed phase develops 3 minutes after injection [38]. Before contrasting, classical HCC is hypointense in T1-weighted and hyperintense in T2-weighted images. Contrasting reveals similar enhancement pattern as in CT with arterial enhancement and subsequent washout [18]. In addition, MRI can be applied to disclose tumour thrombus in portal venous system [39].

Most metastases show mild-to moderate high signal intensity on T2-WI. In some cases, e.g., in cystic or necrotic metastases, T2 signal increases.

The sensitivity of MRI can be further improved by diffusion-weighted imaging, based on the assessment of Brownian motion of water molecules and water diffusion within a voxel (a tridimensional pixel). Cell membranes limit the diffusion, therefore greater cellularity, seen also in malignant tumours, results in diffusion restriction [40]. However, the fibrosis also decreases the mobility of water molecules. By different modalities, diffusion-weighted imaging can increase the sensitivity for HCC detection, the liver-to-lesion contrast and the specificity in the differential diagnosis with benign cirrhotic nodules [27].

Another advance in liver pathology is represented by hepatobiliary phase MRI using contrast agents that are absorbed by hepatocytes and excreted in biliary system, e.g., gadoxetate disodium and gadobenate dimeglumine. These agents undergo dual elimination via biliary excretion (50%) and renal glomerular filtration, while the traditional agents, as gadopentetic acid, are almost completely excreted via kidneys [41]. The hepatobiliary phase of MRI corresponds to the peak parenchymal enhancement due to contrast uptake in hepatocytes. Depending on the agent, the hepatobiliary phase develops either 10–20 (gadoxetate) or 60 (gadobenate dimeglumine) minutes after injection [42]. Most of HCCs are hypointense in hepatobiliary phase [18].

MRI can be applied to distinguish between HCC and benign lesion in non-cirrhotic liver. In such patients, HCCs are hypointense in T1, hypo- or hyperintense in T2, lack central enhancement in the tumour, exhibit satellite lesions and do not uptake liver-specific contrast agents [43].

Positron emission tomography (PET) is a non-invasive radiologic visualisation that demonstrates metabolic activity in normal or pathological tissue. It is usually performed in combination with CT to ensure both anatomical imaging and metabolic evaluation. 18-fluorodeoxyglucose (FDG) is one of the radiopharmaceuticals used in PET/CT. It discloses areas of high glucose uptake as many tumours including HCC are characterised by aerobic glycolysis: the Warburg effect [44].

The significance of FDG PET/CT in HCC evaluation is not unequivocal. The distinction between small, well-differentiated HCC *versus* regenerative or dysplastic nodules can be difficult. The positive aspect of PET/CT is the ability to detect extrahepatic metastases of HCC. Considering that PET/CT provides whole-body examination, it is recommended before liver transplantation [45, 46]. Hypothetically, prognostic role of PET/CT in HCC has been discussed as well as the ability to predict response to treatment [46]. Other radiopharmaceuticals are also under discussion, including lipid radiotracer on choline base, like 11C-choline or 18F-fluorocholine [47]. 68Ga-labelled prostate-specific membrane antigen, that is used to diagnose prostate cancer, is present in other tumours, including HCC [48].

3. Pathology

Needle biopsies followed by morphologic and immunohistochemical examination can be invaluable for the characterisation of liver masses. However, nowadays clear-cut radiologic diagnostic criteria have been established for the non-invasive diagnostics of HCC; therefore, the advantages and indications of the biopsy should be considered against the risks and contraindications. Liver biopsy is recommended only in selected patients, thoughtfully evaluating the diagnostic yield [6].

Currently, three general groups of indications (see **Table 2**) for liver biopsy are known: to establish the diagnosis, to assess the prognosis and/or to assist in the management of patient

Diagnosis:

- Identification and staging of parenchymal and cholestatic liver diseases (alcohol-induced liver disease; non-alcoholic steatohepatitis; primary biliary cirrhosis; primary sclerosing cholangitis; Wilson's disease, haemochromatosis)
- Evaluation of persistent abnormal liver biochemical tests
- Evaluation of the type and extent of drug-induced liver injury
- Diagnosis of multisystem infiltrative disorders
- Identification and determination of the nature of focal/diffuse intrahepatic abnormalities on imaging studies

Prognosis and management:

- Pre-treatment evaluation and staging of chronic hepatitis, e.g. chronic viral hepatitis B and C
- Evaluation of pre-transplant living-related donor
- Evaluation of post-transplant patient with abnormal liver tests (rejection *versus* infection)
- Evaluation of treatment efficacy for liver diseases

Table 2. Indications for liver biopsy [49].

with known liver disease [49]. Percutaneous liver core biopsy is most frequently performed to evaluate the presence and activity of inflammation and extent of fibrosis/stage of frequent liver diseases, mostly chronic viral hepatitis, alcohol-induced liver disease and NAFLD. Regarding focal liver lesions, biopsy can yield the diagnosis. Molecular analyses of tissue may help determine the most appropriate individual treatment strategy for the patient with HCC [50] but are still under development for HCC. At present, biopsy from a nodule in cirrhotic liver is indicated if the findings of radiological imaging are controversial [6].

Although biopsy is often essential, sometimes it may be difficult to undertake because of associated risks (see **Table 3**). Percutaneous, ultrasound-guided liver biopsy (the Menghini method) has become the worldwide standard [51]. However, it is appropriate only in cooperative patients. Thus, if the patient refuses from the procedure, it is absolutely contraindicated. Although precise blood clotting parameters are unsettled, coagulopathies should be mentioned as a serious contraindication [49]. In this case, mini-laparoscopy or transjugular liver biopsy might be considered [51]. Among relative contraindications, ascites should be pointed out, as it may prevent adequate sampling of tissue, as well as increase the risk of bleeding [49]. Biopsies of malignant liver lesions also carry a low risk of tumour seeding.

Significant complications due to liver biopsy arise in about 1% of cases, with less than 0.1% mortality [51]. The main complications are post-interventional haemorrhage and bile leakage; others, like injuries to gall bladder, lung, kidney, as well as bacteraemia are rare [49, 51].

The initial assessment of liver tissue starts with the overall evaluation of parenchymal architecture. Haematoxylin and eosin represents the generally accepted standard stain in liver pathology [6]. Helpful additional visualisation methods in liver pathology include Masson's trichrome to assess fibrosis, Gordon and Sweets reticulin to evaluate lobular architecture and hepatocyte plate thickness, Perl's iron to detect hemosiderin deposits and periodic acid-Schiff (PAS) stain to identify glycogen, mucus or chitin of certain liver parasites.

Microscopically, cells of classical HCC resemble normal hepatocytes. The similarity to normal liver is most notable in well to moderately differentiated tumours. In such cases, the loss of the normal liver cell plates and plate thickness change from 1 to 2 cell nuclei to 3 or more nuclei

Absolute contraindications

- Uncooperative patient
- History of unexplained bleeding
- Tendency to bleed (prothrombin time more than 3–4 seconds over control; platelet count <50,000 mm^3; prolonged bleeding time (≥10 minutes))
- Unavailability of blood transfusion support
- Recurrent use of aspirin or other non-steroidal anti-inflammatory drugs within last 7–10 days

Relative contraindications

- Ascites
- Morbid obesity
- Infection in the right pleural cavity or below the right hemidiaphragm
- Suspected haemangioma or other vascular tumour
- Suspected hydatid disease (Echinococcal cysts)

Table 3. Contraindications of liver biopsy [49].

across a single neoplastic cord is a feature of malignancy. In healthy liver, narrow cords of hepatocytes are running in parallel, but even well-differentiated HCC shows a disorganised pattern secondary to the increased thickness of the hepatocyte cords (usually more than 3 cells thick), that can be highlighted by reticulin staining. The invasive growth of HCC disrupts and destroys the liver plate architecture, leading to decreased amount of reticulin and disorganised pattern of it. However, the loss of reticulin is not complete. HCC is characterised by the absence of normal portal tracts and/or naked or unaccompanied arteries in accordance with the radiologic hypervascularity and high contrast in the arterial phase of contrast-enhanced CT [6]. Invasion in connective tissues is diagnostic. However, except scirrhous and fibrolamellar HCC, stroma is usually scant in HCC. Loss of perinodular ductular proliferation is a manifestation of invasive growth [6]. Vascular invasion is diagnostic if evident.

Cytologically, HCC shows both signs of hepatocellular differentiation that serves as the clue to hepatocellular origin of the tumour and atypia indicating malignant behaviour. Regarding tumour differentiation, bile production is a reliable indicator of hepatocellular origin. Bile can be found in the cytoplasm of neoplastic cells or in lumina of acinar complexes. Similarly to benign counterparts, steatosis, Mallory bodies and hyaline globules can develop in cytoplasm of tumour cells. HCC cells can have intranuclear inclusions and/or optically clear cytoplasm. Giant cells are occasionally present. Iron accumulation in cells of hepatocellular carcinoma is not seen, even in the setting of hereditary hemochromatosis. In hepatocytes, nuclear pleomorphism can be a feature of regenerative changes; therefore, mitotic activity is more suspicious of malignancy, and the presence of atypical mitoses definitively confirms the presence of a malignant tumour. However, in well-differentiated HCC, abnormal mitoses are rare and are not mandatory for diagnosis [6].

The histologic patterns of HCC include trabecular (the most common pattern), acinar (pseudoglandular), solid and scirrhous patterns. Trabecular HCC resembles normal liver architecture. In acinar or pseudoglandular HCC, the neoplastic cells are arranged in gland-like tubules containing bile or fibrin. Solid HCC is characterised by compact, sheet-like arrangement of neoplastic cells. Scirrhous HCC exhibit marked desmoplasia; it will be described in detail later. HCC is characterised by significant inter- and intratumoural heterogeneity, manifesting as variability of grade and growth patterns [3]. Grade progression can be present even in a single patient and, in fact, reflects the biology of HCC. Hepatocellular carcinoma frequently develops in foci with equivocal biological potential, e.g., dysplastic cirrhotic nodule. Such early HCC typically is well differentiated. Over the disease course, well-differentiated HCC progresses to advanced dedifferentiated tumour. The heterogeneity can lead to diagnostic problems and failures in biopsy due to sampling errors. For instance, if a small suspicious nodule was evident by radiological imaging and a biopsy was obtained, the differential diagnosis between dysplastic nodule and HCC will frequently imply the necessity to distinguish between premalignant process and well-differentiated tumour, usually lacking marked cell atypia or clear-cut invasion. In addition, both processes can be adjacent in the tissues.

HCC has several histologic variants, including fibrolamellar, sarcomatoid, scirrhous, steatohepatitic and clear cell HCC, presenting with peculiar morphological features. Some cases display lymphoepithelioma-like morphology. In addition, correlations between histological and molecular subtypes have been reported [52].

Fibrolamellar HCC is a rare subtype accounting for less than 1% of HCC. Typically, fibrolamellar carcinoma is diagnosed in young adults lacking liver cirrhosis or other known predisposing factors [3]. The mean age of diagnosis is 26 years [53]. Association with germline pathogenic variants of *TP53* gene has been reported suggesting that some cases of fibrolamellar HCC might represent Li-Fraumeni syndrome. Interestingly, in the case described by Andrade et al., a germline mutation of *TP53* was identified not only in proband affected by fibrolamellar HCC but also in her asymptomatic mother [54].

The presence of fibrous septae and central scar with possible calcification leads to architectural similarity with focal nodular hyperplasia [3, 6]. Histologically, the neoplastic cells are arranged in trabeculae and sheets, separated by collagen fibres that undergo hyalinisation and show the typical lamellar pattern [3]. Fibrolamellar HCC is defined by triad of histologic features: (1) large, polygonal neoplastic hepatocytes with wide eosinophilic granular cytoplasm. Ground glass pale bodies and PAS-positive cytoplasmic globules can be present [3, 53] but are neither sufficient nor necessary for diagnosis. (2) Prominent single eosinophilic macronucleoli should be present, and frequently are seen on the background of vesicular chromatin structure [3, 6]. (3) Lamellar fibrosis, usually present in at least half of the tumour tissue [53].

The immunophenotype of fibrolamellar HCC is also unusual, showing expression of hepatocellular markers in combination with biliary, progenitor and stem cell features as well as macrophage markers (CD68). The granular or dot-like expression of CD68 in association with appropriate morphology is helpful in diagnosing fibrolamellar HCC [6].

Prognosis of fibrolamellar HCC is poor. The 5-year survival is similar to conventional HCC arising in non-cirrhotic liver [53]; however, it is better than for classical HCC arising in cirrhotic liver [3].

Sarcomatoid HCC can occur either primarily or within classical HCC [3]. This subtype, comprising 1.8–3.9% of HCC, is partially or fully composed of malignant spindle-shaped cells, occasionally showing heterologous (rhabdoid, osteoid or chondroid) differentiation [53]. If there is no adjacent area of classical HCC, it is difficult to distinguish sarcomatous HCC from true sarcomas, including primary or metastatic tumours, e.g., metastatic gastrointestinal stromal tumour, leiomyosarcoma or fibrosarcoma. Haematoxylin-eosin stain alone can be insufficient, necessitating immunohistochemistry [3]. Considering the high grade and remarkable anaplasia of sarcomatoid HCC, hepatocellular markers should be supplemented with pancytokeratin and specific markers for sarcoma, including CD117, DOG, actin, desmin, S-100, CD34 and CD31. Hepatocellular antigens are frequently negative, and even pancytokeratin is expressed only in 23–63% cases of sarcomatoid HCC [53]; therefore, complex assessment of morphology is mandatory along with clinical history and IHC for sarcoma.

Scirrhous HCC is a rare type, accounting for 0.2% to 4.6% of HCC. It can develop beneath liver capsule leading to pedunculated gross view [3, 53]. Microscopically, scirrhous HCC is characterised by diffuse fibrosis surrounding thin trabeculae of neoplastic cells. Such fibrosis can occur either after various regimens of oncologic treatment (chemotherapy, transarterial chemoembolization, irradiation) or in untreated patients [3]. However, HCC exhibiting post-treatment fibrosis should not be classified as scirrhous [53]. The marked desmoplasia and morphology of the tumour cells, displaying clusters, strands and tubules, can lead to misdiagnosis as cholangiocarcinoma or metastasis both in biopsy and in preoperative imaging. While conventional HCC is characterised by CT enhancement in the arterial phase and washout in the venous phase, scirrhous HCC can present with peripheral ring-like enhancement in the arterial phase and delayed central enhancement in the venous phase [53]. In addition, expression of cytokeratin 19 is frequent [52]. Haemorrhage or necrosis is usually absent. Marked CD8-positive lymphocytic infiltrate can be present [3, 53]. Regarding molecular profile, scirrhous HCC is associated with mutations in *TSC1/TSC2* genes, lack of *CTNNB1* mutations, presence of epithelial to mesenchymal transformation and stem cell profile [52].

Lymphoepithelioma-like carcinoma is characterised by the presence of rich lymphocytic infiltrate surrounding pleomorphic, small, polygonal neoplastic cells that might show syncytial growth [1].

Steatohepatitic HCC is remarkable for similarity to steatohepatitis that can even lead to missed diagnosis in well-differentiated cases [53]. This subtype HCC is characterised by the presence of fat vacuoles in more than 5% of the tumour. The neoplastic cells also show Mallory bodies and ballooning degeneration. The stroma features pericellular and trabecular fibrosis as well as inflammatory infiltrate, consisting of neutrophils, plasma cells and lymphocytes [3]. Infiltrative borders are characteristic. Within the tumour, fibrosis can be prominent [53]. The patients can have underlying steatohepatitis due to metabolic syndrome/NASH [3] or alcohol-induced liver disease [53]. However, this phenotype of carcinoma is also seen in patients without steatohepatitic changes in the non-neoplastic liver tissue [3]. Molecularly, IL6/JAK/STAT molecular pathway is frequently activated along with immunohistochemical C-reactive protein expression. In contrast, mutations in *CTNNB1* gene or activation of Wnt/Beta-catenin pathway are not evident. Regarding immunophenotype, low expression of glutamine synthetase has been observed [52].

Clear cell HCC features optically clear cytoplasm due to the presence of glycogen and fat vesicles in the neoplastic cells. The architecture is mostly trabecular [3].

The differential diagnosis of HCC includes benign pathological processes, for instance, dysplastic nodule in a cirrhotic liver while hepatic adenoma, focal nodular hyperplasia and bile duct adenoma should be considered in non-cirrhotic liver. Parasitic infestations, e.g., echinococcosis and infrequent benign tumours, e.g., angiomyolipoma occasionally need to be ruled out. The malignant tumours that enter the spectrum of differential diagnoses of hepatocellular carcinoma include metastases of extrahepatic tumours as well as cholangiocarcinoma, hepatoblastoma and non-epithelial liver tumours.

3.1. Immunohistochemistry and differential diagnosis

Benign and malignant liver tumours may share morphologic similarities; thus, immunohistochemical assessment is crucial to set the correct diagnosis. The two challenging tasks are (1) to distinguish low-grade/early HCC from benign lesions like liver adenoma, focal nodular hyperplasia or dysplastic nodule and (2) to differentiate high-grade HCC from metastatic tumours in the liver.

The differential diagnosis of HCC varies also depending on the underlying liver pathology. In cirrhotic liver, primary tumours such as HCC and cholangiocarcinoma are much more common than secondary tumours [3]. In contrast, in non-cirrhotic liver, HCC accounts only for about 2% of tumours and metastatic lesions predominate over primary liver neoplasms. Metastasis can mimic HCC, especially in case of clear cell renal cancer, clear cell adenocarcinoma of the female genital organs, hepatoid gastric carcinoma, adrenal carcinoma and melanoma. Metastatic gastrointestinal neuroendocrine tumours can be challenging to differentiate from HCC, especially if trabecular architecture is present [3]. In the evaluation of HCC diagnosis, arginase-1, hepatocyte paraffin-1 antigen, glypican-3, carcinoembryonic antigen by polyclonal primary antibody, CD10, glutamine synthetase and CD34 are frequently assessed. Alfa-fetoprotein is partially replaced by new markers showing higher expression frequency and less background. However, it is still helpful in some cases. Clathrin and bile salt export pump protein represent promising novel targets.

Arginase-1 (Arg1) is occasionally considered the most sensitive and specific marker of hepatocellular differentiation [55], characterised by sensitivity and specificity of approximately 90% [55]. Arginase-1 represents manganese metalloenzyme involved in the urea cycle [56]. It catalyses the hydrolysis of arginine to ornithine and urea. Arg1 is expressed in normal human liver [6] and hepatocellular tumours, including HCC. Arg1 shows better sensitivity and specificity diagnosing HCC, compared to HepPar1 and glypican 3 [55], although other researchers prefer HepPar1 (see further) to identify hepatocellular differentiation [3]. Regarding the types of HCC that might cause diagnostic difficulties—high-grade HCC and scirrhous HCC—Arg1 is characterised by sensitivity of 85 and 85%, exceeding the sensitivity of HepPar1 (64 and 26%, respectively). Arg1 displays diffuse nuclear and cytoplasmic expression pattern in HCC [6, 55]. Most other tumours are negative for Arg1, but focal or weak expression can occur in colorectal, pancreatic, breast and prostatic carcinomas, cholangiocarcinoma or hepatoid tumours [55].

Hepatocyte paraffin-1 (HepPar1) antigen is another marker of hepatocellular differentiation. Some authors prefer HepPar1 as the best marker to confirm the hepatocellular origin of a tumour [3]. HepPar1 is a carbamoyl phosphate synthetase 1: another enzyme involved in urea synthesis. In contrast to Arg1, it is expressed not only in the liver but also in non-neoplastic small intestinal mucosa and Barrett's oesophagus [56]. HepPar1 has diffuse granular cytoplasmic staining pattern. The sensitivity and specificity in HCC reaches 80%. HepPar1 is expressed in almost all well-differentiated HCCs. However, only less than 50% of high-grade cases express HepPar1 [3]. Most of metastatic and/or non-hepatocellular tumours, including adenocarcinomas, neuroendocrine tumours, renal cell carcinoma, adrenocortical carcinoma, melanoma and angiomyolipoma, are negative for HepPar1. However, focal reactivity is occasionally observed. Strong expression can be present in cholangiocarcinomas and metastatic oesophageal, gastric and pulmonary adenocarcinomas [55]. Positive reaction has also been reported in non-ampullary small intestinal adenocarcinomas (60%) and ampullary adenocarcinomas with intestinal (73%) differentiation while expression in ampullary adenocarcinomas exhibiting pancreatobiliary (14%) morphology or colonic (9%) adenocarcinomas is rare [56].

Glypican-3 (GPC3) is a member of the glypican family of heparan sulphate proteoglycans. It is bound to the external surface of plasma membrane through a glycosyl-phosphatidyl-inositol anchor. Glypicans regulate signalling via Wnt, Hedgehog, fibroblast growth factor and bone morphogenetic protein pathways. Thus, glypicans are involved in the control of cell proliferation. In HCC, GPC3 promotes cancer growth by stimulating Wnt signalling. The GPC3 molecule can be released to extracellular environment after it has been cleaved off by lipase [57]. Hence, the functional activity of GPC3 explains its role as possible serum marker or treatment target for HCC. GPC3 is normally found in foetal liver and placenta but is absent from healthy adult liver and benign hepatocellular lesions including focal nodular hyperplasia and liver adenoma [55]. Thus, expression of GPC3 in liver biopsy is highly suggestive of HCC. The staining pattern is (1) granular or diffuse cytoplasmic, possibly with membranous enhancement; (2) membranous or (3) Golgi complex-related [6, 55]. Heterogeneity can lead to focal lack of expression; therefore, negative result in biopsy does not exclude HCC. The sensitivity of GPC3 ranges from 56 to 62% in low grade (G1) HCC to 80–83% in intermediate grade (G2) HCC, 85–89% in high grade (G3) HCC and 79% in scirrhous HCC [55]. GPC3 is expressed in many extrahepatic tumours that can spread to the liver, including metastatic adenocarcinoma, squamous cell carcinoma, non-seminomatous germ cell tumours (choriocarcinoma, yolk sac tumour) and malignant melanoma (5%). Cholangiocarcinoma can be positive (5%) as well [6, 55]. The strong advantages of GPC3 include the absence of it from non-malignant liver as well as high sensitivity in high-grade HCC. Lack of specificity is the greatest pitfall [55].

Carcinoembryonic antigen (CEA) family represents a class of different glycoproteins belonging to immunoglobulin superfamily. Within CEA family, adhesion molecules and pregnancy-specific glycoproteins are distinguished. The functions of CEA family include cell adhesion, as well as cell interaction in pregnancy, immune reactions and angiogenesis [58]. By immunohistochemistry, CEA is found in foetal and adult epithelial cells [6]. In liver pathology, CEA assessment by polyclonal antibody (pCEA) is strongly advised. In HCC, distinct specific canalicular or so called chicken-wire fence pattern can be observed. Metastatic adenocarcinomas show diffuse membranous, luminal and/or cytoplasmic positivity [55]. In higher grade HCC, the specific canalicular pattern is progressively lost and replaced by unspecific membranous expression [6].

CD10 is a zinc-dependent metalloproteinase, located in cell surface membranes. It exhibits neutral endopeptidase activity: cleavage of peptides at the amino side of hydrophobic residues. CD10 inactivates several hormones, as glucagon, oxytocin and bradykinin. In HCC, CD10 shows canalicular expression similarly to pCEA. However, the sensitivity of CD10 for HCC is lower, around 50% [55].

Alpha-fetoprotein (AFP), the protein encoded by *AFP* gene on 4q25, is the major plasma protein in developing foetus. It is produced by liver and yolk sac and might represent the foetal analogue of albumin. AFP can bind metal ions, fats and bilirubin. In adults, AFP is found in HCC and germ cell tumours but normal liver tissue does not express AFP [3]. Although the sensitivity of AFP for HCC is only 30–50% and high background can frequently limit the interpretation [55], truly positive cases in our experience were easy to recognise. In contrast to HepPar1 and pCEA, AFP positivity increases with dedifferentiation of HCC [3].

Glutamine synthetase (GS) is an enzyme that catalyses the condensation reaction between glutamate and ammonia resulting in glutamine. GS is regulated by beta-catenin molecular pathway. In normal liver tissue, immunohistochemical expression of glutamine synthetase is found only in a thin central perivenular (zone 3) area. In contrast, extensive diffuse cytoplasmic expression is present in 70% of HCC [6].

CD34 has multiple diagnostic roles. Within its wide expression spectrum, endothelial cells are also positive. Sinusoidal expression of CD34 is increased in both benign and malignant hepatocellular lesions, contrasting with limited expression in periportal sinusoids within normal liver [55] or in parenchymal capillaries close to fibrous septa within cirrhotic tissues [6]. In HCC, the endothelial expression of CD34 increases, until capillarisation of the sinusoids becomes complete. The capillarisation develops due to higher oxygen tension in HCC. Although incomplete CD34 expression does not exclude HCC, diffuse positive reaction is strongly suggestive of HCC. However, limited sampling in biopsy can lead to pitfalls as foci of complete CD34 expression are seen in adenomas and in periphery of cirrhotic nodules. If such foci are predominantly sampled within the biopsy, false overestimation of CD34 reactivity is possible [6].

Clathrin is one of the novel markers appearing in the differential diagnostics between malignant and non-malignant hepatocellular nodules. Clathrin is a protein that forms airscrew-like triskelion consisting of three light chains and three heavy chains. When these molecules assemble between themselves, clathrin-coated vesicles arise and participate in endocytosis and exocytosis. Thus, clathrin participates in cell communication and signalling, in the transport of nutrients, receptors and other macromolecules. During mitosis, clathrin stabilises mitotic spindle. The heavy chain of clathrin is significantly upregulated in HCC. In the initial reports, striking contrast in the immunohistochemical staining was found between tumour and surrounding tissues suggesting high affinity and low background. The expression pattern was cytoplasmic and membranous. Expression of the heavy chain of clathrin was tested for the distinction between HCC and benign nodules. The sensitivity and specificity of the heavy chain of clathrin was 41.2 and 77.2%, and the sensitivity increased to 61.1% in combination with glypican-3 [59].

Bile salt export pump protein is a transport molecule that is present in bile canaliculi. By immunohistochemistry, bile salt export pump protein was expressed in 89.6% HCC, mostly (76.7%) in canalicular pattern. In comparison with cholangiocarcinomas and metastatic tumours, expression of bile salt export pump protein had 90% sensitivity and 100% specificity for HCC. The performance of bile salt export pump protein was comparable to arginase-1 showing both sensitivity and specificity of 94% and slightly better than HepPar1 characterised by sensitivity 90% and specificity 97% [60].

3.2. Well-differentiated hepatocellular carcinoma *versus* adenoma

Hepatocellular adenoma (HCA) is defined as benign monoclonal proliferation of well-differentiated hepatocytes. The most common risk factor for HCA is exposure to high oestrogen levels in oral contraceptives, thus the disease has strong female predominance (9:1). Adenomas are typically small, solitary lesions in non-cirrhotic liver. Occasionally, multiple tumours are observed [61]. In HCA, the neoplastic hepatocytes are arranged in cords and sheets, typically two layers thick [3, 62]. The portal triads and interlobular bile ducts are absent from adenoma tissue [63]. Pseudoglandular architecture can be observed, especially in adenomas associated with anabolic use. HCA cells appear larger due to intracellular glycogen or fat accumulation. Nuclear atypia is absent [3].

Several molecular subtypes of hepatocellular adenomas are known [62, 64], including hepatocyte nuclear factor 1α (HNF1α) inactivated type (H-HCA); β-catenin activated type (B-HCA); inflammatory HCA (I-HCA) and the unclassifiable type (U-HCA). Not surprisingly, beta-catenin activated subtype is associated with malignant transformation [62]. Beta-catenin mutations are reported in 20% of HCCs, especially in patients with underlying hepatitis C virus infection. HCC arising from B-HCA is usually well to moderately differentiated and lacks vascular invasion or satellite nodules [3]. Mutations lead to remarkable overexpression of *GLUL* gene (coding for glutamine synthase), thus beta-catenin activation can be assessed by intense homogeneous cytoplasmic expression of glutamine synthase and by aberrant nuclear localisation of beta-catenin [62, 63]. H-HCA shows decreased expression of liver fatty acid-binding protein, and presence of fat in neoplastic cells can be seen histologically. I-HCA is characterised by immunohistochemical positivity for serum amyloid A and C-reactive protein. Marked inflammatory infiltrate, ductular reactions and sinusoid dilation can be present in the tissue as well. U-HCA lacks gene mutations or specific immunohistochemical findings, but is diagnosed as HCA by histology [61]. Liver adenomas express hepatocellular markers and have lower proliferation activity than HCC [63]. To discriminate between adenoma and HCC, the following parameters are of importance: (1) clinical history in order to disclose risk factors that might indicate either HCA or HCC; (2) structure of surrounding liver as presence of cirrhosis favours HCC; (3) expression of HCA subtype-specific proteins; (4) presence or absence of cell atypia and invasion; (5) hepatocyte plate thickness and (6) expression of malignancy-associated HCC markers, e.g., GPC3.

3.3. Well-differentiated hepatocellular carcinoma *versus* focal nodular hyperplasia

Focal nodular hyperplasia (FNH) is a hyperplastic hepatocellular proliferation resulting from blood flow abnormalities. It is a pathological focus characterised by nodular architecture, hypervascular central scar associated with thick fibrous septa between hepatocyte nodules, inflammatory infiltrate, presence of ductular reaction and sinusoid dilation [55, 61–63].

To distinguish FNH from HCC, GPC3, heat shock protein 70 (HSP70) and reticulin network can be assessed. Loss of reticulin framework, immunohistochemical expression of GPC3 and/or diffuse nuclear expression of HSP70 favours HCC. Such immunohistochemical evaluation has 100% specificity for HCC although the sensitivity is only 43–46%. Typical "map-like" pattern of GS expression is evident in FNH. It is characterised by wide central positive areas in the middle of nodules. The positive foci interconnect between themselves, while periseptal areas remain negative. This reactivity pattern contrasts with normal liver showing limited perivenular reactivity in the middle of lobules [55].

3.4. Well-differentiated hepatocellular carcinoma *versus* high-grade dysplastic cirrhotic nodule

Dysplastic cirrhotic nodules (DNs) are characteristic precursors of HCC in the setting of chronic liver disease and/or liver cirrhosis. Most but not all dysplastic nodules are small, not exceeding the diameter of 1 cm [6]. Morphologically DNs are classified into high-grade DN and low-grade DN. Low-grade DN, carrying low risk of transformation to HCC, is generally characterised by monotonous cell population when compared with the surrounding cirrhotic liver, mildly increased cell density and minimal cell atypia. The nuclear/cytoplasmic ratio is mildly increased, nuclear atypia is slight, mitoses are absent and cell plates are 1–2 cells thick. The reticulin network is retained. The borders of low-grade dysplastic nodule are rounded, but the adjacent liver parenchyma is not compressed [3]. In contrast, high-grade dysplastic nodules can have many of classical HCC features. The nuclear/cytoplasmic ratio is increased. Nuclei show hyperchromasia and irregular borders and can be peripherally located. Occasional mitoses can be present. Cell plates are thicker than 2 cells. Cytoplasm switches to basophilic staining. Pseudoglandular structures start to appear. Occasional unpaired arteries have been observed. Lack of invasion is the most reliable criterion in the differential diagnosis with early HCC [3]. This trait is both important and biologically substantiated as the invasion is the hallmark of malignant tumours. However, it can be notoriously difficult to apply practically. In early HCC, invasion can be absent from biopsy due to sampling error. Regarding high-grade dysplastic nodule, entrapment of perinodular hepatocytes into fibrous tissues mimics invasion. To classify the entrapped hepatocytes correctly, immunohistochemical investigation of ductular proliferation can be helpful, as further described, because these non-neoplastic intraseptal hepatocytes and ductular proliferation stem from common progenitors [3].

Expression of GPC3 points towards malignant hepatocellular tumour, as it was previously noted. However, GPC3 expression has been reported in 3–76% of dysplastic nodules. Glutamine synthetase is expressed in 69.8% of HCC contrasting with 13.6% in high-grade DN. Heat shock protein 70 is found in 73.5% of HCC and only exceptional dysplastic nodules [3]. To distinguish high-grade DN from early HCC, immunohistochemical panel comprising heat shock protein 70, glypican-3 and glutamine synthetase has been recommended. Expression of one marker is compatible with DN, while HCC expresses at least two markers. The sensitivity of this panel is estimated as 60–78% [55].

In addition, cytokeratin (CK) 7 and/or CK19 and CD34 can be useful in the assessment of architecture and reactive changes. HCC is characterised by more diffuse expression of CD34 and loss of ductular reaction at the nodule interface. Dysplastic nodule shows only focal CD34 expression in the periphery of the nodule and more marked proliferation of CK7-positive ductules surrounding DN [55]. In the ductular reaction, CK7 and CK19 usually are coexpressed. Thus, gradual loss of CK7 and CK19 positive ductular reaction in perinodular stroma correlates with progression of cirrhotic to dysplastic nodule and further to HCC. Ductular reaction is present around ≥50% of perimeter of a DN, while it is almost lost in HCC [3].

Different systems for complex evaluation of the biological potential of hepatocellular nodule have been proposed. Integrated evaluation of haematoxylin-eosin findings together with reticulin stain and immunohistochemistry for CD34 has been suggested. A hepatocellular nodule should be classified as HCC if at least three features from the following are present: necrosis; cellular atypia; thickness of trabeculae more than 4 cells; mitotic activity or diffuse expression of CD34 in the sinusoidal endothelium [6]. Alternatively, stromal invasion, loss of reticulin network and positivity for at least two out of three markers (HSP70, GS, GPC3) are considered the strongest parameters discriminating HCC from high-grade dysplastic nodule [3].

3.5. Hepatocellular carcinoma *versus* metastasis

If high-grade malignant tumour is found in the liver, the differential diagnosis includes metastatic malignancy *versus* HCC and cholangiocarcinoma. Any malignant tumour can ultimately spread to the liver via bloodstream, lymphogeneous dissemination or transperitoneal spread. In some biopsy series, metastatic lung, colorectal, pancreatic and breast carcinomas have been the most common secondary liver tumours [3]. However, frequency of different metastatic malignant tumours in liver biopsies depends on many factors, including the biological potential of the tumour and its incidence in the population as well as institutional approach to liver biopsy in different oncological patients. This, in turn, may depend on the patient's general status, presence of contraindications for biopsy or significant oncological treatment and the availability of effective treatment.

In order to distinguish HCC from metastatic tumours, it is advisable to combine at least two hepatocellular markers and at least two antigens that are more frequently seen in adenocarcinomas. Among hepatocellular markers, Arg1 should be combined with either HepPar1 or GPC3. Most of adenocarcinomas express cytokeratin (CK) 19, MOC-31 and CK7 [55]. The spectrum of immunohistochemical panel should be planned in accordance with tissue availability within the biopsy. The suggested minimal panel includes ARG1 and CK19 [55], while maximal investigation might include several HCC markers accounting for different grades of HCC, several adenocarcinoma markers and antigens that are characteristic for certain tissues (neuroendocrine or melanocytic differentiation) or epithelia of specific organs, e.g., breast, large bowel, lung, thyroid, kidney and others. Panels of immunohistochemical markers can disclose the location of primary tumour giving rise to metastasis. Thus, CK20 and CXD2 are typical for metastatic colorectal carcinoma; CDX2 and CK7 for gastric carcinoma; TTF-1 and napsin A for lung adenocarcinoma and oestrogen receptor, mammaglobin, GATA3 or GCDFP-15 for breast cancer [65]. The expression frequencies of different tissue- and organ-specific antigens in metastases and corresponding primary tumours are further outlined in **Table 4**.

Antigen	Tumour	Frequency, %	References
CDX2	Colorectal carcinoma	100	[66]
CDX2	Metastatic colorectal carcinoma	96.7–100	[67, 68]
SATB2	Primary colorectal carcinoma	96.0	[68]
SATB2	Metastatic colorectal carcinoma	92.2	[68]
CK20	Metastatic colorectal carcinoma	97.1	[68]
TTF-1	Lung adenocarcinoma	83.3	[69]
Napsin A	Lung adenocarcinoma	86.7	[69]
HMB-45	Metastatic melanoma	76–81	[70, 71]
MART-1	Melanoma	48.4–83	[72, 73]

Antigen	Tumour	Frequency, %	References
MART-1	Metastatic melanoma	63–82	[70, 72, 73]
Tyrosinase	Melanoma	71	[72]
Tyrosinase	Metastatic melanoma	63	[72]
PAX-8	Ovarian cancer	80	[69]
PAX-8	Endometrial cancer	100	[69]
PAX-8	Renal cancer	83–93.3	[69, 74]
PAX-8	Metastatic renal cancer	93.9	[74]
Napsin A	Renal cancer	50	[69]
Gross cystic disease fluid protein-15	Breast carcinoma	23.9–60	[75, 76]
Gross cystic disease fluid protein-15	Primary triple negative breast carcinoma	10–14	[75, 77]
Gross cystic disease fluid protein-15	Primary non-triple negative breast carcinoma	69	[77]
Gross cystic disease fluid protein-15	Metastatic triple negative breast carcinoma	21	[75]
Mammaglobin	Breast carcinoma	46.6–80	[75, 76]
Mammaglobin	Primary triple negative breast carcinoma	17–25	[75, 77]
Mammaglobin	Primary non-triple negative breast carcinoma	61	[77]
Mammaglobin	Metastatic triple negative breast carcinoma	41	[75]
GATA3	Invasive breast cancer	82.5–94	[76, 78]
GATA3	Primary triple negative breast carcinoma	20.2–87	[77–80]
GATA3	Metastatic triple negative breast carcinoma	44	[79]
GATA3	Luminal A breast carcinoma	99.5	[80]
GATA3	Luminal B breast carcinoma	97.7	[80]
GATA3	HER2-positive breast carcinoma	59.6–68.5	[76, 80]

CDX2, caudal type homeobox 2; SATB2, special adenosine-thymidine-rich-binding protein 2; CK, cytokeratin; TTF-1, thyroid transcription factor 1; HMB-45, melanosome protein human melanoma black 45; MART-1, melanoma antigen recognized by T cells 1; PAX-8, paired box gene 8; GATA3, guanosine-adenosine -thymidine -adenosine nucleotide sequences binding protein 3.

Table 4. Frequency of immunohistochemical expression of selected tissue- or organ-specific markers [66–80].

When differentiating between HCC and metastasis, the peculiar immunophenotype of fibrolamellar HCC must be recognised promptly. Fibrolamellar HCC expresses hepatocellular proteins, such as HepPar1, GPC3 or pCEA; biliary (CK7), progenitor and stem cell (CK19, CD44) antigens and macrophage markers (CD68). The granular or dot-like expression of CD68 in a tumour featuring appropriate morphology is helpful in diagnosing fibrolamellar HCC [6].

4. Molecular analysis

The molecular classification of hepatocellular carcinoma is still developing. Thus, different approaches have been proposed. Although the present tools of molecular analysis assure the

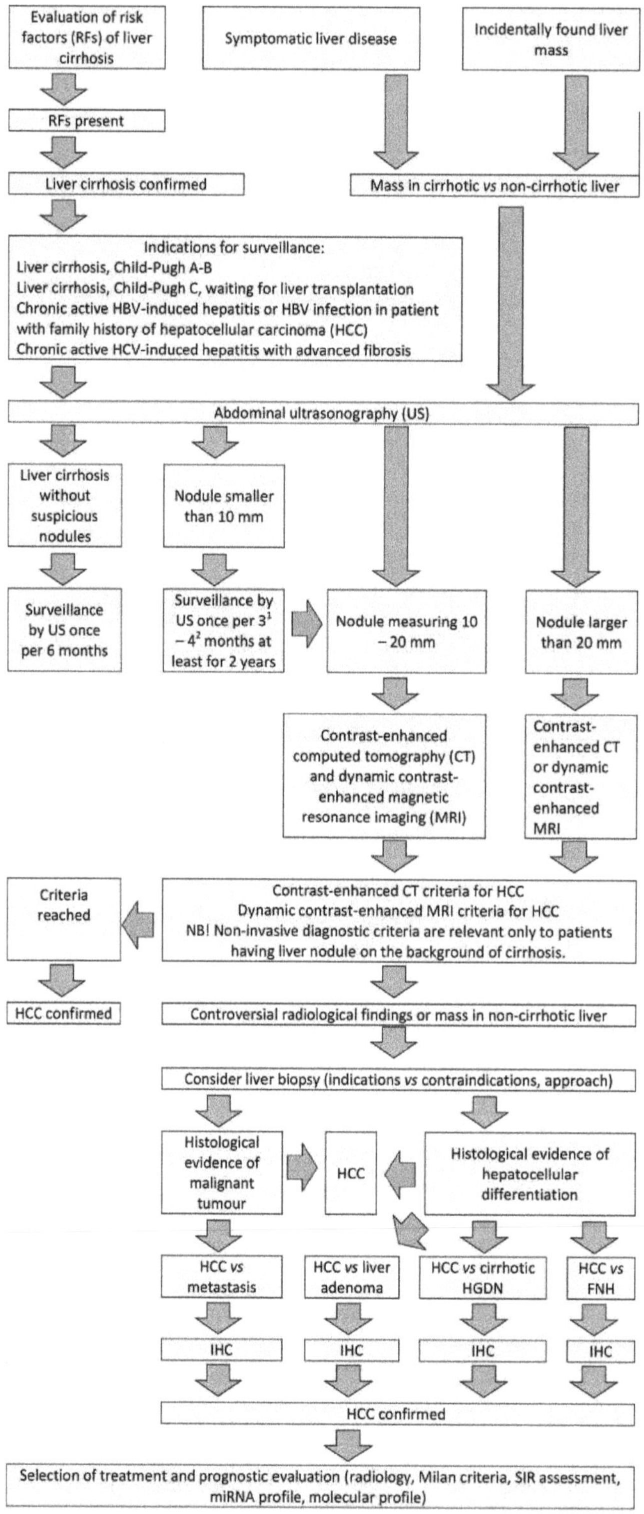

Figure 1. Diagnostic algorithm of hepatocellular carcinoma. 1—Recommended by the American Association for the Study of the Liver diseases (AASLD). 2—Recommended by the European Association for the Study of the Liver (EASL). Abbreviations: RFs, risk factors; *vs*, versus; HBV, hepatitis B virus; HCC, hepatocellular carcinoma; HCV, hepatitis C virus; US, ultrasonography; CT, computed tomography; MRI, magnetic resonance imaging; HGDN, high-grade dysplastic nodule; FNH, focal nodular hyperplasia; IHC, immunohistochemistry; SIR, systemic inflammatory response; mi, micro; RNA; ribonucleic acid.

technical background for in-depth studies, HCC might be more difficult target for the systematisation of molecular findings than other tumours. The problems are associated with heterogeneity of etiological factors and their geographic distribution in different populations with diverse genetic background [81].

A trans-ancestry study has been carried out involving 608 cases of HCC. The cohort was created to reflect both etiological and geographic/genetic diversity of HCC. The main identified molecular targets were TP53–Rb pathway, Wnt pathway, modulators of chromatin and transcription, mTOR–PIK3CA pathway and mutations in genes regulating telomere maintenance [82].

French research team has recently proposed molecular classification into six subtypes, designated as G1–G6. The first three subtypes are characterised by *TP53* mutations and are high-grade tumours. G1–G2 share *AXIN1* and *ATM* mutations, while G1 also possesses *RPS6KA3* mutations. G3 is characterised by mutations in *TSC1/TSC2* and *FGF19*. G3 is also associated with haemochromatosis, macrovascular invasion, macrotrabecular and compact histological pattern as well as presence of multinucleated and pleomorphic cells. Sarcomatoid changes are more frequent in G1–G2, but clear cells—in G1. G4–G6 lack *TP53* mutations and are low-grade tumours. G5–G6 exhibit mutations in *CTNNB1* gene, while G4 lacks both mutations in *TP53* and *CTNNB1*. G4 tumours are more frequently characterised by small size, steatohepatitic morphology and inflammatory infiltrates as well as absence of satellite nodules and vascular invasion. G5–G6 carcinomas display microtrabecular pattern, cholestasis and lack inflammatory infiltrates. By immunohistochemistry, these HCCs are characterised by nuclear expression of beta catenin and strong positivity for glutamine synthetase [52].

5. Diagnostic algorithm of hepatocellular carcinoma

Nowadays, the classic diagnostic algorithm of HCC (see **Figure 1**) includes the evaluation of risk factors in a given patient to assess the need for surveillance. Cirrhotic patients are referred to ultrasound examination once per 6 months. Suspicious nodules are further evaluated by CT and MRI. Characteristic findings by CT and MRI including arterial hypervascularisation represent the basis of non-invasive diagnostics. In controversial and non-cirrhotic cases, biopsy is indicated that might need supplementation by immunohistochemistry according to the morphological features. Innovations are expected in the field of miRNA-based liquid biopsy to support radiological diagnosis, addition of SIR assessment and miRNA profile to select the optimal treatment, e.g. possibly broadening Milan criteria (see also chapter "Innovative Blood Tests for Hepatocellular Carcinoma: Liquid Biopsy and Evaluation of Systemic Inflammatory Reaction"), and novel immunohistochemical markers for cases that still remain ambiguous.

6. Conclusions

HCC is a frequent and aggressive malignant tumour, estimated to range sixth by incidence and second by mortality in the global cancer statistics. The high ratio of mortality to incidence (0.95) and the close geographic correlation between incidence and mortality reflects the dismal prognosis. However, longer survival can be reached in early diagnosed and properly treated cases.

Awareness of the risk factors of HCC is helpful both in diagnostics and in order to set up the surveillance. Liver cirrhosis is the main risk factor; surveillance is indicated in these patients. A tumour found in cirrhotic liver is more likely to be HCC than metastasis or liver adenoma. However, the differential diagnosis includes a dysplastic cirrhotic nodule.

The other risk factors act mainly through inducing cirrhosis although a fraction of HCC can precede the development of cirrhosis in a patient affected by chronic liver disease or develop in non-fibrotic liver. Thus, the complete list of the risk factors of HCC includes chronic active hepatitis B or C, liver damage by alcohol and/or aflatoxins, as well as NASH. The risk factors can act synergistically. Evaluating the HCC risk in any patient, the relative risk must be considered in accordance to the risk factors that are identified in that individual. However, to estimate the expected cancer burden in the population, population attributable fractions are of importance; these parameters depend both on relative risk and population frequency of each particular factor.

Non-invasive radiological approach is the gold standard in the diagnostics of HCC in contrast with most of other malignant tumours necessitating confirmation by a biopsy. Biopsy is indicated only in radiologically controversial cases or to prove HCC in non-cirrhotic liver.

Ultrasonography is used for surveillance and the initial step of diagnostics. For surveillance of cirrhotic patient, US is carried out once in 6 months. If a suspicious focus is disclosed, the further approach is based on the size. Either CT or MRI is indicated for mass lesions larger than 20 mm, while both methods are recommended for a nodule measuring between 10 and 20 mm. Nodules that are smaller than 1 cm are followed up by US once in 4 months. Hypervascularity is a characteristic trait of HCC in CT and MRI. PET and CEUS may have additional role in HCC diagnostics.

If biopsy is carried out, HCC can be diagnosed if both signs of hepatocellular differentiation and cellular atypia or invasion are present. Low-grade tumours must be differentiated from dysplastic nodule, focal nodular hyperplasia and adenoma while high-grade HCC must be distinguished from metastasis. Mass lesion in cirrhotic liver is most probably a dysplastic nodule or HCC while adenomas and metastases usually develop in non-cirrhotic liver. In a Western patient, clearly malignant tumour in a non-cirrhotic liver has higher probability to represent a metastatic carcinoma.

Regarding immunohistochemistry, arginase-1 and HepPar antigen are reasonable hepatocellular markers that are used to distinguish HCC from metastases. Novel immunohistochemical markers of HCC include bile salt export pump protein and heavy chain of clathrin. Glypican should be used with caution due to the reported expression in a wide range of extrahepatic tumours. In order to discriminate between low-grade HCC and FNH, reticulin network, glypican-3 and heat shock protein 70 can be assessed. The differential diagnosis between high grade dysplastic nodule and low grade HCC can be very complicated as both processes share several morphological features and can coexist, biologically representing subsequent stages of HCC development. The features favouring malignancy over dysplastic nodule, include (1) expression of at least two markers in a panel consisting from glypican-3, heat shock protein 70 and glutamine synthetase; (2) diffuse expression of CD34 due to higher oxygen tension in HCC and (3) loss of perifocal CK7- and CK19-positive ductular reaction as a sign of invasive growth.

Regarding molecular classification of HCC, reasonable success has been reached by French research group and trans-ancestry study team. However, no unified classification has been established yet. Molecular profile can have both diagnostic and prognostic value.

Acknowledgements

BS was financially supported by post-doctoral research project 1.1.1.2./VIAA/1/16/242.

Author details

Dzeina Mezale[1], Ilze Strumfa[1]*, Andrejs Vanags[2], Arturs Kalva[1], Dainis Balodis[1], Boriss Strumfs[3], Ilze Fridrihsone[1], Arnis Abolins[1] and Janis Gardovskis[2]

*Address all correspondence to: ilze.strumfa@rsu.lv

1 Department of Pathology, Riga Stradins University, Riga, Latvia

2 Department of Surgery, Riga Stradins University, Riga, Latvia

3 Latvian Institute of Organic Synthesis, Riga, Latvia

References

[1] Bosman FT, Carneiro F, Hruban RH, Theise ND. WHO Classification of Tumours of the Digestive System. IARC: Lyon; 2010. 417 p

[2] Ryerson AB, Eheman CR, Altekruse SF, Ward JW, Jemal A, Sherman RL, Henley SJ, Holtzman D, Lake A, Noone AM, Anderson RN, Ma J, Ly KN, Cronin KA, Penberthy L, Kohler BA. Annual report to the nation on the status of cancer, 1975–2012, featuring the increasing incidence of liver cancer. Cancer. 2016;**122**(9):1312-1337. DOI: 10.1002/cncr.29936

[3] Schlageter M, Terracciano LM, D'Angelo S, Sorrentino P. Histopathology of hepatocellular carcinoma. World Journal of Gastroenterology. 2014;**20**(43):15955-15964. DOI: 10.3748/wjg.v20.i43.15955

[4] Mezale D, Strumfa I, Vanags A, Mezals M, Fridrihsone I, Strumfs B, Balodis D. Non-alcoholic steatohepatitis, liver cirrhosis and hepatocellular carcinoma: The molecular pathways. In: Tsoulfas G, editor. Liver Cirrhosis – Update and Current Challenges. Rijeka: IntechOpen; 2017. pp. 1-34. DOI: 10.5772/intechopen.68771

[5] Andreana L, Isgro G, Pleguezuelo M, Germani G, Burroughs AK. Surveillance and diagnosis of hepatocellular carcinoma in patients with cirrhosis. World Journal of Hepatology. 2009;**1**(1):48-61. DOI: 10.4254/wjh.v1.i1.48

[6] Pittman ME, Brunt EM. Anatomic pathology of hepatocellular carcinoma: Histopathology using classic and new diagnostic tools. Clinical Liver Disease. 2015;**19**(2):239-259. DOI: 10.1016/j.cld.2015.01.003

[7] Serra C, Righi S, De Molo C, Felicani C. Current role of contrast-enhanced ultrasound in the diagnosis of hepatocellular carcinoma. Journal of Hepatology and Gastrointestinal Disorders. 2015;**1**:102. DOI: 10.4172/2475-3181.1000102

[8] Ferlay J, Soerjomataram I, Dikshit R, Eser S, Mathers C, Rebelo M, Parkin DM, Forman D, Bray F. Cancer incidence and mortality worldwide: Sources, methods and major patterns in GLOBOCAN 2012. International Journal of Cancer. 2015;**136**(5):E359-E386. DOI: 10.1002/ijc.29210

[9] Njei B, Rotman Y, Ditah I, Lim JK. Emerging trends in hepatocellular carcinoma incidence and mortality. Hepatology. 2015;**61**(1):191-199. DOI: 10.1002/hep.27388

[10] Ghouri YA, Mian I, Rowe JH. Review of hepatocellular carcinoma: Epidemiology, etiology, and carcinogenesis. Journal of Carcinogenesis. 2017;**16**(1). DOI: 10.4103/jcar.JCar_9_16. https://www.ncbi.nlm.nih.gov/pmc/articles/PMC5490340/

[11] El-Serag HB, Mason AC. Rising incidence of hepatocellular carcinoma in the United States. The New England Journal of Medicine. 1999;**340**(10):745-750. DOI: 10.1056/NEJM199903113401001

[12] Herbst DA, Reddy KR. Risk factors for hepatocellular carcinoma. Clinical Liver Disease. 2012;**1**(6):180-182. DOI: 10.1002/cld.111

[13] Janevska D, Chaloska-Ivanova V, Janevski V. Hepatocellular carcinoma: Risk factors, diagnosis and treatment. Open Access Macedonian Journal of Medical Sciences. 2015; **3**(4):732-736. DOI: 10.3889/oamjms.2015.111

[14] Liu Y, Wu F. Global burden of aflatoxin-induced hepatocellular carcinoma: A risk assessment. Environmental Health Perspectives. 2010;**118**(6):818-824. DOI: 10.1289/ehp.0901388

[15] Bagnardi V, Rota M, Botteri E, Tramacere I, Islami F, Fedirko V, Scotti L, Jenab M, Turati F, Pasquali E, Pelucchi C, Galeone C, Bellocco R, Negri E, Corrao G, Boffetta P, La Vecchia C. Alcohol consumption and site specific cancer risk: A comprehensive dose-response meta-analysis. British Journal of Cancer. 2015;**112**(3):580-593. DOI: 10.1038/bjc.2014.579

[16] Stickel F, Hellerbrand C. Non-alcoholic fatty liver disease as a risk factor for hepatocellular carcinoma: Mechanisms and implications. Gut. 2010;**59**(10):1303-1307. DOI: 10.1136/gut.2009.199661

[17] Razumilava N, Gores GJ, Lindor KD. Cancer surveillance in patients with primary sclerosing cholangitis. Hepatology. 2011;**54**(5):1842-1852. DOI: 10.1002/hep.24570

[18] Nowicki TK, Markiet K, Szurowska E. Diagnostic imaging of hepatocellular carcinoma – A pictorial essay. Current Medical Imaging Reviews. 2017;**13**(2):140-153. DOI: 10.2174/1573405612666160720123748

[19] Sherman M, Llovet JM. Smoking, hepatitis B virus infection, and development of hepatocellular carcinoma. Journal of the National Cancer Institute. 2011;**103**(22):1642-1643. DOI: 10.1093/jnci/djr430

[20] Fingas CD, Best J, Sowa JP, Canbay A. Epidemiology of nonalcoholic steatohepatitis and hepatocellular carcinoma. Clinical Liver Disease. 2016;**8**(5):119-122. DOI:10.1002/cld.585

[21] Baffy G, Brunt EM, Caldwell SH. Hepatocellular carcinoma in non-alcoholic fatty liver disease: An emerging menace. Journal of Hepatology. 2012;**56**(6):1384-1391. DOI: 10.1016/j.jhep.2011.10.027

[22] Younossi ZM, Koenig AB, Abdelatif D, Fazel Y, Henry L, Wymer M. Global epidemiology of non-alcoholic fatty liver disease – Meta-analytic assessment of prevalence, incidence and outcomes. Hepatology. 2016;**64**(1):73-84. DOI: 10.1002/hep.28431

[23] Mittal S, El-Serag HB. Epidemiology of hepatocellular carcinoma: Consider the population. Journal of Clinical Gastroenterology. 2013;**47**(Suppl):S2-S6. DOI: 10.1097/MCG.0b013e3182872f29

[24] Qian GS, Ross RK, Yu MC, Yuan JM, Gao YT, Henderson BE, Wogan GN, Groopmen JD. A follow-up study of urinary markers of aflatoxin exposure and liver cancer risk in Shanghai, People's Republic of China. Cancer Epidemiology, Biomarkers & Prevention. 1994;**3**(1):3-10

[25] Welzel TM, Graubard BI, Quraishi S, Zeuzem S, Davila JA, El-Serag HB, McGlynn KA. Population-attributable fractions of risk factors for hepatocellular carcinoma in the United States. The American Journal of Gastroenterology. 2013;**108**(8):1314-1321. DOI: 10.1038/ajg.2013.160

[26] Lin MT, Wang CC, Cheng YF, Eng HL, Yen YH, Tsai MC, Tseng PL, Chang KC, Wu CK, Hu TH. Comprehensive comparison of multiple-detector computed tomography and dynamic magnetic resonance imaging in the diagnosis of hepatocellular carcinoma with varying degrees of fibrosis. PLoS One. 2016;**11**(11):e0166157. DOI: 10.1371/journal.pone.0166157

[27] Schraml C, Kaufmann S, Rempp H, Syha R, Ketelsen D, Notohamiprodjo M, Nikolaou K. Imaging of HCC – Current state of the art. Diagnostics (Basel). 2015;**5**(4):513-545. DOI: 10.3390/diagnostics5040513

[28] Yu SJ. A concise review of updated guidelines regarding the management of hepatocellular carcinoma around the world: 2010–2016. Clinical and Molecular Hepatology. 2016;**22**(1):7-17. DOI: 10.3350/cmh.2016.22.1.7

[29] Bennett GL, Krinsky GA, Abitbol RJ, Kim SY, Theise ND, Teperman LW. Sonographic detection of hepatocellular carcinoma and dysplastic nodules in cirrhosis: Correlation of

pretransplantation sonography and liver explant pathology in 200 patients. American Journal of Roentgenology. 2002;**179**(1):75-80. DOI: 10.2214/ajr.179.1.1790075

[30] Martie A, Sporea I, Popescu A, Sirli R, Danila M, Serban C, Ardelean M, Bota S, Sendroiu M, Chisevescu D. Contrast enhanced ultrasound for the characterization of hepatocellular carcinoma. Medical Ultrasonography. 2011;**13**(2):108-113

[31] Omata M, Cheng AL, Kokudo N, Kudo M, Lee JM, Jia J, Tateishi R, Han KH, Chawla YK, Shiina S, Jafri W, Payawal DA, Ohki T, Ogasawara S, Chen PJ, Lesmana CRA, Lesmana LA, Gani RA, Obi S, Dokmeci AK, Sarin SK. Asia-Pacific clinical practice guidelines on the management of hepatocellular carcinoma: A 2017 update. Hepatology International. 2017; **11**(4):317-370. DOI: 10.1007/s12072-017-9799-9

[32] Elsayed EE, Koryem EM, Mohammed SA. Multidetector computed tomography in the detection of hepatocellular carcinomas meeting the Milan criteria before liver transplantation. Menoufia Medical Journal. 2016;**29**(2):291-296. DOI: 10.4103/1110-2098.192448

[33] Herzen J, Willner MS, Fingerle AA, Noel PB, Kohler T, Drecoll E, Rummeny EJ, Pfeiffer F. Imaging liver lesions using grating-based phase-contrast computed tomography with bilateral filter post-processing. PLoS One. 2014;**9**(1):e83369. DOI: 10.1371/journal.pone.0083369

[34] Senturk S, Cetin B, Cengiz M, Bilici A, Ozekinci S. Dynamic multidetector computed tomography findings of hepatocellular carcinoma of hepatitis B virus-positive and -negative patients. Cancer Imaging. 2014;**14**:9. DOI: 10.1186/1470-7330-14-9

[35] Ariff B, Lloyd CR, Khan S, Shariff M, Thillainayagam AV, Bansi DS, Khan SA, Taylor-Robinson SD, Lim AK. Imaging of liver cancer. World Journal of Gastroenterology. 2009; **15**(11):1289-1300. DOI: 10.3748/wjg.15.1289

[36] Lee YJ, Lee JM, Lee JS, Lee HY, Park BH, Kim YH, Han JK, Choi BI. Hepatocellular carcinoma: Diagnostic performance of multidetector CT and MR imaging – A systematic review and meta-analysis. Radiology. 2015;**275**(1):97-109. DOI: 10.1148/radiol.14140690

[37] Jhaveri K, Cleary S, Audet P, Balaa F, Bhayana D, Burak K, Chang S, Dixon E, Haider M, Molinari M, Reinhold C, Sherman M. Consensus statements from a multidisciplinary expert panel on the utilization and application of a liver-specific MRI contrast agent (gadoxetic acid). American Journal of Roentgenology. 2015;**204**(3):498-509. DOI: 10.2214/AJR.13.12399

[38] Niendorf E, Spilseth B, Wang X, Taylor A. Contrast enhanced MRI in the diagnosis of HCC. Diagnostics (Basel). 2015;**5**(3):383-398. DOI: 10.3390/diagnostics5030383

[39] Sandrasegaran K, Tahir B, Nutakki K, Akisik FM, Bodanapally U, Tann M, Chalasani N. Usefulness of conventional MRI sequences and diffusion-weighted imaging in differentiating malignant from benign portal vein thrombus in cirrhotic patients. American Journal of Roentgenology. 2013;**201**(6):1211-1219. DOI: 10.2214/AJR.12.10171

[40] Guimaraes MD, Hochhegger B, Benveniste MF, Odisio BC, Gross JL, Zurstrassen CE, Tyng CC, Bitencourt AG, Marchiori E. Improving CT-guided transthoracic biopsy of mediastinal

lesions by diffusion-weighted magnetic resonance imaging. Clinics (São Paulo, Brazil). 2014; **69**:787-791. DOI: 10.6061/clinics/2014(11)13

[41] Fowler KJ, Linehan DC, Menias CO. Colorectal liver metastases: State of the art imaging. Annals of Surgical Oncology. 2013;**20**(4):1185-1193. DOI: 10.1245/s10434-012-2730-7

[42] Strumfa I, Vasko E, Vanags A, Simtniece Z, Trapencieris P, Gardovskis J. Hepatic surgery for colorectal cancer metastasis — Possibilities and prerequisites. In: Abdeldayem H, editor. Recent Advances in Liver Diseases and Surgery. Rijeka: InTech; 2015. pp. 169-203 DOI: 10.5772/60971

[43] Fischer MA, Raptis DA, Donati OF, Hunziker R, Schade E, Sotiropoulos GC, McCall J, Bartlett A, Bachellier P, Frilling A, Breitenstein S, Clavien PA, Alkadhi H, Patak MA. MR imaging features for improved diagnosis of hepatocellular carcinoma in the non-cirrhotic liver: Multi-center evaluation. European Journal of Radiology. 2015;**84**(10):1879-1887. DOI: 10.1016/j.ejrad.2015.06.029

[44] Iansante V, Choy PM, Fung SW, Liu Y, Chai JG, Dyson J, Del Rio A, D'Santos C, Williams R, Chokshi S, Anders RA, Bubici C, Papa S. PARP14 promotes the Warburg effect in hepatocellular carcinoma by inhibiting JNK1-dependent PKM2 phosphorylation and activation. Nature Communications. 2015;**6**:7882. DOI: 10.1038/ncomms8882

[45] Talbot JN, Fartoux L, Balogova S, Nataf V, Kerrou K, Gutman F, Huchet V, Ancel D, Grange JD, Rosmorduc O. Detection of hepatocellular carcinoma with PET/CT: A prospective comparison of 18F-fluorocholine and 18F-FDG in patients with cirrhosis or chronic liver disease. Journal of Nuclear Medicine. 2010;**51**(11):1699-1706. DOI: 10.2967/jnumed.110.075507

[46] Kim YI, Paeng JC, Cheon GJ, Suh KS, Lee DS, Chung JK, Kang KW. Prediction of posttransplantation recurrence of hepatocellular carcinoma using metabolic and volumetric indices of 18F-FDG PET/CT. Journal of Nuclear Medicine. 2016;**57**(7):1045-1051. DOI: 10.2967/jnumed.115.170076

[47] Talbot JN, Michaud L, Grange JD, Rosmorduc O, Balogova A. Use of choline PET for studying hepatocellular carcinoma. Clinical and Translational Imaging. 2014;**2**:103-113. DOI: 10.1007/s40336-014-0055-1

[48] Sasikumar A, Joy A, Nanabala R, Pillai MR, Thomas B, Vikraman KR. (68)Ga-PSMA PET/CT imaging in primary hepatocellular carcinoma. European Journal of Nuclear Medicine and Molecular Imaging. 2016;**43**(4):795-796. DOI: 10.1007/s00259-015-3297-x

[49] Randazzo C, Licata A, Almasio PL. Liver biopsy – Indications, procedures, results. In: Tagaya N, editor. Liver Biopsy – Indications, Procedures, Results. Rijeka: InTech; 2012. pp. 3-22. DOI: 10.5772/52616

[50] Venkatesh SK, Chandan V, Roberts LR. Liver masses: A clinical, radiologic, and pathologic perspective. Clinical Gastroenterology and Hepatology. 2014;**12**(9):1414-1429. DOI: 10.1016/j.cgh.2013.09.017

[51] Tannapfel A, Dienes HP, Lohse AW. The indications for liver biopsy. Deutsches Ärzteblatt International. 2012;**109**(27–28):477-483. DOI: 10.3238/arztebl.2012.0477

[52] Calderaro J, Couchy G, Imbeaud S, Amaddeo G, Letouze E, Blanc JF, Laurent C, Hajji Y, Azoulay D, Bioulac-Sage P, Nault JC, Zucman-Rossi J. Histological subtypes of hepatocellular carcinoma are related to gene mutations and molecular tumour classification. Journal of Hepatology. 2017;**67**(4):727-738. DOI: 10.1016/j.jhep.2017.05.014

[53] Shafizadeh N, Kakar S. Hepatocellular carcinoma: Histologic subtypes. Surgical Pathology Clinics. 2013;**6**(2):367-384. DOI: 10.1016/j.path.2013.03.007

[54] Andrade RC, de Lima MAFD, de Faria PAS, Vargas FR. TP53 germline and somatic mutations in a patient with fibrolamellar hepatocellular carcinoma. Familial Cancer. 2017;**17**(1):119-122. DOI: 10.1007/s10689-017-9998-5

[55] Choi WT, Kakar S. Immunohistochemistry in the diagnosis of hepatocellular carcinoma. Gastroenterology Clinics of North America. 2017;**46**(2):311-325. DOI: 10.1016/j.gtc.2017.01.006

[56] Lagana S, Hsiao S, Bao F, Sepulveda A, Moreira R, Lefkowitch J, Remotti H. HepPar-1 and Arginase-1 immunohistochemistry in adenocarcinoma of the small intestine and ampullary region. Archives of Pathology & Laboratory Medicine. 2015;**139**(6):791-795. DOI: 10.5858/arpa.2013-0249-OA

[57] Filmus J, Capurro M, Rast J. Glypicans. Genome Biology. 2008;**9**(5):224. DOI: 10.1186/gb-2008-9-5-224.

[58] Pavlopoulou A, Scorilas A. A comprehensive phylogenetic and structural analysis of the carcinoembryonic antigen (CEA) gene family. Genome Biology and Evolution. 2014;**6**(6):1314-1326. DOI: 10.1093/gbe/evu103

[59] Seimiya M, Tomonaga T, Matsushita K, Sunaga M, Oh-Ishi M, Kodera Y, Maeda T, Takano S, Togawa A, Yoshitomi H, Otsuka M, Yamamoto M, Nakano M, Miyazaki M, Nomura F. Identification of novel immunohistochemical tumor markers for primary hepatocellular carcinoma; clathrin heavy chain and formiminotransferase cyclodeaminase. Hepatology. 2008;**48**(2):519-530. DOI: 10.1002/hep.22364

[60] Lagana SM, Salomao M, Remotti HE, Knisely AS, Moreira RK. Bile salt export pump: A sensitive and specific immunohistochemical marker of hepatocellular carcinoma. Histopathology. 2015;**66**(4):598-602. DOI: 10.1111/his.12601

[61] Kondo F, Fukusato T, Kudo M. Pathological diagnosis of benign hepatocellular nodular lesions based on the new World Health Organization classification. Oncology. 2014;**87** (Suppl 1):37-49. DOI: 10.1159/000368144

[62] Nault JC, Mallet M, Pilati C, Calderaro J, Bioulac-Sage P, Laurent C, Laurent A, Cherqui D, Balabaud C, Zucman-Rossi J. High frequency of telomerase reverse-transcriptase promoter somatic mutations in hepatocellular carcinoma and preneoplastic lesions. Nature Communications. 2013;**4**:2218. DOI: 10.1038/ncomms3218

[63] Strumfa I, Vilmanis J, Vanags A, Vasko E, Sulte D, Simtniece Z, Abolins A, Gardovskis J. Primary and metastatic tumours of the liver: Expanding scope of morphological and immunohistochemical details in the biopsy. In: Tagaya N, editor. Liver Biopsy – Indications, Procedures, Results. Rijeka: InTech; 2012. pp. 115-159. DOI: 10.5772/52838

[64] Bioulac-Sage P, Balabaud C, Zucman-Rossi J. Subtype classification of hepatocellular adenoma. Digestive Surgery. 2010;**27**(1):39-45. DOI: 10.1159/000268406

[65] Park SY, Kim BH, Kim JH, Lee S, Kang GH. Panels of immunohistochemical markers help determine primary sites of metastatic adenocarcinoma. Archives of Pathology & Laboratory Medicine. 2007;**131**(10):1561-1567

[66] Sen A, Mitra S, Das RN, Dasgupta S, Saha K, Chatterjee U, Mukherjee K, Datta C, Chattopadhyay BK. Expression of CDX-2 and Ki-67 in different grades of colorectal adenocarcinomas. Indian Journal of Pathology & Microbiology. 2015;**58**(2):158-162. DOI: 10.4103/0377-4929.155304

[67] Saad RS, Ghorab Z, Khalifa MA, Xu M. CDX2 as a marker for intestinal differentiation: Its utility and limitations. World Journal of Gastrointestinal Surgery. 2011;**3**(11):159-166. DOI: 10.4240/wjgs.v3.i11.159

[68] Zhang YJ, Chen JW, He XS, Zhang HZ, Ling YH, Wen JH, Deng WH, Li P, Yun JP, Xie D, Cai MY. SATB2 is a promising biomarker for identifying a colorectal origin for liver metastatic adenocarcinomas. eBioMedicine. 2018;**28**:62-69. DOI: 10.1016/j.ebiom.2018.01.001

[69] El-Maqsoud NM, Tawfiek ER, Abdelmeged A, Rahman MF, Moustafa AA. The diagnostic utility of the triple markers Napsin A, TTF-1, and PAX8 in differentiating between primary and metastatic lung adenocarcinomas. Tumour Biology. 2016;**37**(3):3123-3134. DOI: 10.1007/s13277-015-3964-3

[70] Zubovits J, Buzney E, Yu L, Duncan LM. HMB-45, S-100, NK1/C3, and MART-1 in metastatic melanoma. Human Pathology. 2004;**35**(2):217-223. DOI: https://doi.org/10.1016/j.humpath.2003.09.019

[71] Spanknebel K, Coit DG, Bieligk SC, Gonen M, Rosai J, Klimstra DS. Characterization of micrometastatic disease in melanoma sentinel lymph nodes by enhanced pathology: Recommendations for standardizing pathologic analysis. The American Journal of Surgical Pathology. 2005;**29**(3):305-317. DOI: 10.1097/01.pas.0000152134.36030.b7

[72] Reinke S, Koniger P, Herberth G, Audring H, Wang H, Ma J, Guo Y, Sterry W, Trefzer U. Differential expression of MART-1, tyrosinase, and SM5-1 in primary and metastatic melanoma. The American Journal of Dermatopathology. 2005;**27**(5):401-406. DOI: 10.1097/01.dad.0000180076.17932.ee

[73] Plaza JA, Suster D, Perez-Montiel D. Expression of immunohistochemical markers in primary and metastatic malignant melanoma: A comparative study in 70 patients using a tissue microarray technique. Applied Immunohistochemistry & Molecular Morphology. 2007;**15**(4):421-425. DOI: 10.1097/PAI.0b013e318032ea5d

[74] Barr ML, Jilaveanu LB, Camp RL, Adeniran AJ, Kluger HM, Shuch B. PAX-8 expression in renal tumours and distant sites: A useful marker of primary and metastatic renal cell carcinoma? Journal of Clinical Pathology. 2015;**68**(1):12-17. DOI: 10.1136/jclinpath-2014-202259

[75] Huo L, Zhang J, Gilcrease MZ, Gong Y, Wu Y, Zhang H, Resetkova E, Hunt KK, Deavers MT. Gross cystic disease fluid protein-15 and mammaglobin A expression determined by immunohistochemistry is of limited utility in triple negative breast cancer. Histopathology. 2013;**62**(2):267-274. DOI: 10.1111/j.1365-2559.2012.04344.x

[76] Ni YB, Tsang JYS, Shao MM, Chan SK, Cheung SY, Tong J, To KF, Tse GM. GATA-3 is superior to GCDFP-15 and mammaglobin to identify primary and metastatic breast cancer. Breast Cancer Research and Treatment. 2018;**169**(1):25-32. DOI: 10.1007/s10549-017-4645-2 [Epub ahead of print]

[77] Kandalaft PL, Simon RA, Isacson C, Gown AM. Comparative sensitivities and specificities of antibodies to breast markers GCDFP-15, mammaglobin A, and different clones of antibodies to GATA-3: A study of 338 tumours using whole sections. Applied Immunohistochemistry & Molecular Morphology. 2016;**24**(9):609-614. DOI: 10.1097/PAI.00000 00000000237

[78] Peng Y, Butt YM, Chen B, Zhang X, Tang P. Update on immunohistochemical analysis in breast lesions. Archives of Pathology & Laboratory Medicine. 2017;**141**(8):1033-1051. DOI: 10.5858/arpa.2016-0482-RA

[79] Huo L, Gong Y, Guo M, Gilcrease MZ, Wu Y, Zhang H, Zhang J, Resetkova E, Hunt KK, Deavers MT. GATA-binding protein 3 enhances the utility of gross cystic disease fluid protein-15 and mammaglobin A in triple-negative breast cancer by immunohistochemistry. Histopathology. 2015;**67**(2):245-254. DOI: 10.1111/his.12645

[80] Shaoxian T, Baohua Y, Xiaoli X, Yufan C, Xiaoyu T, Hongfen L, Rui B, Xiangjie S, Ruohong S, Wentao Y. Characterisation of GATA3 expression in invasive breast cancer: Differences in histological subtypes and immunohistochemically defined molecular subtypes. Journal of Clinical Pathology. 2017;**70**(11):926-934. DOI: 10.1136/jclinpath-2016-204137

[81] Fakhri B, Lim KH. Molecular landscape and sub-classification of gastrointestinal cancers: A review of literature. Journal of Gastrointestinal Oncology. 2017;**8**(3):379-386. DOI: 10.21037/jgo.2016.11.01

[82] Totoki Y, Tatsuno K, Covington KR, Ueda H, Creighton CJ, Kato M, Tsuji S, Donehower LA, Slagle BL, Nakamura H, Yamamoto S, Shinbrot E, Hama N, Lehmkuhl M, Hosoda F, Arai Y, Walker K, Dahdouli M, Gotoh K, Nagae G, Gingras MC, Muzny DM, Ojima H, Shimada K, Midorikawa Y, Goss JA, Cotton R, Hayashi A, Shibahara J, Ishikawa S, Guiteau J, Tanaka M, Urushidate T, Ohashi S, Okada N, Doddapaneni H, Wang M, Zhu Y, Dinh H, Okusaka T, Kokudo N, Kosuge T, Takayama T, Fukayama M, Gibbs RA, Wheeler DA, Aburatani H, Shibata T. Trans-ancestry mutational landscape of hepatocellular carcinoma genomes. Nature Genetics. 2014;**46**(12):1267-1273. DOI: 10.1038/ng.3126

10

The Diagnostic and Prognostic Potential of Micro RNAs for Hepatocellular Carcinoma

Xi-Dai Long, Wei-Zhong Tang, Jun Lu,
Xiao-Ying Huang, Jin-Guang Yao, Tian-Qi Zhang,
Xing-Zhizi Wang, Qun-Ying Su, Chun-Ying Luo,
Xue-Ming Wu, Chao Wang, Li-Xia Zeng,
Qiang Xia and Yun Ma

Abstract

Hepatocellular carcinoma (also termed hepatocarcinoma) is the third cancer-related cause of death worldwide. To our knowledge, markers such as α-fetoprotein display poor performance in the early diagnosis and prognosis prediction of hepatocarcinoma. MicroRNAs are an evolutionarily conserved class of small noncoding single-stranded RNA typically consisting of 18–24 nucleotides. They have been reported to act as tumor suppressors or oncogenes via reversely regulating gene expression. Recent evidence has revealed that microRNAs, especially in body fluids such as the blood and urine, display important diagnostic and prognostic potential for hepatocarcinoma. Here, we reviewed currently available data on microRNAs and hepatocarcinoma, with emphasis on the biogenesis and function of microRNAs and their potential diagnostic and prognostic value for hepatocarcinoma. We also discussed the clinical utility perspectives of microRNAs in hepatocarcinoma and possible challenges.

Keywords: hepatocarcinoma, microRNA, diagnosis, prognosis

1. Introduction

Hepatocarcinoma, also termed as hepatocellular carcinoma (HCC) or liver carcinoma, is the most common primary liver malignant disease in adults [1]. One of the most striking features of this malignant tumor is the wide variation in its incidence in different parts of the world. In areas of high incidence, such as China, hepatocarcinoma is among the leading cause of cancer-correlated deaths in recent years, with an annual incidence of approximately 40 per 100,000 [2, 3]. However, the countries in the low incidence, such as the USA, have only 2.3% of cancer-related deaths in past decades. Globally, hepatocarcinoma is the fifth most common cancer among males and the eighth most common among females [1]. Furthermore, the incidence of this tumor generally increases with age, although there are geographic and gender differences. The precise reasons for this difference is not known, but growing evidence has exhibited that multiple factors including chronic viral hepatitis B (HBV) and C (HCV), aflatoxin (such as aflatoxin B1) exposure, hepatic cirrhosis, obesity, diabetes, and vitamin D deficiency play an important role [4–6]. Although the molecular mechanism of hepatocarcinoma has been unclear, these hepatocarcinoma patients with early diagnosis often have good prognosis with more than 50% of five overall survival rate [6]. This is mainly because they benefit from the curative treatment such as curative resection and orthotropic liver transplantation [6]. However, if patients are lately diagnosed, the cumulative 5-year survival rate remarkably reduces to less than 10%, and tumor recurrence risk noticeably increases (about 70–80% of 5-year recurrence rate). Thus, it is very urgent to identify specific and sensitive markers for early diagnosing hepatocarcinoma at a curative stage, monitoring recurrence of tumor, and predicting prognosis of tumor [6].

Currently, the early diagnosis of hepatocarcinoma is based on the following two classes of methods: imaging examination which mainly consists of ultrasonography, magnetic resonance imaging, and computed tomography and serological tests such as serous α-fetoprotein (AFP) [4, 7]. Although advances in imaging technologies have significantly improved the early screening of hepatocarcinoma, these methods are so costly and unsatisfactory in early diagnosis that is not suitable for daily clinical practice [4, 7]. About serological methods, AFP is the most widely utilized marker for the diagnosis and prognosis prediction of hepatocarcinoma. However, this biomarker is limited because of its modest accuracy (with sensitivity of 40–65% and specificity of 87–96%) and about 30–40% of the false-negative rate for patients with early-stage hepatocarcinoma [8]. Additionally, serum AFP levels of some benign hepatic lesions, such as liver nodular hyperplasia, inflammation lesions of liver, and liver fibrotic cirrhosis, may give false-positive results [8]. Therefore, the reliability of this biomarker to determine hepatocarcinoma is inadequate because of its low sensitivity and specificity.

Emerging evidence has exhibited a correlation between dysregulation of microRNAs and development of hepatocarcinoma. Particularly, microRNAs are characterized by high stability in body fluids (including the blood and urine) and tissue specific in expression patterns, indicative of microRNAs in body fluids acting as potentially novel and ideal biomarkers for hepatocarcinoma diagnosis and prognosis prediction [8–16].

This review attempts to briefly review currently available data on microRNAs and hepatocarcinoma, with emphasis on (1) the biogenesis and function of microRNA, (2) potential diagnostic and prognostic value for hepatocarcinoma, and (3) the different value for hepatocarcinoma induced by different causes. Additionally, we summarized the clinical applicative perspectives and potential challenges of microRNAs in hepatocarcinoma.

2. MicroRNA biogenesis and function

Previous several reports have thoroughly reviewed biogenesis and function of microRNAs [8, 11, 17–29]. In brief, microRNAs are an evolutionarily conserved class of small noncoding single-stranded RNA typically consisting of 18–24 nucleotides. Originally, they are first transcribed by the RNA polymerase enzyme II into a kind of primary production named as primary microRNA that is characterized by long nucleotide sequences, 5′-cap structure, and 3′-poly-A tail, resembling protein-coding mRNAs. Then, primary microRNAs form a hairpin-shaped stem-loop structure and are processed into microRNA precursors (usually containing 60–70 nucleotides) by the microprocessor complex (consisting of DGCR8/Pasha and Drosha). After that, their precursors are transported to the cytoplasm and treated into a short double-strand duplex structure by another RNase endonuclease III (also called Dicer). Finally, the duplex structure (also called microRNA-microRNA*) is unwound into mature microRNAs by helicases. To date, it has been identified that there are more than 1800 microRNAs in the mammalian genome (miRDatabase) (**Figure 1**) [30]. Functionally, microRNAs are involved in regulating the expression of their

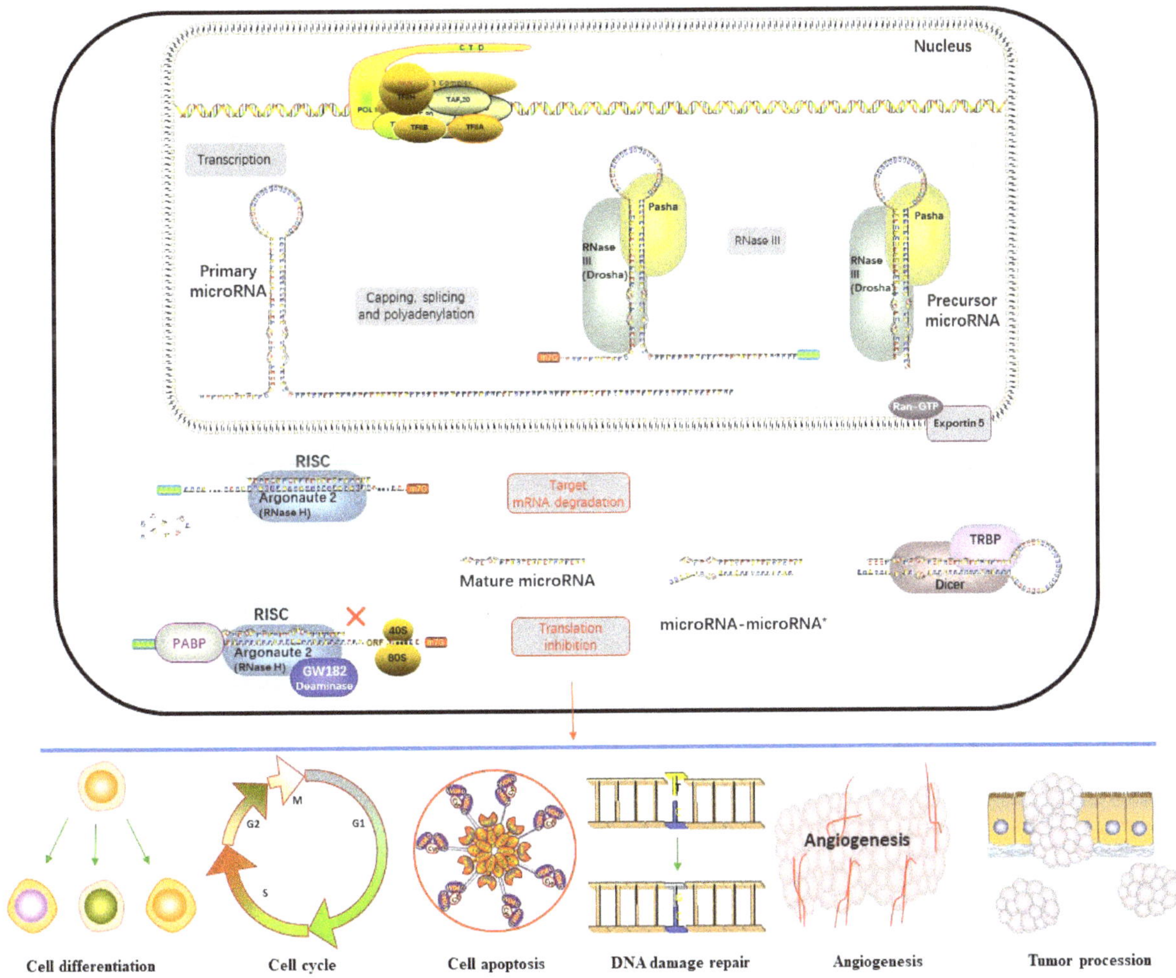

Figure 1. Biosynthesis and functions of microRNA. In the nucleus, the microRNA genes are transcribed into primary microRNAs by RNA polymerase II (Pol II). The primary microRNAs are then cleaved by Drosha and DGCR8 and produce their precursor molecules (also named as precursor microRNA). After that, the precursor molecules are transported to the cytoplasm by Exportin-5 and Ran-GTP and undergo final processing step including the cleavage by Dicer and the formation of stem-loop duplex molecule structure which contains the single-stranded mature microRNA molecule and a microRNA* fragment. Finally, the duplex molecule structure is incorporated into the RNA-induced silencing complex (RISC), the microRNA* fragments are degraded, and mature microRNA molecules are formed. The mature microRNAs can display genic regulation role via recognizing and binding to the 3′-untranslated region of their target genes' mRNAs. *Note*: This figure is plotted according to ScienceSlides (version#2016).

targeting genes via recognizing and integrating into the 3′-untranslated region of these genes' mRNAs. On the basis of perfect or imperfect base-base complementarity of microRNAs-their targeting mRNA binding, one microRNA specifically regulates the expression of multiple mRNAs, and at the same time, one mRNA might be inhibited by multiple microRNAs. This indicates the specificity and diversity of microRNAs regulating gene expression. In the past decades, microRNAs are emerged as important players in a very wide range of physiological processes including cell differentiation, cell proliferation and apoptosis, cycle regulation, survival, detoxification, physiological timing, metabolism, angiogenesis, hormone secretion, and DNA damage repair (**Figure 1**). Furthermore, growing evidence has shown that microRNAs can also display a role in the etiology and pathogenesis of various cancers by targeting many oncogenes or tumor inhibitive genes (**Figure 1**) [24, 27, 29–32]. Recent several reports have exhibited that some microRNAs involve in the tumorigenesis and procession of hepatocarcinoma and may become new potential markers for hepatocarcinoma diagnosis and prognosis [24, 27, 29, 31, 32].

3. MicroRNAs as novel biomarkers for hepatocarcinoma diagnosis

3.1. Diagnostic potential of single microRNA for hepatocarcinoma

With increasing incidence and death rate of hepatocarcinoma, it is very expected to identify one or several diagnostic biomarkers (with both high sensitivity and specificity) such as microRNAs for this malignancy. Growing evidence has shown that the expression change of all microRNAs in the peripheral blood may have a unique advantage because they exhibit tissue specificity and relative stability and can also provide some specific cues for early and small hepatocarcinoma [8–14]. Until now, more than 30 circulating microRNAs have been identified to have diagnostic potential for hepatocarcinoma (**Table 1**). For example, microRNA-122 has been reported as a hepatic-specific microRNA, accounting for 70% of the total microRNAs in hepatic tissues. This microRNA, a high conservative microRNA between vertebrate species, is indicative of a regulator of fatty acid metabolism and playing a critical role in liver homeostasis and tumorigenesis [19, 33, 34]. Increasing evidence has shown that elevated serum amount of microRNA-122 is positively associated with the severity of hepatic diseases including hepatitis, fatty- and alcohol-related liver damage, and drug-induced hepatotoxicity [35–39]. Interestingly, this increasing serum expression of microRNA-122 is noticeable and indicated that it could serve as a potential biomarker for the detection of patients with hepatocarcinoma from healthy controls with about 85% of the area under the receiver operating characteristic curve (AUC), 80% of sensitivity, and 80% of specificity [40, 41]. These results indicate that the dysregulated miR-122 in the peripheral blood may be used as a potential marker for hepatocarcinoma diagnosis. Results from retrospective studies have suggested that the microRNA-200 family (consisting of microRNA-200a and microRNA -200b) is also a promising biochemical biomarker for hepatocarcinoma diagnosis because of its deregulation during the development of both hepatic fibrosis and hepatocarcinoma [42, 43]. The elevated plasma levels of microRNA-21 can distinguish patients with hepatocarcinoma from cases with chronic hepatitis (with 61.1% of sensitivity and 83.3% of specificity) or healthy controls (the corresponding sensitivity and specificity are 87.3 and 92.0%, respectively) [44]. This suggests that this biomarker may have higher diagnostic potential than AFP. Some

MicroRNAs	Source	Diagnostic relevance	Expression level	AUC (95% CI)	Sen (%)	Spe (%)	Refs
miR-12	Serum	HCCs (n = 101) vs. HCs (n = 89)	Upregulated	0.87 (0.81–0.93)	84.0	75.3	[41]
miR-122	Serum	HCCs (n = 101) vs. HCs (n = 89)	Upregulated	0.79 (0.71–0.86)	70.7	69.1	[41]
miR-223	Serum	HCCs (n = 101) vs. CHCs (n = 89)	Upregulated	0.86 (0.80–0.92)	80.0	76.5	[41]
miR-12	Serum	HCCs (n = 101) vs. HCs (n = 48)	Upregulated	0.91 (0.84–0.97)	80.0	95.6	[41]
miR-122	Serum	HCCs (n = 101) vs. HCs (n = 48)	Upregulated	0.93 (0.88–0.98)	80.0	91.2	[41]
miR-223	Serum	HCCs (n = 101) vs. HCs (n = 48)	Upregulated	0.88 (0.81–0.94)	80.0	75.0	[41]
miR-122	Serum	HCCs (n = 70) vs. HCs (n = 34)	Upregulated	0.87 (0.79–0.95)	81.6	83.3	[40]
miR-122	Serum	HCCs (n = 70) vs. CHCs (n = 45)	Upregulated	0.63 (0.52–0.74)	77.6	57.8	[40]
miR-21	Plasma	HCCs (n = 126) vs. HCs (n = 50)	Upregulated	0.77	61.1	83.3	[44]
miR-21	Plasma	HCCs (n = 126) vs. CHCs (n = 30)	Upregulated	0.95	87.3	92.0	[44]
miR-143	Serum	HCCs (n = 95) vs. CTLs (n = 245)	Upregulated	0.80 (0.68–0.92)	73.0	83.0	[46]
miR-215	Serum	HCCs (n = 95) vs. CTLs (n = 245)	Upregulated	0.82 (0.72–0.97)	80.0	91.0	[46]
miR-10b	Serum	HCCs (n = 27) vs. HCs (n = 50)	Upregulated	0.85 (0.76–0.94)	/	/	[51]
miR-10b	Serum	HCCs (n = 27) vs. CLDs (n = 31)	Upregulated	0.73 (0.60–0.86)	/	/	[51]
miR-106b	Serum	HCCs (n = 27) vs. HCs (n = 50)	Upregulated	0.82 (0.72–0.91)	/	/	[51]
miR-106b	Serum	HCCs (n = 27) vs. CLDs (n = 31)	Upregulated	0.71 (0.57–0.84)	/	/	[51]
miR-181a	Serum	HCCs (n = 27) vs. HCs (n = 50)	Upregulated	0.89 (0.81–0.97)	/	/	[51]
miR-181a	Serum	HCCs (n = 27) vs. CLDs (n = 31)	Upregulated	0.81 (0.70–0.92)	/	/	[51]
miR-206	Serum	HCCs (n = 261) vs. HCs (n = 173)	Upregulated	0.62 (0.55–0.68)	48.1	78.8	[52]
miR-143-3p	Serum	HCCs (n = 261) vs. HCs (n = 173)	Upregulated	0.76 (0.70–0.80)	68.1	83.3	[52]
miR-433-3p	Serum	HCCs (n = 261) vs. HCs (n = 173)	Upregulated	0.74 (0.67–0.80)	79.3	64.4	[52]
miR-1228-5p	Serum	HCCs (n = 261) vs. HCs (n = 173)	Upregulated	0.55 (0.44–0.60)	79.3	27.8	[52]
miR-199a-5p	Serum	HCCs (n = 261) vs. HCs (n = 173)	Downregulated	0.64 (0.57–0.71)	59.3	66.7	[52]

MicroRNAs	Source	Diagnostic relevance	Expression level	AUC (95% CI)	Sen (%)	Spe (%)	Refs
miR-122-5p	Serum	HCCs (n = 261) vs. HCs (n = 173)	Downregulated	0.70 (0.63–0.77)	48.9	82.2	[52]
miR-192-5p	Serum	HCCs (n = 261) vs. HCs (n = 173)	Downregulated	0.70 (0.62–0.77)	71.9	75.6	[52]
miR-26a-5p	Serum	HCCs (n = 261) vs. HCs (n = 173)	Downregulated	0.76 (0.70–0.82)	68.9	74.4	[52]
miR-206	Serum	HCCs (n = 261) vs. CCs (n = 233)	Upregulated	0.69 (0.62–0.77)	77.8	68.9	[52]
miR-143-3p	Serum	HCCs (n = 261) vs. CCs (n = 233)	Upregulated	0.66 (0.60–0.73)	60.7	72.7	[52]
miR-433-3p	Serum	HCCs (n = 261) vs. CCs (n = 233)	Upregulated	0.64 (0.58–0.71)	56.4	67.4	[52]
miR-1228-5p	Serum	HCCs (n = 261) vs. CCs (n = 233)	Upregulated	0.54 (0.47–0.61)	66.7	47	[52]
miR-199a-5p	Serum	HCCs (n = 261) vs. CCs (n = 233)	Downregulated	0.59 (0.52–0.66)	59.3	57.6	[52]
miR-122-5p	Serum	HCCs (n = 261) vs. CCs (n = 233)	Downregulated	0.75 (0.69–0.81)	48.9	90.2	[52]
miR-192-5p	Serum	HCCs (n = 261) vs. CCs (n = 233)	Downregulated	0.69 (0.62–0.75)	54.8	83.3	[52]
miR-26a-5p	Serum	HCCs (n = 261) vs. CCs (n = 233)	Downregulated	0.74 (0.68–0.81)	60.7	90.9	[52]
miR-16	Serum	HCCs (n = 105) vs. CTLs (n = 188)	Downregulated	/	72.1	88.8	[14]
miR-199	Serum	HCCs (n = 105) vs. CTLs (n = 188)	Downregulated	/	62.9	93.5	[14]
miR-199a	Serum	HCCs (n = 105) vs. CTLs (n = 188)	Downregulated	/	78.1	64.5	[14]
miR-375	Serum	HCCs (n = 78) vs. HCs (n = 156)	Downregulated	0.64 (0.56–0.74)	/	/	[53]
miR-199a-3p	Serum	HCCs (n = 78) vs. HCs (n = 156)	Downregulated	0.88 (0.83–0.94	/	/	[53]
miR-30c-5p	Plasma	HCCs (n = 8) vs. CTLs (n = 86)	Upregulated	/	/	/	[54]
miR-223-3p	Plasma	HCCs (n = 8) vs. CTLs (n = 86)	Downregulated	/	/	/	[54]
miR-202c-3p	Plasma	HCCs (n = 8) vs. CTLs (n = 86)	Upregulated	/	/	/	[54]
miR-17-57	Plasma	HCCs (n = 8) vs. CTLs (n = 86)	Upregulated	/	/	/	[54]
miR-4651	Serum	AHCCs (n = 279) vs. HCs (n = 338)	Upregulated	0.89 (0.86–0.92)	78.1	99.1	[55]
miR-4651	Serum	AHCCs (n = 279) vs. AHCs (n = 292)	Upregulated	0.82 (0.78–0.85)	78.1	85.3	[55]
miR-4651	Serum	AHCCs (n = 279) vs. ALCs (n = 32)	Upregulated	0.80 (0.71–0.88)	78.1	81.2	[55]

MicroRNAs	Source	Diagnostic relevance	Expression level	AUC (95% CI)	Sen (%)	Spe (%)	Refs
miR-4651	Serum	AHCCs (n = 279) vs. CTLs (n = 662)	Upregulated	0.85 (0.82–0.88)	78.1	92.1	[55]
miR-143	Serum	HCCs (n = 131) vs. HCs (n = 122)	Downregulated	0.83	80.3	82.4	[56]
miR-125b	Plasma	HCCs (n = 64) vs. HCs (n = 56)	Downregulated	0.89	90.0	80.0	[57]
miR-125b	Plasma	HCCs (n = 64) vs. CHBs (n = 63)	Downregulated	0.96	90.0	90.0	[57]
miR-125b	Plasma	HCCs (n = 64) vs. CCs (n = 59)	Downregulated	0.96	90.0	90.0	[57]
miR-150	Serum	HCCs (n = 120) vs. CHBs (n = 110)	Downregulated	0.88 (0.84–0.93)	79.1	76.5	[58]
miR-150	Serum	HCCs (n = 120) vs. HCs (n = 120)	Downregulated	0.93 (0.90–0.96)	82.5	83.7	[58]
miR-106b	Plasma	HCCs (n = 47) vs. CTLs (n = 61)	Upregulated	0.81	0.7	0.8	[59]
miR-200a	Serum	HCCs (n = 22) vs. HCs (n = 15)	Downregulated	0.82 (0.69–0.97)	/	/	[60]
miR-200a	Serum	HCCs (n = 22) vs. CCs (n = 22)	Downregulated	0.73 (0.56–0.89)	/	/	[60]
miR-143	Serum	HCCs (n = 95) vs. CHCs (n = 118)	Upregulated	0.62 (0.51–0.76)	78.0	64.0	[46]
miR-215	Serum	HCCs (n = 95) vs. CHCs (n = 118)	Upregulated	0.80 (0.67–0.95)	78.0	89.0	[46]
miR-143	Serum	HCCs (n = 95) vs. HCs (n = 127)	Upregulated	0.80 (0.68–0.92)	78.0	89.0	[46]
miR-215	Serum	HCCs (n = 95) vs. HCs (n = 127)	Upregulated	0.82 (0.72–0.97)	80.0	91.0	[46]
miR-101	Serum	HCCs (n = 67) vs. HCs (n = 30)	Downregulated	0.79 (0.69–0.87)	76.1	70.0	[61]
miR-483-5p	Serum	HCCs (n = 49) vs. HCs (n = 49)	Upregulated	0.91	75.5	89.8	[62]
miR-122a	Plasma	HCCs (n = 85) vs. HCs (n = 85)	Downregulated	0.71	70.6	67.1	[63]
miR-618	Urine	HCCs (n = 32) vs. CTLs (n = 74)	Upregulated	0.66	64.0	68.0	[47]
miR-650	Urine	HCCs (n = 32) vs. CTLs (n = 74)	Downregulated	0.65	72.0	58.0	[47]
miR-126	tumor tissue	HCCs vs. CAs	Upregulated	/	/	/	[48]

Abbreviation: miR, microRNA; HCCs, cases with hepatocarcinoma; CTLs, non-HCC controls (including healthy control and other nontumor controls); HCs, healthy controls; CCs, controls with liver cirrhosis; CHBs, patients with chronic hepatitis B; CLDs, cases with nontumor chronic liver diseases; Sen, sensitivity; Spe, specificity; AUC, the area under the receiver operating characteristic curve; CI, confidence interval; Refs, references.

Table 1. The microRNAs as diagnostic biomarkers for hepatocarcinoma.

other serum microRNAs, such as microRNA-15b, microRNA-130b, miR-143, and miR-215, are additional potential biomarkers that are significantly dysregulated in hepatocarcinoma [45, 46]. Noticeably, these biomarkers also exhibit their diagnostic potential for patients with early-stage hepatocarcinoma and/or negative-status AFP [45, 46].

Recently, some evidence has also exhibited that microRNAs in urine samples and liver tissues have screening potential for hepatocarcinoma (**Table 1**). Actually, the detection of five deregulated microRNAs, including microR-618, microRNA-625, microRNA-650, microRNA-532, and miR-516-5P, in the urine samples has already been used for screening patients with the early and small hepatocarcinoma from these with risk factors such as chronic virus hepatitis, liver cirrhosis, and dysplasia [47]. Barshack et al. [48] investigated differential diagnosis potential of microRNAs for discriminating hepatocarcinoma from metastatic tumors in the liver using custom microarray expression technique. In their study, they tested the distributed features of microRNAs among 144 tumor samples with or without metastatic adenocarcinoma and similar hepatocarcinoma in the morphology and immune types and found that microR-141 and microR-200c can promote non-hepatic epithelial phenotypes while microRNA-126 displays hepatic epithelial phenotypes. Higher expression of microRNA-126 is further shown in these tissue samples with hepatocarcinoma. Therefore, the change profiles of microRNAs in body fluids (such as urine) and tumor tissues may represent a kind of gold biomarkers for such cancers as liver carcinoma.

However, the specificity of a single microRNA identifying hepatocarcinoma is relatively poor. For example, the serum level of aforementioned liver-specific microRNA-122 is upregulated not only among cases with hepatocarcinoma but also among these with chronic virus hepatitis, liver cirrhosis, and fatty liver diseases caused by alcohol or non-alcohol [49, 50]. Evidence has shown that serum microRNA-122 does not discriminate patients with hepatocarcinoma from these with chronic hepatitis, although higher expression is observed among cancer cases [40, 41]. This indicates that more investigations on the basis of large size of samples and the prospective randomized controlled trials should help us for addressing these concerns.

3.2. Diagnostic potential of microRNA panel for hepatocarcinoma

Because hepatocarcinoma is a multifactor-induced highly complex malignant disease with heterogeneous feature, a combination of multiple microRNAs in place of a single microRNA may have higher accuracy for hepatocarcinoma discrimination. Several circulating microRNA panels have been reported to have higher early diagnostic value for hepatocarcinoma (**Table 2**) [47, 51, 52, 64–70]. For example, Lin et al. [70] preformed a three-stage study consisting of the discovery stage (including 6 cases with hepatocarcinoma and 8 cases with chronic hepatitis B), the training stage (including 108 cases with hepatocarcinoma, 51 cases with chronic hepatitis B, 47 cases with liver cirrhosis, and 51 healthy controls), and the validation stage (including 229 patients with hepatocarcinoma and 424 controls with or with nontumor liver diseases). In the first stage, they identified 31 different serum microRNAs between individuals with hepatocarcinoma and those with chronic hepatitis B using the TaqMan Array technique. Next, they validated these different microRNAs and constructed diagnostic panel containing miR-29a, miR-29c, miR-133a, miR-143, miR-145, miR-192, and miR-505 on the basis of logistic regression model. Finally, the established serum microRNA panel was tested among

MicroRNA panel	Source	AUC (95% CI)	Sen (%)	Spe (%)	Diagnostic relevance	Refs
miR-10b + miR-106b + miR-181a	Serum	0.94 (0.89–0.99)	/	/	HCCs (n = 27) vs. HCs (n = 50)	[51]
miR-10b + miR-106b + miR-181a	Serum	0.91 (0.80–0.97)	/	/	HCCs (n = 27) vs. CLDs (n = 31)	[51]
miR-206 + miR-143-3p + miR-433-3p + miR-1228-5p + miR-199a-5p + miR-122-5p + miR-192-5p + miR-26a-5p	Serum	0.89 (0.85–0.94)	82.8	83.3	HCCs (n = 261) vs. HCs (n = 173)	[52]
miR-206 + miR-143-3p + miR-433-3p + miR-1228-5p + miR-199a-5p + miR-122-5p + miR-192-5p + miR-26a-5p	Serum	0.89 (0.84–0.94)	81.6	84.6	HCCs (n = 261) vs. CCs (n = 233)	[52]
miR-122 + miR-192 + miR-21 + miR-223 + miR-26a + miR-27a + miR-801	Plasma	0.86 (0.83–0.90)	68.6	90.1	HCCs (n = 204) vs. CTLs (n = 303)	[64]
miR-122 + miR-192 + miR-21 + miR-223 + miR-26a + miR-27a + miR-801	Plasma	0.89 (0.85–0.92)	81.8	83.5	HCCs (n = 196) vs. CTLs (n = 194)	[64]
miR-27b-3p + miR-192-5p	Serum	0.84 (0.78–0.89)	0.7	0.9	HCCs (n = 91) vs. CTLs (n = 91)	[65]
miR-92-3p + miR-107 + miR-3126-5p	Serum	0.97 (0.95–0.99)	/	/	HCCs (n = 115) vs. HCs (n = 40)	[66]
88-miRNA	Serum	1.00 (0.97–1.00)	100.0	99.2	HCCs (n = 261) vs. CCs (n = 233)	[67]
miR214-5p + miR-125b + miR-1269 + miR-375	Serum	0.95	96.9	83.2	HCCs (n = 224) vs. HCs (n = 84)	[68]
miR-122 + miR-885-5p + miR-29b	Serum	1.00	/	/	HCCs (n = 192) vs. HCs (n = 96)	[69]
miR-29a + miR-29c + miR-133a + miR-143 + miR-145 + miR-192 + miR-505	Serum	0.82 (0.77–0.87)	74.5	89.9	HCCs (n = 153) vs. CTLs (n = 199)	[70]
miR-29a + miR-29c + miR-133a + miR-143 + miR-145 + miR-192 + miR-505	Serum	0.88 (0.82–0.95)	85.7	91.1	HCCs (n = 49) vs. CTLs (n = 90)	[70]
miR-618 + miR-650	Urine	0.69	58.0	75.0	HCCs (n = 32) vs. CTLs (n = 74)	[47]

Abbreviation: miR, microRNA; HCCs, cases with hepatocarcinoma; CTLs, non-HCC controls (including healthy control and other nontumor controls); HCs, healthy controls; CCs, controls with liver cirrhosis; CHBs, patients with chronic hepatitis B; CLDs, cases with nontumor chronic liver diseases; Sen, sensitivity; Spe, specificity; AUC, the area under the receiver operating characteristic curve; CI, confidence interval; Refs, references.

Table 2. The microRNA panel as diagnostic biomarkers for hepatocarcinoma.

individuals from the training and validation cohorts. These data identified seven microRNAs and constructed a serum microRNA panel with an increasing diagnostic accuracy for hepatocarcinoma [AUC = 0.826 (0.771–0.880) for training set and 0.817 (0.769–0.865) and 0.884 (0.818–0.951) for two different validation sets, respectively]. Interestingly, a nest case-control study has further proved that this panel could be used to detect preclinical hepatocarcinoma as well as small-size, early-stage, and α-fetoprotein-negative disease.

Similarly, Jiang et al. [59] and Zhou et al. [64] also attempted to identify possible combination of different microRNAs for increasing diagnostic accuracy of hepatocarcinoma on the basis of different controls with or without liver diseases. They found that the panel consisting of miR-10b, miR-106b, and miR-181a as well as the combination of miR-122, miR-192, miR-21, miR-223, miR-26a, miR-27a, and miR-801 can improve detection of hepatocarcinoma. These reports indicate that the panel of microRNAs may have better performance than a single-microRNA assay.

3.3. Diagnostic potential of microRNAs binding with AFP for hepatocarcinoma

AFP has been regarded as the most important marker for hepatocarcinoma screening and diagnosis, ever since it was identified in the peripheral blood samples from patients with hepatocarcinoma in 1964 [8, 71, 72]. However, this marker is relatively unsatisfactory because of its low sensitivity and specificity. This is mainly because only 60–80% of cases with hepatocarcinoma show positive AFP, whereas about 40% of cirrhotic patients also exhibit different degree increasing level of serum AFP [73, 74]. Thus, AFP may not be a reliable hepatocarcinoma marker, especially for early-stage and/or AFP-negative hepatocarcinoma. On the basis of low sensitivity and specificity of AFP for hepatocarcinoma diagnosis, the American Association for the Study of Liver Disease Practice Guidelines has thrown it away for prognostic surveillance and tumor diagnosis [75]. However, recent studies have displayed that the combination of AFP in the peripheral blood and microRNAs in body fluids may improve the sensitivity and specificity of hepatocarcinoma diagnosis and increase their diagnostic potential [14, 47, 55, 58, 65–67, 69, 70, 76].

For example, Wu et al. [55] investigated the joint diagnostic value of serum microRNA-4651 and AFP for hepatocarcinoma in 279 hepatocarcinoma patients, 324 controls with liver injury, and 338 healthy controls. Their results imply that serum microRNA-4651 has higher expression level among cases with hepatocarcinoma (AUC of 0.85; sensitivity of 78.1% and specificity of 92.1%); this increasing expression also displays higher diagnostic potential than AFP at cutoff of 20 ng/mL (AFP20) (AUC = 0.80, sensitivity = 61.3%, and specificity = 98.8%) and of 400 ng/mL (AFP400) (AUC = 0.72, sensitivity = 43.0%, and specificity = 100.0%). Noticeably, the combination of serum microRNA-4651 with AFP significantly improves the discrimination power between patients with hepatocarcinoma and with chronic nontumor liver injury (AUC = 0.90, sensitivity = 83.2%, and specificity = 97.1%). Similar findings have also been observed in the analyses of combination of serum AFP and other microRNAs, such as miR-29a, miR-29c, miR-133a, miR-143, miR-145, miR-192, miR-505, miR-16, miR-195, and miR-199a [14, 47, 58, 65–67, 69, 70, 76]. Altogether, these data suggest that the combination of microRNAs with AFP may improve diagnostic potential of hepatocarcinoma.

4. Prognostic potential of microRNA for hepatocarcinoma

In the past decades, growing evidence has exhibited that microRNAs can act as prognostic biomarkers for hepatocarcinoma [56, 77–101], and **Table 3** summarizes these significantly affecting hepatocarcinoma outcomes. Functionally, the microRNAs affect hepatocarcinoma prognosis

MicroRNAs	Source	Expression level	Prognostic significance	HR (95%CI)	Refs
miR-122	Serum	Upregulated	Increasing levels correlate with poor OS	OS, 0.08 (0.03–0.22)	[120]
miR-1	Serum	Upregulated	Increasing levels correlate with poor OS	OS, 0.45 (0.23–0.86)	[121]
miR-122	Serum	Upregulated	Correlated with clinical chemistry parameters of hepatic necroinflammation, liver function, and synthetic capacity	/	[121]
miR-221	Serum	Upregulated	(1) Correlated with tumor size, cirrhosis, and tumor stage; (2) increasing levels decreased survival rate	/	[122]
miR-4651	Serum	Upregulated	Increasing levels correlate with poor OS and RFS	OS, 2.67 (1.61–4.42) RFS, 3.62 (1.49–8.81)	[55]
miR-1268a	Tumor tissues	Upregulated	Increasing levels correlate with poor OS and RFS	OS, 2.44 (1.82–3.23) RFS, 2.86 (2.08–3.85)	[115]
miR-24	Tumor tissues	Upregulated	Increasing levels correlate with poor OS and RFS	OS, 3.58 (2.34–5.46) RFS, 4.75 (2.66–8.47)	[77]
miR-429	Tumor tissues	Upregulated	Increasing levels correlate with poor OS and RFS	OS, 4.64 (2.56–8.41) RFS, 6.94 (3.19–15.08)	[78]
miR-143	Serum	Downregulated	Decreasing levels correlate with poor OS and RFS	/	[56]
miR-9	Tumor tissues	Upregulated	Increasing levels correlate with poor OS and RFS	/	[123]
miR-92b	Tumor tissues, serum	Upregulated	Increasing levels promoting tumor metastasis	/	[102]
miR-150	Serum	Downregulated	Increasing levels correlate with poor OS	0.45 (0.23–0.85)	[58]
miR-21	Serum	Upregulated	Increasing levels correlate with poor OS	2.23 (1.33–3.74)	[76]
20-miRNA signature	Tumor tissues	10 downregulated and 20 upregulated miRNAs	6 were risk factors and 14 were protective factors	OS, 2.75 (1.58–4.79)	[124]
miR-221	Tumor tissues	Upregulated	Increasing expression promotes metastasis-free survival	/	[125]

MicroRNAs	Source	Expression level	Prognostic significance	HR (95%CI)	Refs
miR-96	Tumor tissues	Upregulated	Increasing expression correlates with poor RFS	/	[126]
miR-92a	Tumor tissues	Downregulated	Decreasing expression correlates with poor RFS	RFS, 1.60 (1.00–2.50)	[79]
miR-22	Tumor tissues	Downregulated	Decreasing expression correlates with poor RFS	/	[80]
miR-500	Serum	Upregulated	Decreasing expression correlates with tumor resected	/	[127]
miR-375	Tumor tissues	/	Decreasing expression correlates with poor RFS	RFS, 3.273	[81]
miR-148b	Tumor tissues	Downregulated	Decreasing expression correlates with poor OS	OS, 1.86 (1.23–2.98)	[82]
miR-101	Tumor tissues	Downregulated	Decreasing expression correlates with poor OS and RFS	RFS, 2.56 (1.32–5.69) OS, 3.27 (1.18–6.92)	[83]
miR-19a	Tumor tissues	Downregulated	Decreasing expression correlates with poor OS and RFS	/	[84]
miR-210	Tumor tissues	Upregulated	Increasing expression correlates with poor OS	/	[80]
miR-224	Tumor tissues	Upregulated	Increasing expression correlates with poor OS and RFS	/	[85]
miR-29	Tumor tissues	Downregulated	Decreasing expression correlates with poor and RFS	/	[86]
miR-139-5p	Tumor tissues	Downregulated	Decreasing expression correlates with poor OS	/	[87]
miR-1	Tumor tissues	Downregulated	Decreasing expression correlates with poor OS and RFS	OS, 2.79	[88]
miR-199b-5p	Tumor tissues	Downregulated	Decreasing expression correlates with poor OS	/	[89]
miR-130b	Tumor tissues	Upregulated	Increasing expression correlates with poor OS and RFS	RFS, 4.00 (1.58–7.90) OS, 2.52 (1.02–7.90)	[90]
miR-9	Tumor tissues	Upregulated	Increasing expression correlates with poor OS and RFS	/	[91]
miR-25	Tumor tissues	Upregulated	Increasing expression correlates with poor OS and RFS	RFS, 1.62 OS, 2.18	[92]
let-7	Tumor tissues	Upregulated	Increasing expression correlates with poor OS	/	[93]

MicroRNAs	Source	Expression level	Prognostic significance	HR (95%CI)	Refs
miR-30a	Tumor tissues	Downregulated	Decreasing expression correlates with poor RFS	RFS, 3.2 (1.5–6.8)	[94]
miR-99a	Tumor tissues	Downregulated	Decreasing expression correlates with poor RFS	RFS, 1.60 (1.00–2.50)	[79]
miR-106b	Tumor tissues	Upregulated	Increasing expression correlates with poor OS	OS, 2.00 (1.13–6.98)	[95]
miR-130a	Tumor tissues	Downregulated	Decreasing expression correlates with poor OS	OS, 2.22 (1.10–4.46)	[96]
miR-19b	Tumor tissues	/	Increasing expression correlates with good OS	OS, 0.45 (0.24–0.85)	[97]
miR-148a	Tumor tissues	Downregulated	Decreasing expression correlates with poor OS	/	[98]
miR-372	Tumor tissues	Upregulated	Increasing expression correlates with poor OS and RFS	RFS, 6.83 OS, 9.53	[99]
miR-630	Tumor tissues	Downregulated	Increasing expression correlates with good OS and RFS	OS, 0.71 (0.26–1.92) RFS, 0.66 (0.33–1.35)	[100]
miR-100	Tumor tissues	Downregulated	Decreasing expression correlates with poor OS	OS, 1.66 (1.32–2.82)	[101]

Abbreviation: miR, microRNA; OS, overall survival; RFS, tumor recurrence-free survival; HR, hazard ratio; CI, confidence interval; Refs, references.

Table 3. The microRNAs as prognostic biomarkers for hepatocarcinoma.

via the following pathways: (1) promoting cancerous growth and proliferation [77, 78, 80, 83, 89, 98, 99, 102–113], (2) inhibiting cancerous apoptosis [77, 78, 86, 99, 101, 107–109, 111, 112, 114], (3) increasing microvessel density in the tumor tissues [77, 115], (4) affecting cell cycles [24, 25, 27, 28, 116–119], (5) increasing the risk of tumor metastasis [77, 115], and (6) decreasing the sensitivity of cancer cells to anticancer drugs [115]. For example, Lu et al. [115] investigated the prognostic potential of microRNA-1268a for hepatocarcinoma in 411 patients with hepatocarcinoma. Their results imply that microRNA-1268a expression in the cancerous tissues is significantly related to tumor features including tumor volume, stage and grade, and microvessel density. Results from multivariable factors analyses based on Cox regression models show that microRNA-1268a expression is independent of other known prognostic factors for hepatocarcinoma. Furthermore, transarterial chemoembolization (TACE) treatment can improve the prognosis of hepatocarcinoma patients with low microRNA-1268a expression, but not for those with high microRNA-1268e expression. These data imply that the dysregulation of microRNA-1268a can modify the response of cancer cells to antidrugs. Their following studies prove that upregulated microRNA-1268a inhibited while its downregulation enhanced doxorubicin (an anticancer drug)-induced the death of tumor cells. Similarly, Liu et al. [77] and Huang et al. [78] investigated the roles of microRNAs, such as microRNA-24 and microRNA-429, in the tumorigenesis of liver cancer on the basis of analyses of hepatocarcinoma samples and genic toxicity induced by aflatoxin B1 and found the dysregulation of these microRNAs increased microvessel density and mutation frequency of TP53 gene possibly resulting from the loss of DNA repair capacity. Taken together, these reports indicate that microRNAs in body fluids and cancerous tissues may be important candidate biomarkers for hepatocarcinoma prognosis.

5. Further direction

In the past decades, the advance in pathological mechanisms of microRNAs regulating tumorigenesis and procession of hepatocarcinoma holds great promise for identifying whether microRNAs in body fluids (such as blood and urine) act as novel early diagnostic and prognostic biomarkers for this malignancy. However, we are still far from a comprehensive view of this kind of potentials. Although some hepato-specific microRNAs have been identified, microRNAs in body fluids may be from hemocytes and vascular endothelial cells and others from tissues and organs with high blood flow as well as hepatocarcinoma. This kind of heterogeneous origin indicates that the dysregulation of tumor-specific microRNA signatures may be concealed by microRNAs from other origins. Furthermore, well-standardized protocols of testing microRNAs have not been constructed or confirmed on the basis of the prospective, randomized controlled trials. Disclosing the different diagnostic and prognostic potential of microRNAs will greatly benefit our constructing high accurate diagnostic and prognostic models for hepatocarcinoma and will shed important light on the early diagnosis, tumor monitoring, and prognosis prediction for individuals with risk factors.

6. Summary

To conclude, the advances in technologies, including microarray PCR technology, high-throughput sequencing, and mass spectrometry, make it possible to identify new markers for hepatocarcinoma diagnosis and prognosis. On the whole, the microRNAs are a class of attractive markers and may replace known traditional serum markers such as AFP on the basis of the following reasons. First, because many circulating microRNAs is highly stable and readily detected in patients with hepatocarcinoma, they may have higher diagnostic potential (with high AUCs, sensitivity, and specificity) for hepatocarcinoma than AFP. Second, some microRNAs appear in the urine and can be utilized for screening patients with high-risk factors of hepatocarcinoma. Third, some dysregulated microRNAs in the body fluids can change with the different stages of hepatocarcinoma, indicative of their potential in monitoring tumor recurrence. Finally, different expressions of microRNAs are useful for treatment strategies such as TACE selection. Taken together, the dysregulated microRNAs in body fluids (including urine and blood) may be a kind of promised biomarkers for liver carcinoma diagnosis and prognosis because they are early detected and easily monitored.

However, there are several issues to be noted. First, research on the diagnostic and prognostic potential of microRNAs is still in the early stages, and challenges are noticeable in the clinical utilization of significant microRNAs. Second, in spite of these biomarkers that are discussed well, their therapeutic potential still remains unclear. Finally, although the diagnostic and prognostic potential of microRNAs is well evaluated on the basis of retrospective case-control studies, results from the prospective, randomized controlled trials are absent. Finally, because of the polygenic feature for hepatocarcinoma development, it is essential for a panel of biomarkers to determine high-risk individuals. Thus, the advances in the fields of microRNAs including their origins, stability, detection strategies, variant characteristics, and biofunctions in hepatocarcinoma will progress microRNAs in body fluids to become possible tools for hepatocarcinoma diagnosis and prognosis in the future.

Conflicts of interest and source of funding

The authors declare no competing financial interests. This study was supported in part by the National Natural Science Foundation of China (nos. 81760502, 81572353, 81372639, 81472243, 81660495, and 81460423), the Innovation Program of Guangxi Municipal Education Department (nos. 201204LX674 and 201204LX324), Innovation Program of Guangxi Health Department (no. Z2013781), the Natural Science Foundation of Guangxi (nos. 2017GXNSFGA198002, 2017GXNSFAA198002, 2016GXNSFDA20380003, 2015GXNSFAA139223, 2013GXNSFAA019251, 2014GXNSFDA20118021, and 2014GXNSFAA118144), the Youth Natural Science Foundation of Guangxi Medical University (no. GXMUYSF201522), Research Program of Guangxi "Zhouyue Scholar" (no. 2017–38), Research Program of Guangxi Specially Invited Expert (no. 2017-6th), Research Program of Guangxi Clinic Research Center of Hepatobiliary Diseases (no. AD17129025), and Open Research Program from Molecular Immunity Study Room Involving in Acute & Severe Diseases in Guangxi Colleges and Universities (nos. kfkt20160062 and kfkt20160063).

Abbreviations

AFP α-fetoprotein

AFB1 aflatoxin B1

AUC the area under the receiver operating characteristic curve

CT computed tomography

HBV hepatitis virus B

HCC hepatocellular carcinoma

HCV hepatitis virus C

MRI magnetic resonance imaging

Author details

Xi-Dai Long[1,2*†], Wei-Zhong Tang[3†], Jun Lu[2†], Xiao-Ying Huang[1†], Jin-Guang Yao[1,4†], Tian-Qi Zhang[1†], Xing-Zhizi Wang[1†], Qun-Ying Su[1†], Chun-Ying Luo[1], Xue-Ming Wu[1], Chao Wang[5], Li-Xia Zeng[6], Qiang Xia[2] and Yun Ma[6]

*Address all correspondence to: sjtulongxd@263.net or yunandama@hotmail.com

1 Department of Pathology, the Affiliated Hospital of Youjiang Medical University for Nationalities, Baise, PR China

2 Department of Liver Surgery, Ren Ji Hospital, School of Medicine, Shanghai Jiao Tong University, Shanghai, PR China

3 Department of Gastrointestinal Surgery, the Affiliated Tumor Hospital, Guangxi Medical University, Nanning, PR China

4 Department of Medicine, Guangxi Scientific Technological University School of Medicine, Liuzhou, PR China

5 Department of Medicine, the Affiliated Hospital of Youjiang Medical University for Nationalities, Baise, PR China

6 Department of Pathology, the Affiliated Tumor Hospital, Guangxi Medical University, Nanning, PR China

† These authors contributed equally

References

[1] Siegel RL, Miller KD, Jemal A. Cancer statistics, 2017. CA: a Cancer Journal for Clinicians. 2017;**67**:7-30. DOI: 10.3322/caac.21387

[2] Chen W, Zheng R, Baade PD, Zhang S, Zeng H, Bray F, Jemal A, XQ Y, He J. Cancer statistics in China, 2015. CA: a Cancer Journal for Clinicians. 2016;**66**:115-132. DOI: 10.3322/caac.21338

[3] Long J, Luo GP, Xiao ZW, Liu ZQ, Guo M, Liu L, Liu C, Xu J, Gao YT, Zheng Y, Wu C, Ni QX, Li M, Yu X. Cancer statistics: Current diagnosis and treatment of pancreatic cancer in shanghai, China. Cancer Letters. 2014. DOI: 10.1016/j.canlet.2014.01.004

[4] Page AJ, Cosgrove DC, Philosophe B, Pawlik TM. Hepatocellular Carcinoma: Diagnosis, Management, and Prognosis. Surgical Oncology Clinics of North America. 2014;**23**:289-311. DOI: 10.1016/j.soc.2013.10.006

[5] Njei B, Rotman Y, Ditah I, Lim JK. Emerging trends in hepatocellular carcinoma incidence and mortality. Hepatology. 2014. DOI: 10.1002/hep.27388

[6] Giannini EG, Farinati F, Ciccarese F, Pecorelli A, Rapaccini GL, Di Marco M, Caturelli E, Zoli M, Borzio F, Trevisani F, Cancer g IL. Prognosis of untreated hepatocellular carcinoma. Hepatology. 2014. DOI: 10.1002/hep.27443

[7] Nault JC. Pathogenesis of hepatocellular carcinoma according to aetiology. Best Practice & Research. Clinical Gastroenterology. 2014;**28**:937-947. DOI: 10.1016/j.bpg.2014.08.006

[8] Tsuchiya N, Sawada Y, Endo I, Saito K, Uemura Y, Nakatsura T. Biomarkers for the early diagnosis of hepatocellular carcinoma. World Journal of Gastroenterology. 2015;**21**: 10573-10583. DOI: 10.3748/wjg.v21.i37.10573

[9] Hung CH, TH H, SN L, Kuo FY, Chen CH, Wang JH, Huang CM, Lee CM, Lin CY, Yen YH, Chiu YC. Circulating microRNAs as biomarkers for diagnosis of early hepatocellular carcinoma associated with hepatitis B virus. International Journal of Cancer. 2016;**138**:714-720. DOI: 10.1002/ijc.29802

[10] Huang JT, Liu SM, Ma H, Yang Y, Zhang X, Sun H, Zhang X, Xu J, Wang J. Systematic review and meta-analysis: Circulating miRNAs for diagnosis of Hepatocellular carcinoma. Journal of Cellular Physiology. 2016;**231**:328-335. DOI: 10.1002/jcp.25135

[11] Zhang YC, Xu Z, Zhang TF, Wang YL. Circulating microRNAs as diagnostic and prognostic tools for hepatocellular carcinoma. World Journal of Gastroenterology. 2015; **21**:9853-9862. DOI: 10.3748/wjg.v21.i34.9853

[12] Chang-Hao Tsao S, Behren A, Cebon J, Christophi C. The role of circulating microRNA in hepatocellular carcinoma. Frontiers in Bioscience (Landmark Ed). 2015;**20**:78-104

[13] Yang Y, Zhu R. Diagnostic value of circulating microRNAs for hepatocellular carcinoma. Molecular Biology Reports. 2014;**41**:6919-6929. DOI: 10.1007/s11033-014-3578-7

[14] KZ Q, Zhang K, Li H, Afdhal NH, Albitar M. Circulating microRNAs as biomarkers for hepatocellular carcinoma. Journal of Clinical Gastroenterology. 2011;**45**:355-360. DOI: 10.1097/MCG.0b013e3181f18ac2

[15] Wong KF, Xu Z, Chen J, Lee NP, Luk JM. Circulating markers for prognosis of hepatocellular carcinoma. Expert Opinion on Medical Diagnostics. 2013;**7**:319-329. DOI: 10.1517/17530059.2013.795146

[16] Zhao X, Yang Z, Li G, Li D, Zhao Y, Wu Y, Robson SC, He L, Xu Y, Miao R, Zhao H. The role and clinical implications of microRNAs in hepatocellular carcinoma. Science China. Life Sciences. 2012;**55**:906-919. DOI: 10.1007/s11427-012-4384-x

[17] Lyra-Gonzalez I, Flores-Fong LE, Gonzalez-Garcia I, Medina-Preciado D, Armendariz-Borunda J. MicroRNAs dysregulation in hepatocellular carcinoma: Insights in genomic medicine. World Journal of Hepatology. 2015;**7**:1530-1540. DOI: 10.4254/wjh.v7.i11.1530

[18] Cardin R, Piciocchi M, Bortolami M, Kotsafti A, Barzon L, Lavezzo E, Sinigaglia A, Rodriguez-Castro KI, Rugge M, Farinati F. Oxidative damage in the progression of chronic liver disease to hepatocellular carcinoma: An intricate pathway. World Journal of Gastroenterology. 2014;**20**:3078-3086. DOI: 10.3748/wjg.v20.i12.3078

[19] Lagos-Quintana M, Rauhut R, Yalcin A, Meyer J, Lendeckel W, Tuschl T. Identification of tissue-specific microRNAs from mouse. Current Biology. 2002;**12**:735-739

[20] Saunders MA, Liang H, Li WH. Human polymorphism at microRNAs and microRNA target sites. Proceedings of the National Academy of Sciences of the United States of America. 2007;**104**:3300-3305. DOI: 10.1073/pnas.0611347104

[21] Griffiths-Jones S. The microRNA registry. Nucleic Acids Research. 2004;**32**:D109-D111. DOI: 10.1093/nar/gkh023

[22] Griffiths-Jones S, Grocock RJ, van Dongen S, Bateman A, Enright AJ. miRBase: microRNA sequences, targets and gene nomenclature. Nucleic Acids Research. 2006;**34**:D140-D144. DOI: 10.1093/nar/gkj112

[23] Zhang B, Pan X, Cobb GP, Anderson TA. microRNAs as oncogenes and tumor suppressors. Developmental Biology. 2007;**302**:1-12. DOI: 10.1016/j.ydbio.2006.08.028

[24] Wojcicka A, de la Chapelle A, Jazdzewski K. MicroRNA-related sequence variations in human cancers. Human Genetics. 2014;**133**:463-469. DOI: 10.1007/s00439-013-1397-x

[25] van Rooij E. The art of microRNA research. Circulation Research. 2011;**108**:219-234. DOI: 10.1161/CIRCRESAHA.110.227496

[26] Sontheimer EJ. Assembly and function of RNA silencing complexes. Nature Reviews. Molecular Cell Biology. 2005;**6**:127-138. DOI: 10.1038/nrm1568

[27] Schwabe RF, Wang TC. Targeting liver cancer: First steps toward a miRacle? Cancer Cell. 2011;**20**:698-699. DOI: 10.1016/j.ccr.2011.11.021

[28] Ranganathan K, Sivasankar V. MicroRNAs - biology and clinical applications. Journal of Oral and Maxillofacial Pathology. 2014;**18**:229-234. DOI: 10.4103/0973-029X.140762

[29] Lynam-Lennon N, Maher SG, Reynolds JV. The roles of microRNA in cancer and apoptosis. Biological Reviews of the Cambridge Philosophical Society. 2009;**84**:55-71. DOI: 10.1111/j.1469-185X.2008.00061.x

[30] Bartel DP. MicroRNAs: Genomics, biogenesis, mechanism, and function. Cell. 2004;**116**: 281-297. DOI: S0092867404000455 [pii]

[31] Kumar A. MicroRNA in HCV infection and liver cancer. Biochimica et Biophysica Acta. 1809;**2011**:694-699. DOI: 10.1016/j.bbagrm.2011.07.010

[32] Boeri M, Pastorino U, Sozzi G. Role of microRNAs in lung cancer: microRNA signatures in cancer prognosis. Cancer Journal. 2012;**18**:268-274. DOI: 10.1097/PPO.0b013e318258b743

[33] Celton-Morizur S, Desdouets C. Liver physiological polyploidization: MicroRNA-122 a key regulator. Clinics and Research in Hepatology and Gastroenterology. 2017;**41**:123-125. DOI: 10.1016/j.clinre.2016.07.006

[34] Hsu SH, Delgado ER, Otero PA, Teng KY, Kutay H, Meehan KM, Moroney JB, Monga JK, Hand NJ, Friedman JR, Ghoshal K, Duncan AW. MicroRNA-122 regulates polyploidization in the murine liver. Hepatology. 2016;**64**:599-615. DOI: 10.1002/hep.28573

[35] Cho HJ, Kim JK, Nam JS, Wang HJ, Lee JH, Kim BW, Kim SS, Noh CK, Shin SJ, Lee KM, Cho SW, Cheong JY. High circulating microRNA-122 expression is a poor prognostic marker in patients with hepatitis B virus-related hepatocellular carcinoma who undergo radiofrequency ablation. Clinical Biochemistry. 2015;**48**:1073-1078. DOI: 10.1016/j.clinbiochem.2015.06.019

[36] Kumar S, Chawla YK, Ghosh S, Chakraborti A. Severity of hepatitis C virus (genotype-3) infection positively correlates with circulating microRNA-122 in patients sera. Disease Markers. 2014;**2014**:435476. DOI: 10.1155/2014/435476

[37] van der Meer AJ, Farid WR, Sonneveld MJ, de Ruiter PE, Boonstra A, van Vuuren AJ, Verheij J, Hansen BE, de Knegt RJ, van der Laan LJ, Janssen HL. Sensitive detection of hepatocellular injury in chronic hepatitis C patients with circulating hepatocyte-derived microRNA-122. Journal of Viral Hepatitis. 2013;**20**:158-166. DOI: 10.1111/jvh.12001

[38] Arataki K, Hayes CN, Akamatsu S, Akiyama R, Abe H, Tsuge M, Miki D, Ochi H, Hiraga N, Imamura M, Takahashi S, Aikata H, Kawaoka T, Kawakami H, Ohishi W, Chayama K. Circulating microRNA-22 correlates with microRNA-122 and represents viral replication and liver injury in patients with chronic hepatitis B. Journal of Medical Virology. 2013;**85**:789-798. DOI: 10.1002/jmv.23540

[39] Ding X, Ding J, Ning J, Yi F, Chen J, Zhao D, Zheng J, Liang Z, Hu Z, Du Q. Circulating microRNA-122 as a potential biomarker for liver injury. Molecular Medicine Reports. 2012;**5**:1428-1432. DOI: 10.3892/mmr.2012.838

[40] Qi P, Cheng SQ, Wang H, Li N, Chen YF, Gao CF. Serum microRNAs as biomarkers for hepatocellular carcinoma in Chinese patients with chronic hepatitis B virus infection. PLoS One. 2011;**6**:e28486. DOI: 10.1371/journal.pone.0028486

[41] Xu J, Wu C, Che X, Wang L, Yu D, Zhang T, Huang L, Li H, Tan W, Wang C, Lin D. Circulating microRNAs, miR-21, miR-122, and miR-223, in patients with hepatocellular carcinoma or chronic hepatitis. Molecular Carcinogenesis. 2011;**50**:136-142. DOI: 10.1002/mc.20712

[42] Murakami Y, Yasuda T, Saigo K, Urashima T, Toyoda H, Okanoue T, Shimotohno K. Comprehensive analysis of microRNA expression patterns in hepatocellular carcinoma and non-tumorous tissues. Oncogene. 2006;**25**:2537-2545. DOI: 10.1038/sj.onc.1209283

[43] Hung CS, Liu HH, Liu JJ, Yeh CT, Chang TC, CH W, Ho YS, Wei PL, Chang YJ. MicroRNA-200a and -200b mediated hepatocellular carcinoma cell migration through the epithelial to mesenchymal transition markers. Annals of Surgical Oncology. 2013;**20**(Suppl 3):S360-S368. DOI: 10.1245/s10434-012-2482-4

[44] Tomimaru Y, Eguchi H, Nagano H, Wada H, Kobayashi S, Marubashi S, Tanemura M, Tomokuni A, Takemasa I, Umeshita K, Kanto T, Doki Y, Mori M. Circulating microRNA-21 as a novel biomarker for hepatocellular carcinoma. Journal of Hepatology. 2012;**56**:167-175. DOI: 10.1016/j.jhep.2011.04.026

[45] Liu AM, Yao TJ, Wang W, Wong KF, Lee NP, Fan ST, Poon RT, Gao C, Luk JM. Circulating miR-15b and miR-130b in serum as potential markers for detecting hepatocellular carcinoma: A retrospective cohort study. BMJ Open. 2012;**2**:e000825. DOI: 10.1136/bmjopen-2012-000825

[46] Zhang ZQ, Meng H, Wang N, Liang LN, Liu LN, SM L, Luan Y. Serum microRNA 143 and microRNA 215 as potential biomarkers for the diagnosis of chronic hepatitis and hepatocellular carcinoma. Diagnostic Pathology. 2014;**9**:135. DOI: 10.1186/1746-1596-9-135

[47] Abdalla MA, Haj-Ahmad Y. Promising candidate urinary MicroRNA biomarkers for the early detection of Hepatocellular carcinoma among high-risk hepatitis C virus Egyptian patients. Journal of Cancer. 2012;**3**:19-31

[48] Barshack I, Meiri E, Rosenwald S, Lebanony D, Bronfeld M, Aviel-Ronen S, Rosenblatt K, Polak-Charcon S, Leizerman I, Ezagouri M, Zepeniuk M, Shabes N, Cohen L, Tabak S, Cohen D, Bentwich Z, Rosenfeld N. Differential diagnosis of hepatocellular carcinoma from metastatic tumors in the liver using microRNA expression. The International Journal of Biochemistry & Cell Biology. 2010;**42**:1355-1362. DOI: 10.1016/j.biocel.2009.02.021

[49] Vliegenthart ADB, Berends C, Potter CMJ, Kersaudy-Kerhoas M, Dear JW. MicroRNA-122 can be measured in capillary blood which facilitates point-of-care testing for drug-induced liver injury. British Journal of Clinical Pharmacology. 2017;**83**:2027-2033. DOI: 10.1111/bcp.13282

[50] Qiao DD, Yang J, Lei XF, Mi GL, Li SL, Li K, CQ X, Yang HL. Expression of microRNA-122 and microRNA-22 in HBV-related liver cancer and the correlation with clinical features. European Review for Medical and Pharmacological Sciences. 2017;**21**:742-747

[51] Jiang L, Cheng Q, Zhang BH, Zhang MZ. Circulating microRNAs as biomarkers in hepatocellular carcinoma screening: A validation set from China. Medicine (Baltimore). 2015;**94**:e603. DOI: 10.1097/MD.0000000000000603

[52] Tan Y, Ge G, Pan T, Wen D, Chen L, Yu X, Zhou X, Gan J. A serum microRNA panel as potential biomarkers for hepatocellular carcinoma related with hepatitis B virus. PLoS One. 2014;**9**:e107986. DOI: 10.1371/journal.pone.0107986

[53] Yin J, Hou P, Wu Z, Wang T, Nie Y. Circulating miR-375 and miR-199a-3p as potential biomarkers for the diagnosis of hepatocellular carcinoma. Tumour Biology. 2015;**36**:4501-4507. DOI: 10.1007/s13277-015-3092-0

[54] Oksuz Z, Serin MS, Kaplan E, Dogen A, Tezcan S, Aslan G, Emekdas G, Sezgin O, Altintas E, Tiftik EN. Serum microRNAs; miR-30c-5p, miR-223-3p, miR-302c-3p and miR-17-5p could be used as novel non-invasive biomarkers for HCV-positive cirrhosis and hepatocellular carcinoma. Molecular Biology Reports. 2015;**42**:713-720. DOI: 10.1007/s11033-014-3819-9

[55] XM W, Xi ZF, Liao P, Huang HD, Huang XY, Wang C, Ma Y, Xia Q, Yao JG, Long XD. Diagnostic and prognostic potential of serum microRNA-4651 for patients with hepatocellular carcinoma related to aflatoxin B1. Oncotarget. 2017. DOI: 10.18632/oncotarget.16027

[56] Zhang J, Lin H, Wang XY, Zhang DQ, Chen JX, Zhuang Y, Zheng XL. Predictive value of microRNA-143 in evaluating the prognosis of patients with hepatocellular carcinoma. Cancer Biomarkers. 2017;**19**:257-262. DOI: 10.3233/CBM-160357

[57] Chen S, Chen H, Gao S, Qiu S, Zhou H, Yu M, Tu J. Differential expression of plasma microRNA-125b in hepatitis B virus-related liver diseases and diagnostic potential for hepatitis B virus-induced hepatocellular carcinoma. Hepatology Research. 2017;**47**:312-320. DOI: 10.1111/hepr.12739

[58] Yu F, Lu Z, Chen B, Dong P, Zheng J. microRNA-150: A promising novel biomarker for hepatitis B virus-related hepatocellular carcinoma. Diagnostic Pathology. 2015;**10**:129. DOI: 10.1186/s13000-015-0369-y

[59] Jiang L, Li X, Cheng Q, Zhang BH. Plasma microRNA might as a potential biomarker for hepatocellular carcinoma and chronic liver disease screening. Tumour Biology. 2015;**36**:7167-7174. DOI: 10.1007/s13277-015-3446-7

[60] Dhayat SA, Husing A, Senninger N, Schmidt HH, Haier J, Wolters H, Kabar I. Circulating microRNA-200 family as diagnostic marker in Hepatocellular carcinoma. PLoS One. 2015;**10**:e0140066. DOI: 10.1371/journal.pone.0140066

[61] Xie Y, Yao Q, Butt AM, Guo J, Tian Z, Bao X, Li H, Meng Q, Lu J. Expression profiling of serum microRNA-101 in HBV-associated chronic hepatitis, liver cirrhosis, and hepatocellular carcinoma. Cancer Biology & Therapy. 2014;**15**:1248-1255. DOI: 10.4161/cbt.29688

[62] Shen J, Wang A, Wang Q, Gurvich I, Siegel AB, Remotti H, Santella RM. Exploration of genome-wide circulating microRNA in hepatocellular carcinoma: MiR-483-5p as a potential biomarker. Cancer Epidemiology, Biomarkers & Prevention. 2013;**22**:2364-2373. DOI: 10.1158/1055-9965.EPI-13-0237

[63] Luo J, Chen M, Huang H, Yuan T, Zhang M, Zhang K, Deng S. Circulating microRNA-122a as a diagnostic marker for hepatocellular carcinoma. OncoTargets and Therapy. 2013;**6**:577-583. DOI: 10.2147/OTT.S44215

[64] Zhou J, Yu L, Gao X, Hu J, Wang J, Dai Z, Wang JF, Zhang Z, Lu S, Huang X, Wang Z, Qiu S, Wang X, Yang G, Sun H, Tang Z, Wu Y, Zhu H, Fan J. Plasma microRNA panel to diagnose hepatitis B virus-related hepatocellular carcinoma. Journal of Clinical Oncology. 2011;**29**:4781-4788. DOI: 10.1200/JCO.2011.38.2697

[65] Zhu HT, Liu RB, Liang YY, Hasan AME, Wang HY, Shao Q, Zhang ZC, Wang J, He CY, Wang F, Shao JY. Serum microRNA profiles as diagnostic biomarkers for HBV-positive hepatocellular carcinoma. Liver International. 2017;**37**:888-896. DOI: 10.1111/liv.13356

[66] Zhang Y, Li T, Qiu Y, Zhang T, Guo P, Ma X, Wei Q, Han L. Serum microRNA panel for early diagnosis of the onset of hepatocellular carcinoma. Medicine (Baltimore). 2017;**96**:e5642. DOI: 10.1097/MD.0000000000005642

[67] Long XR, Zhang YJ, Zhang MY, Chen K, Zheng XFS, Wang HY. Identification of an 88-microRNA signature in whole blood for diagnosis of hepatocellular carcinoma and other chronic liver diseases. Aging (Albany NY). 2017;**9**:1565-1584. DOI: 10.18632/aging.101253

[68] Elemeery MN, Badr AN, Mohamed MA, Ghareeb DA. Validation of a serum microRNA panel as biomarkers for early diagnosis of hepatocellular carcinoma post-hepatitis C infection in Egyptian patients. World Journal of Gastroenterology. 2017;**23**:3864-3875. DOI: 10.3748/wjg.v23.i21.3864

[69] Zekri AN, Youssef AS, El-Desouky ED, Ahmed OS, Lotfy MM, Nassar AA, Bahnassey AA. Serum microRNA panels as potential biomarkers for early detection of hepatocellular carcinoma on top of HCV infection. Tumour Biology. 2016;**37**:12273-12286. DOI: 10.1007/s13277-016-5097-8

[70] Lin XJ, Chong Y, Guo ZW, Xie C, Yang XJ, Zhang Q, Li SP, Xiong Y, Yuan Y, Min J, Jia WH, Jie Y, Chen MS, Chen MX, Fang JH, Zeng C, Zhang Y, Guo RP, Wu Y, Lin G, Zheng L, Zhuang SM. A serum microRNA classifier for early detection of hepatocellular carcinoma: A multicentre, retrospective, longitudinal biomarker identification study with a nested case-control study. The Lancet Oncology. 2015;**16**:804-815. DOI: 10.1016/S1470-2045(15)00048-0

[71] Gupta S, Bent S, Kohlwes J. Test characteristics of alpha-fetoprotein for detecting hepatocellular carcinoma in patients with hepatitis C. A systematic review and critical analysis. Annals of Internal Medicine. 2003;**139**:46-50

[72] Trevisani F, D'Intino PE, Morselli-Labate AM, Mazzella G, Accogli E, Caraceni P, Domenicali M, De Notariis S, Roda E, Bernardi M. Serum alpha-fetoprotein for diagnosis of hepatocellular carcinoma in patients with chronic liver disease: Influence of HBsAg and anti-HCV status. Journal of Hepatology. 2001;**34**:570-575

[73] Marrero JA, Feng Z, Wang Y, Nguyen MH, Befeler AS, Roberts LR, Reddy KR, Harnois D, Llovet JM, Normolle D, Dalhgren J, Chia D, Lok AS, Wagner PD, Srivastava S, Schwartz M. Alpha-fetoprotein, des-gamma carboxyprothrombin, and lectin-bound alpha-fetoprotein in early hepatocellular carcinoma. Gastroenterology. 2009;**137**:110-118. DOI: 10.1053/j.gastro.2009.04.005

[74] Spangenberg HC, Thimme R, Blum HE. Serum markers of hepatocellular carcinoma. Seminars in Liver Disease. 2006;**26**:385-390. DOI: 10.1055/s-2006-951606

[75] Zinkin NT, Grall F, Bhaskar K, Otu HH, Spentzos D, Kalmowitz B, Wells M, Guerrero M, Asara JM, Libermann TA, Afdhal NH. Serum proteomics and biomarkers in hepatocellular carcinoma and chronic liver disease. Clinical Cancer Research. 2008;**14**:470-477. DOI: 10.1158/1078-0432.CCR-07-0586

[76] Wang X, Zhang J, Zhou L, Lu P, Zheng ZG, Sun W, Wang JL, Yang XS, Li XL, Xia N, Zhang N, Dou KF. Significance of serum microRNA-21 in diagnosis of hepatocellular carcinoma (HCC): Clinical analyses of patients and an HCC rat model. International Journal of Clinical and Experimental Pathology. 2015;**8**:1466-1478

[77] Liu YX, Long XD, Xi ZF, Ma Y, Huang XY, Yao JG, Wang C, Xing TY, Xia Q. MicroRNA-24 modulates aflatoxin B1-related hepatocellular carcinoma prognosis and tumorigenesis. BioMed Research International. 2014;**2014**:482926. DOI: 10.1155/2014/482926

[78] Huang XY, Yao JG, Huang HD, Wang C, Ma Y, Xia Q, Long XD. MicroRNA-429 modulates hepatocellular carcinoma prognosis and tumorigenesis. Gastroenterology Research and Practice. 2013;**2013**:804128. DOI: 10.1155/2013/804128

[79] Li D, Liu X, Lin L, Hou J, Li N, Wang C, Wang P, Zhang Q, Zhang P, Zhou W, Wang Z, Ding G, Zhuang SM, Zheng L, Tao W, Cao X. MicroRNA-99a inhibits hepatocellular carcinoma growth and correlates with prognosis of patients with hepatocellular carcinoma. The Journal of Biological Chemistry. 2011;**286**:36677-36685. DOI: 10.1074/jbc.M111.270561

[80] Zhang J, Yang Y, Yang T, Liu Y, Li A, Fu S, Wu M, Pan Z, Zhou W. microRNA-22, down-regulated in hepatocellular carcinoma and correlated with prognosis, suppresses cell proliferation and tumourigenicity. British Journal of Cancer. 2010;**103**:1215-1220. DOI: 10.1038/sj.bjc.6605895

[81] Zhou N, Wu J, Wang X, Sun Z, Han Q, Zhao L. Low-level expression of microRNA-375 predicts poor prognosis in hepatocellular carcinoma. Tumour Biology. 2016;**37**:2145-2152. DOI: 10.1007/s13277-015-3841-0

[82] Zhang Z, Zheng W, Hai J. MicroRNA-148b expression is decreased in hepatocellular carcinoma and associated with prognosis. Medical Oncology. 2014;**31**:984. DOI: 10.1007/s12032-014-0984-6

[83] Zhang Y, Guo X, Xiong L, Kong X, Xu Y, Liu C, Zou L, Li Z, Zhao J, Lin N. MicroRNA-101 suppresses SOX9-dependent tumorigenicity and promotes favorable prognosis of human hepatocellular carcinoma. FEBS Letters. 2012;**586**:4362-4370. DOI: 10.1016/j.febslet.2012.10.053

[84] Zhang Y, Guo X, Li Z, Li B, Li Z, Li R, Guo Q, Xiong L, Yu L, Zhao J, Lin N. A systematic investigation based on microRNA-mediated gene regulatory network reveals that dysregulation of microRNA-19a/Cyclin D1 axis confers an oncogenic potential and a worse prognosis in human hepatocellular carcinoma. RNA Biology. 2015;**12**:643-657. DOI: 10.1080/15476286.2015.1022702

[85] Zhan M, Li Y, Hu B, He X, Huang J, Zhao Y, Fu S, Lu L. Serum microRNA-210 as a predictive biomarker for treatment response and prognosis in patients with hepatocellular carcinoma undergoing transarterial chemoembolization. Journal of Vascular and Interventional Radiology. 2014;**25**:1279-1287 e1271. DOI: 10.1016/j.jvir.2014.04.013

[86] Xiong Y, Fang JH, Yun JP, Yang J, Zhang Y, Jia WH, Zhuang SM. Effects of microRNA-29 on apoptosis, tumorigenicity, and prognosis of hepatocellular carcinoma. Hepatology. 2010;**51**:836-845. DOI: 10.1002/hep.23380

[87] Wang Z, Ding Q, Li Y, Liu Q, Wu W, Wu L, Yu H. Reanalysis of microRNA expression profiles identifies novel biomarkers for hepatocellular carcinoma prognosis. Tumour Biology. 2016;**37**:14779-14787. DOI: 10.1007/s13277-016-5369-3

[88] Wang X, Huang Y, Zhuang H, Qian Y, Zhao Q, Yang L, Gu H, Chen J, Guo R, Liu Y. Downregulation of MicroRNA-1 is associated with poor prognosis in Hepatocellular carcinoma. Clinical Laboratory. 2015;**61**:1331-1336

[89] Wang C, Song B, Song W, Liu J, Sun A, Wu D, Yu H, Lian J, Chen L, Han J. Underexpressed microRNA-199b-5p targets hypoxia-inducible factor-1alpha in hepatocellular carcinoma and predicts prognosis of hepatocellular carcinoma patients. Journal of Gastroenterology and Hepatology. 2011;**26**:1630-1637. DOI: 10.1111/j.1440-1746.2011.06758.x

[90] Wang WY, Zhang HF, Wang L, Ma YP, Gao F, Zhang SJ, Wang LC. High expression of microRNA-130b correlates with poor prognosis of patients with hepatocellular carcinoma. Diagnostic Pathology. 2014;**9**:160. DOI: 10.1186/s13000-014-0160-5

[91] Sun J, Fang K, Shen H, Qian Y. MicroRNA-9 is a ponderable index for the prognosis of human hepatocellular carcinoma. International Journal of Clinical and Experimental Medicine. 2015;**8**:17748-17756

[92] ZX S, Zhao J, Rong ZH, Geng WM, YG W, Qin CK. Upregulation of microRNA-25 associates with prognosis in hepatocellular carcinoma. Diagnostic Pathology. 2014;**9**:47. DOI: 10.1186/1746-1596-9-47

[93] Shi W, Zhang Z, Yang B, Guo H, Jing L, Liu T, Luo Y, Liu H, Li Y, Gao Y. Overexpression of microRNA let-7 correlates with disease progression and poor prognosis in hepatocellular carcinoma. Medicine (Baltimore). 2017;**96**:e7764. DOI: 10.1097/MD.0000000000007764

[94] Liu Z, Tu K, Liu Q. Effects of microRNA-30a on migration, invasion and prognosis of hepatocellular carcinoma. FEBS Letters. 2014;**588**:3089-3097. DOI: 10.1016/j.febslet.2014.06.037

[95] Li BK, Huang PZ, Qiu JL, Liao YD, Hong J, Yuan YF. Upregulation of microRNA-106b is associated with poor prognosis in hepatocellular carcinoma. Diagnostic Pathology. 2014;**9**:226. DOI: 10.1186/s13000-014-0226-4

[96] Li B, Huang P, Qiu J, Liao Y, Hong J, Yuan Y. MicroRNA-130a is down-regulated in hepatocellular carcinoma and associates with poor prognosis. Medical Oncology. 2014;**31**:230. DOI: 10.1007/s12032-014-0230-2

[97] Hung CL, Yen CS, Tsai HW, YC S, Yen CJ. Upregulation of MicroRNA-19b predicts good prognosis in patients with hepatocellular carcinoma presenting with vascular invasion or multifocal disease. BMC Cancer. 2015;**15**:665. DOI: 10.1186/s12885-015-1671-5

[98] Heo MJ, Kim YM, Koo JH, Yang YM, An J, Lee SK, Lee SJ, Kim KM, Park JW, Kim SG. microRNA-148a dysregulation discriminates poor prognosis of hepatocellular carcinoma in association with USP4 overexpression. Oncotarget. 2014;**5**:2792-2806. DOI: 10.18632/oncotarget.1920

[99] Gu H, Guo X, Zou L, Zhu H, Zhang J. Upregulation of microRNA-372 associates with tumor progression and prognosis in hepatocellular carcinoma. Molecular and Cellular Biochemistry. 2013;**375**:23-30. DOI: 10.1007/s11010-012-1521-6

[100] Chen WX, Zhang ZG, Ding ZY, Liang HF, Song J, Tan XL, Wu JJ, Li GZ, Zeng Z, Zhang BX, Chen XP. MicroRNA-630 suppresses tumor metastasis through the TGF-beta- miR-630-slug signaling pathway and correlates inversely with poor prognosis in hepatocellular carcinoma. Oncotarget. 2016;**7**:22674-22686. DOI: 10.18632/oncotarget.8047

[101] Chen P, Zhao X, Ma L. Downregulation of microRNA-100 correlates with tumor progression and poor prognosis in hepatocellular carcinoma. Molecular and Cellular Biochemistry. 2013;**383**:49-58. DOI: 10.1007/s11010-013-1753-0

[102] Zhuang LK, Yang YT, Ma X, Han B, Wang ZS, Zhao QY, Wu LQ, Qu ZQ. MicroRNA-92b promotes hepatocellular carcinoma progression by targeting Smad7 and is mediated by long non-coding RNA XIST. Cell Death & Disease. 2016;**7**:e2203. DOI: 10.1038/cddis.2016.100

[103] Zhang H, Sheng C, Yin Y, Wen S, Yang G, Cheng Z, Zhu Q. PABPC1 interacts with AGO2 and is responsible for the microRNA mediated gene silencing in high grade hepatocellular carcinoma. Cancer Letters. 2015;**367**:49-57. DOI: 10.1016/j.canlet.2015.07.010

[104] Yao M, Wang L, Yao Y, HB G, Yao DF. Biomarker-based MicroRNA therapeutic strategies for Hepatocellular carcinoma. Journal of Clinical and Translational Hepatology. 2014;**2**:253-258. DOI: 10.14218/JCTH.2014.00020

[105] Yao M, Wang L, Qiu L, Qian Q, Yao D. Encouraging microRNA-based therapeutic strategies for Hepatocellular carcinoma. Anti-Cancer Agents in Medicinal Chemistry. 2015;**15**:453-460

[106] Wei L, Lian B, Zhang Y, Li W, Gu J, He X, Xie L. Application of microRNA and mRNA expression profiling on prognostic biomarker discovery for hepatocellular carcinoma. BMC Genomics. 2014;**15**(Suppl 1):S13. DOI: 10.1186/1471-2164-15-S1-S13

[107] Miao HL, Lei CJ, Qiu ZD, Liu ZK, Li R, Bao ST, Li MY. MicroRNA-520c-3p inhibits hepatocellular carcinoma cell proliferation and invasion through induction of cell apoptosis by targeting glypican-3. Hepatology Research. 2014;**44**:338-348. DOI: 10.1111/hepr.12121

[108] Lu Y, Yue X, Cui Y, Zhang J, Wang K. MicroRNA-124 suppresses growth of human hepatocellular carcinoma by targeting STAT3. Biochemical and Biophysical Research Communications. 2013;**441**:873-879. DOI: 10.1016/j.bbrc.2013.10.157

[109] Khare S, Zhang Q, Ibdah JA. Epigenetics of hepatocellular carcinoma: Role of microRNA. World Journal of Gastroenterology. 2013;**19**:5439-5445. DOI: 10.3748/wjg.v19.i33.5439

[110] Hu X, Feng Y, Sun L, Qu L, Sun C. Roles of microRNA-330 and its target gene ING4 in the development of aggressive phenotype in Hepatocellular carcinoma cells. Digestive Diseases and Sciences. 2017;**62**:715-722. DOI: 10.1007/s10620-016-4429-2

[111] Hu S, Ran Y, Chen W, Zhang Y, Xu Y. MicroRNA-326 inhibits cell proliferation and invasion, activating apoptosis in hepatocellular carcinoma by directly targeting LIM and SH3 protein 1. Oncology Reports. 2017;**38**:1569-1578. DOI: 10.3892/or.2017.5810

[112] He XX, Chang Y, Meng FY, Wang MY, Xie QH, Tang F, Li PY, Song YH, Lin JS. MicroRNA-375 targets AEG-1 in hepatocellular carcinoma and suppresses liver cancer cell growth in vitro and in vivo. Oncogene. 2012;**31**:3357-3369. DOI: 10.1038/onc.2011.500

[113] Chen SY, Ma DN, Chen QD, Zhang JJ, Tian YR, Wang ZC, Cai H, Lin Y, Sun HC. MicroRNA-200a inhibits cell growth and metastasis by targeting Foxa2 in hepatocellular carcinoma. Journal of Cancer. 2017;**8**:617-625. DOI: 10.7150/jca.17394

[114] Zhang X, Tang W, Chen G, Ren F, Liang H, Dang Y, Rong M. An encapsulation of gene signatures for Hepatocellular carcinoma, MicroRNA-132 predicted target genes and the corresponding overlaps. PLoS One. 2016;**11**:e0159498. DOI: 10.1371/journal.pone.0159498

[115] YL L, Yao JG, Huang XY, Wang C, XM W, Xia Q, Long XD. Prognostic significance of miR-1268a expression and its beneficial effects for post-operative adjuvant transarterial chemoembolization in hepatocellular carcinoma. Scientific Reports. 2016;**6**:36104. DOI: 10.1038/srep36104

[116] Aguda BD. Modeling microRNA-transcription factor networks in cancer. Advances in Experimental Medicine and Biology. 2013;**774**:149-167. DOI: 10.1007/978-94-007-5590-1_9

[117] Rossi JJ. New hope for a microRNA therapy for liver cancer. Cell. 2009;**137**:990-992. DOI: 10.1016/j.cell.2009.05.038

[118] Zhang G, Wang Q, Xu R. Therapeutics based on microRNA: A new approach for liver cancer. Current Genomics. 2010;**11**:311-325. DOI: 10.2174/138920210791616671

[119] Zhu Z, Zhang X, Wang G, Zheng H. Role of MicroRNAs in Hepatocellular carcinoma. Hepatitis Monthly. 2014;**14**:e18672. DOI: 10.5812/hepatmon.18672

[120] Xu Y, Bu X, Dai C, Shang C. High serum microRNA-122 level is independently associated with higher overall survival rate in hepatocellular carcinoma patients. Tumour Biology. 2015;**36**:4773-4776. DOI: 10.1007/s13277-015-3128-5

[121] Koberle V, Kronenberger B, Pleli T, Trojan J, Imelmann E, Peveling-Oberhag J, Welker MW, Elhendawy M, Zeuzem S, Piiper A, Waidmann O. Serum microRNA-1 and microRNA-122 are prognostic markers in patients with hepatocellular carcinoma. European Journal of Cancer. 2013;**49**:3442-3449. DOI: 10.1016/j.ejca.2013.06.002

[122] Li J, Wang Y, Yu W, Chen J, Luo J. Expression of serum miR-221 in human hepatocellular carcinoma and its prognostic significance. Biochemical and Biophysical Research Communications. 2011;**406**:70-73. DOI: 10.1016/j.bbrc.2011.01.111

[123] Liu Y, Liu H, Yang L, Wu Q, Liu W, Fu Q, Zhang W, Zhang H, Xu J, Gu J. Loss of N-Acetylgalactosaminyltransferase-4 orchestrates Oncogenic MicroRNA-9 in Hepatocellular carcinoma. The Journal of Biological Chemistry. 2017;**292**:3186-3200. DOI: 10.1074/jbc.M116.751685

[124] Wei R, Huang GL, Zhang MY, Li BK, Zhang HZ, Shi M, Chen XQ, Huang L, Zhou QM, Jia WH, Zheng XF, Yuan YF, Wang HY. Clinical significance and prognostic value of microRNA expression signatures in hepatocellular carcinoma. Clinical Cancer Research. 2013;**19**:4780-4791. DOI: 10.1158/1078-0432.CCR-12-2728

[125] Yoon SO, Chun SM, Han EH, Choi J, Jang SJ, Koh SA, Hwang S, Yu E. Deregulated expression of microRNA-221 with the potential for prognostic biomarkers in surgically resected hepatocellular carcinoma. Human Pathology. 2011;**42**:1391-1400. DOI: 10.1016/j.humpath.2010.12.010

[126] Sato F, Hatano E, Kitamura K, Myomoto A, Fujiwara T, Takizawa S, Tsuchiya S, Tsujimoto G, Uemoto S, Shimizu K. MicroRNA profile predicts recurrence after resection in patients with hepatocellular carcinoma within the Milan criteria. PLoS One. 2011;**6**:e16435. DOI: 10.1371/journal.pone.0016435

[127] Yamamoto Y, Kosaka N, Tanaka M, Koizumi F, Kanai Y, Mizutani T, Murakami Y, Kuroda M, Miyajima A, Kato T, Ochiya T. MicroRNA-500 as a potential diagnostic marker for hepatocellular carcinoma. Biomarkers. 2009;**14**:529-538. DOI: 10.3109/13547500903150771

Permissions

All chapters in this book were first published in HCADT, by InTech Open; hereby published with permission under the Creative Commons Attribution License or equivalent. Every chapter published in this book has been scrutinized by our experts. Their significance has been extensively debated. The topics covered herein carry significant findings which will fuel the growth of the discipline. They may even be implemented as practical applications or may be referred to as a beginning point for another development.

The contributors of this book come from diverse backgrounds, making this book a truly international effort. This book will bring forth new frontiers with its revolutionizing research information and detailed analysis of the nascent developments around the world.

We would like to thank all the contributing authors for lending their expertise to make the book truly unique. They have played a crucial role in the development of this book. Without their invaluable contributions this book wouldn't have been possible. They have made vital efforts to compile up to date information on the varied aspects of this subject to make this book a valuable addition to the collection of many professionals and students.

This book was conceptualized with the vision of imparting up-to-date information and advanced data in this field. To ensure the same, a matchless editorial board was set up. Every individual on the board went through rigorous rounds of assessment to prove their worth. After which they invested a large part of their time researching and compiling the most relevant data for our readers.

The editorial board has been involved in producing this book since its inception. They have spent rigorous hours researching and exploring the diverse topics which have resulted in the successful publishing of this book. They have passed on their knowledge of decades through this book. To expedite this challenging task, the publisher supported the team at every step. A small team of assistant editors was also appointed to further simplify the editing procedure and attain best results for the readers.

Apart from the editorial board, the designing team has also invested a significant amount of their time in understanding the subject and creating the most relevant covers. They scrutinized every image to scout for the most suitable representation of the subject and create an appropriate cover for the book.

The publishing team has been an ardent support to the editorial, designing and production team. Their endless efforts to recruit the best for this project, has resulted in the accomplishment of this book. They are a veteran in the field of academics and their pool of knowledge is as vast as their experience in printing. Their expertise and guidance has proved useful at every step. Their uncompromising quality standards have made this book an exceptional effort. Their encouragement from time to time has been an inspiration for everyone.

The publisher and the editorial board hope that this book will prove to be a valuable piece of knowledge for researchers, students, practitioners and scholars across the globe.

List of Contributors

Sarwat Fatima, Hiu Yee Kwan and Zhao Xiang Bian
Lab of Brain and Gut Research, Centre of Clinical Research for Chinese Medicine, School of Chinese Medicine, Hong Kong Baptist University, Kowloon Tong, Hong Kong SAR, China
Centre for Cancer and Inflammation Research, School of Chinese Medicine, Hong Kong Baptist University, Kowloon Tong, Hong Kong SAR, China

Nikki Pui-Yue Lee
Department of Surgery, The University of Hong Kong, Pokfulam, Hong Kong SAR, China

Kosuke Kaji and Hitoshi Yoshiji
Third Department of Internal Medicine, Nara Medical University, Shijo-cho, Kashihara, Nara, Japan

Xiao-Ying Huang, Jin-Guang Y ao, Qun-Ying Su, Xue-Min Wu, Juan Wang and Bing-Chen Huang
Department of Pathology, the Affiliated Hospital of Youjiang Medical University for Nationalities, Baise, China

Qiang Xia
Department of Liver Surgery, Ren Ji Hospital, School of Medicine, Shanghai Jiao Tong University, Shanghai, China

Qun-Qing Xu and Xiao-Ying Zhu
Guangxi Clinic Research Center of Hepatobiliary Diseases, Baise, China

Yan Deng
Department of Epidemiology, Youjiang Medical University for Nationalities, Baise, China

Chao Wang
Department of Medicine, the Affiliated Hospital of Youjiang Medical University for Nationalities, Baise, China

Xi-Dai Long
Department of Pathology, the Affiliated Hospital of Youjiang Medical University for Nationalities, Baise, China
Department of Liver Surgery, Ren Ji Hospital, School of Medicine, Shanghai Jiao Tong University, Shanghai, China
Guangxi Clinic Research Center of Hepatobiliary Diseases, Baise, China

Ilze Strumfa, Dzeina Mezale, Arturs Kalva, Dainis Balodis, Ilze Fridrihsone and Arnis Abolins
Department of Pathology, Riga Stradins University, Riga, Latvia

Boriss Strumfs
Latvian Institute of Organic Synthesis, Riga, Latvia

Andrejs Vanags and Janis Gardovskis
Department of Surgery, Riga Stradins University, Riga, Latvia

Xue-Ming Wu, Xing-Zhizi Wang, Tian-Qi Zhang, Xiao-Ying Huang, Jin-Guang Yao, Chun-Ying Luo and Bing-Chen Huang
Department of Pathology, the Affiliated Hospital of Youjiang Medical College for Nationalities (AHYMCN), Baise, China

Zhi-Feng Xi, Jun Lu, Qiang Xia and Xi-Dai Long
Department of Liver Surgery, Ren Ji Hospital, School of Medicine, Shanghai Jiao Tong University, Shanghai, China

Chao Wang
Department of Medicine, AHYMCN, Baise, China

Zhong-Heng Wei
Department of Tumor, AHYMCN, Baise, China

Qun-Qing Xu
Department of Central Test, Youjiang Medical College for Nationalities, Baise, China

Wen-Pei Yang
Department of Basic Medicine, Youjiang Medical College for Nationalities, Baise, China

Andrew W. Ritchey
University of Texas Health Science Center Houston - McGovern Medical School, Houston, Texas, USA

Joshua D. Kuban and Rahul A. Sheth
MD Anderson Cancer Center, Houston, Texas, USA

Matthew Schade, Jacqueline A Sanabria, Milad Modarresi, Bryan Gillon, Zach Hunter, Jacqueline Fannin and Amrita Mallick
Department of Surgery and the Marshall Institute for Interdisciplinary Research, Marshall University Joan Edwards School of Medicine, Huntington, WV, United States

Boriss Strumfs
Latvian Institute of Organic Synthesis, Riga, Latvia

Henri Brunengraber
Department of Nutrition Proteomic & Metabolomic Core Facility at Case Western Reserve University, Cleveland, OH, United States

Juan Sanabria
Department of Surgery and the Marshall Institute for Interdisciplinary Research, Marshall University Joan Edwards School of Medicine, Huntington, WV, United States
Department of Nutrition Proteomic & Metabolomic Core Facility at Case Western Reserve University, Cleveland, OH, United States

Li Wang
Medical School of Nantong University, Affiliated Hospital of Nantong University, Nantong, Jiangsu Province, China

Wenjie Zheng, Miao Fang and Dengfu Yao
Institute of Clinical Oncology, Affiliated Hospital of Nantong University, Nantong, Jiangsu Province, China

Zhizheng Dong
Department of Diagnostics, Affiliated Hospital of Nantong University, Nantong, Jiangsu Province, China

Min Yao
Medical School of Nantong University, Affiliated Hospital of Nantong University, Nantong, Jiangsu Province, China
Institute of Clinical Oncology, Affiliated Hospital of Nantong University, Nantong, Jiangsu Province, China

Dzeina Mezale, Ilze Strumfa, Arturs Kalva, Dainis Balodis, Ilze Fridrihsone and Arnis Abolins
Department of Pathology, Riga Stradins University, Riga, Latvia

Andrejs Vanags and Janis Gardovskis
Department of Surgery, Riga Stradins University, Riga, Latvia

Xiao-Ying Huang, Tian-Qi Zhang, Xing-Zhizi Wang, Qun-Ying Su, Chun-Ying Luo and Xue-Ming Wu
Department of Pathology, the Affiliated Hospital of Youjiang Medical University for Nationalities, Baise, PR China

Jun Lu and Qiang Xia
Department of Liver Surgery, Ren Ji Hospital, School of Medicine, Shanghai Jiao Tong University, Shanghai, PR China

Wei-Zhong Tang
Department of Gastrointestinal Surgery, the Affiliated Tumor Hospital, Guangxi Medical University, Nanning, PR China

Jin-Guang Yao
Department of Pathology, the Affiliated Hospital of Youjiang Medical University for Nationalities, Baise, PR China
Department of Medicine, Guangxi Scientific Technological University School of Medicine, Liuzhou, PR China

Chao Wang
Department of Medicine, the Affiliated Hospital of Youjiang Medical University for Nationalities, Baise, PR China

Li-Xia Zeng and Yun Ma
Department of Pathology, the Affiliated Tumor Hospital, Guangxi Medical University, Nanning, PR China

Xi-Dai Long
Department of Pathology, the Affiliated Hospital of Youjiang Medical University for Nationalities, Baise, PR China
Department of Liver Surgery, Ren Ji Hospital, School of Medicine, Shanghai Jiao Tong University, Shanghai, PR China

Index

www.ingramcontent.com/pod-product-compliance
Lightning Source LLC
LaVergne TN
LVHW081037210926
848485LV00004B/1047
9781639873005